# OUTCOMES ASSESSMENT IN CLINICAL PRACTICE

EDITED BY

## Lloyd I. Sederer, M.D.

Associate Professor of Psychiatry
Harvard Medical School
Boston, Massachusetts
Senior Vice President for Clinical Services
McLean Hospital
Belmont, Massachusetts

## Barbara Dickey, Ph.D.

Associate Professor of Psychology
Department of Psychiatry
Harvard Medical School
Boston, Massachusetts
Director
Department of Mental Health Services Research
McLean Hospital
Belmont, Massachusetts

## Williams & Wilkins

BALTIMORE • PHILADELPHIA • HONG KONG
LONDON • MUNICH • SYDNEY • TOKYO

A WAVERLY COMPANY

*Editor:* David C. Retford
*Managing Editor:* Kathleen Courtney Millet
*Production Coordinator:* Marette D. Magargle
*Typesetter:* Graphic Sciences Corporation
*Printer:* Port City Press
*Binder:* Port City Press

**Library of Congress Cataloging-in-Publication Data**

Outcomes assessment in clinical practice / edited by Lloyd I. Sederer.
 Barbara Dickey.
     p.    cm.
  Includes bibliographical references and index.
  ISBN 0-683-07630-2
  1. Mental health services—Evaluation.    2. Outcome assessment
(Medical care)   I. Sederer, Lloyd I.   II. Dickey, Barbara.
   [DNLM: 1.  Mental Disorders—therapy.   2. Outcome Assessment
(Health Care)—organization & administration.    3. Substance Abuse-
-therapy.    4. Total Quality Management—methods.   WM 400 093 1996]
RC454.4.0855   1995
362.2—dc20
DNLM/DLC
for Library of Congress                                                95-4785
                                                                                        CIP

                                                                       97  98  99
                                                              3  4  5  6  7  8  9  10

RECYCLED

# OUTCOMES
# ASSESSMENT
## IN
# CLINICAL
# PRACTICE

*To our Families*

# FOREWORD

Over the last 20 years, psychiatry has undergone more profound changes than any other area of medicine. During this time, research largely carried out in university-affiliated psychiatry programs has transformed the understanding of severe mental disorders and effected an equal transformation of their treatment.

In the wake of psychodynamic theories of causality that held sway throughout the predominance of this century, empirical studies have shifted the focus of causality toward the brain mechanisms responsible for mental illness. For example, functional and structural brain imaging have disclosed brain abnormalities in schizophrenia, affective disorders, and obsessive compulsive disorder. Studies in molecular genetics have identified loci on the human genome associated with heritable risks for Alzheimer's and Huntington's diseases and bipolar disorder. In addition, the molecular sites of action of neuropsychotropic medications, including antipsychotics, anxiolytics, antidepressants, and lithium, have been characterized in remarkable detail.

More important, this new knowledge has informed and transformed treatment. A second generation of neuropsychotropic medications was developed on the basis of known sites of action. The serotonin-specific reuptake inhibitors and atypical neuroleptics are examples of the products of new knowledge and offer increased efficacy with fewer noxious side effects. New classes of drugs with cognitive enhancing properties (e.g., Tacrine) are becoming available and hold promise for the symptomatic treatment of dementia. Advances in the neurobiology of substance abuse suggest a pharmacological strategy for alleviating "craving," an important cause of relapse in drug-dependent individuals.

Empirical methods of evaluation also have expanded to include the efficacy of psychological interventions. Objective studies have documented the utility of concurrent psychotherapy with pharmacological treatment to reduce relapse in major depression. Family therapy to reduce expressed emotions has been shown to decrease both antipsychotic dosage and relapse rate in young adults suffering from schizophrenia. Notably, behavioral therapy has been shown to correct abnormal forebrain neuronal activity in patients suffering from obsessive compulsive disorder, as has treatment with fluoxetine. In fact, this behavioral work reified in psychiatric treatment what has been elegantly demonstrated in cognitive neuroscience: that psychological processes modify synaptic activity in the human brain. Finally, recent research has demonstrated the efficacy of psychological interventions in reducing psychiatric disturbances in children who are at high risk because a parent suffers from an affective disorder.

The advances in basic knowledge that we are witnessing are occurring in the context of another profound transformation, namely, how mental health services are provided. Fee-for-service practice is being supplanted by managed systems of care. The traditional dichotomy between inpatient treatment and outpatient treatment is being replaced by multitiered levels of care, which permit briefer hospital stays or diversion of severely ill patients to ambulatory settings. Capitated arrangements, in which providers contract to cover the mental health care for large groups of subscribers based on a fixed rate, are gaining in popularity as cost containment measures, thus making external utilization review part of the past.

Many benefits accrue from the managed care model, especially if clinical providers are involved in management (which has been standard practice in HMOs for 20 years). First, prevention or early identification with intervention receives greater emphasis because of the beneficial effect on utilization of more costly forms of care. Second, quality of care improves as attention is focused on the coordination of the patient's treatment across the levels of care. In effect, reimbursement is not tied to individual clinicians or sites but rather to effective continuity of care. Third, quality can be enhanced by specific standards for credentialing and by standardized algorithms for treatment based on current clinical knowledge and advances.

There is, however, justifiable concern that under the rubric of managed care cost reduction will eclipse quality of care. Mental health services are especially vulnerable because of the misperception that few objective standards for quality exist. As a consequence, "management" can be used as a method for "wearing down" providers by only permitting services in small preapproved increments and overemphasizing "counseling" strategies that ignore recent advances in psychiatry. Conversely, if a major mental disorder is diagnosed, "approved" treatment may be limited to drug therapy, thereby neglecting important empirical evidence that demonstrates the value of linking pharmacological and psychosocial interventions.

Managed care threatens to mismanage mental health services because serious lacunae exist in objective measures of outcome and quality of care. Although psychiatry undeniably has developed objective evidence of the efficacy of specific pharmacological and psychological treatments, the information about the efficacy of these interventions in "natural" clinical settings is limited. This limitation is not trivial because issues such as side effects of treatment, convenience, and cost figure significantly into compliance and, consequently, into outcome. Patients with psychiatric disorders may need to be convinced of the benefits of treatment because denial is intrinsic to certain disorders and stigma is often associated with treatment. However, inadequate or "mismanaged" treatment for mental and substance abuse disorders is profoundly costly because it impairs the individual, undermines job performance, damages families, and results in social costs such as disability and welfare.

To redress these critical problems, it is essential that the field of psychiatry develop objective methods to assess the outcome and quality of mental health and substance abuse care. This book represents an important first step by delineating outcome and patient satisfaction measures and reports by providers who are using these measures in clinical practice. The measures may serve as a foundation for "report cards" that compare health care plans. Although cost reduction is an important goal, an overly narrow focus that addresses only the costs of mental health services will be short sighted if the consequences of inadequate services are neglected.

Ironically, psychiatry developed the double-blind placebo-controlled method that has become the "gold standard" for determining drug efficacy and remains at the forefront of medicine in assessing treatment efficacy. Effectiveness research, now being pioneered by psychiatry, tests the quality of care and outcome of treatment in the real world. It is my belief that the assessment of outcomes in psychiatric practice will provide individuals, employers, and government with the ability to make rational choices about treatments and providers based on reliable and valid measures of quality, outcome, and satisfaction.

Joseph T. Coyle, M.D.
Eben S. Draper Professor of Psychiatry and of Neuroscience
Chair of the Consolidated Department of Psychiatry
Harvard Medical School

# PREFACE

This text aims to provide its readers with a comprehensive resource for understanding and applying outcomes assessment. The text is divided into three sections. The first section provides an overview of the field of outcome assessment and offers methods for integrating outcomes assessment into clinical practice. The second section presents detailed information on a variety of instruments used in measuring outcomes. Each chapter follows a specific blueprint that describes the instrument and characterizes its application, utility, and strengths and limitations. The final section discusses expectations for the future.

Section I begins with an overview of outcomes assessment. In this chapter, we demonstrate the reasons that outcomes assessment has become a clinical, economic, and policy imperative and we provide a summary of the domains of outcome assessment. We also discuss the instruments available to measure the perspectives of patients, clinicians, families, or significant others. In the following chapters, Drs. Docherty and McGlynn provide a comprehensive examination of the conceptual bases of outcomes research and assessment, detailing the methodological considerations essential for success. Dr. Waxman then presents an illustrative case study from a nonprofit hospital-based care system that portrays the development of a cost-conscious outcomes assessment program. This case emphasizes the use of information to enhance clinical quality improvement.

In their chapter, Drs. McLellan and Durell draw on the successful experience of veteran researchers of treatment outcome. They examine the reasonable expectations of psychiatric and substance abuse treatments and present ways to use these treatment goals as criteria for evaluation. The authors discuss symptoms, functioning, and aspects of social and health status and burden and emphasize the importance of assessing outpatient and inpatient treatment goals from different perspectives. They conclude with the five "cardinal features" of outcome evaluation.

As Chair of the Group for the Advancement of Psychiatry's (GAP) Committee on Psychopathology, Dr. Dorwart provides a case-based example of how outcomes evaluation can be incorporated into clinical practice. Paul Ellwood defined outcomes management as ". . . a common patient-understood language . . . on clinical, financial and health outcomes that estimates as best as we can the relation between medical interventions and health outcomes, as well as the relation between health outcomes and money; and an opportunity for each decision maker to have access to the analyses that are relevant to the choices they must make" (1). Dr. Dorwart and the GAP Committee demonstrate how this concept may be achieved.

Section I concludes with a chapter by Drs. Dickey and Wagenaar that traces the merger of clinical trials and services research. The authors demonstrate how we can best appreciate the health status of an individual by considering the perspectives of clinicians, patients, and families; by measuring clinical symptomology, self-reports of illness, and functioning; and by inquiring into the family's sense of burden. This chapter serves as an introduction to our next section by conceptually organizing and integrating the various methods of assessing health status and the different perspectives that must be considered.

Section II is a resource manual on 18 outcome instruments for psychiatric and substance abuse services. We asked each author to provide information in the same outline format to make the material more accessible to the reader. Each chapter begins with a description of the instrument, including key references and a profile of the instrument's application. The target population for the instrument, procedures for data collection, language and cultural diversity, and psychometric properties are all provided. Next, the utility of the instrument is examined. Availability of scoring manuals and interpretation, automation, fees, permission for use, and where and when the instrument has been used are all itemized and discussed. Finally, a summary of strengths and limitations of each instrument is provided.

Section III forecasts the direction in which the field of outcomes assessment may be headed and considers how outcomes assessment may become a component of other critical health care initiatives. Dr. McIntyre, Chair of the American Psychiatric Association's (APA) Committee on Practice Guidelines, reviews the essential role of outcomes assessment in the continuous refinement of practice guidelines. Dr. Geraty examines how the managed behavioral health care industry, which now has benefit responsibility for almost 100 million Americans, has incorporated the assessment of outcomes. He also considers the role of assessment in the next generation(s) of managed care.

Dr. Dickey, drawing on the work of the Mental Health Statistics Improvement Program's Task Force on the Design of the Mental Health Component of a Health Plan Report Card under National Reform, and others, describes different approaches to reporting the performance of health care plans in delivering psychiatric and substance abuse services. Dr. Dickey discusses the potential benefits of report cards if existing problems in data collection and reporting can be solved.

Section III continues with a discussion on a major and vital initiative of the APA's Office of Research. Dr. Zarin and Ms. West describe the development of a national network of practicing psychiatrists, in private and public treatment settings, who will provide ongoing data for clinical and health service research under the naturalistic conditions that exist in the community. The Practice Research Network will serve as an important source of clinical effectiveness studies that should influence practice (treatment) guidelines, reimbursement, and policy planning. The section concludes with Dr. Hohmann's thoughtful analysis of how we can improve existing measurement instruments, with particular sensitivity to the sociocultural, economic, and clinical variables affecting outcome assessment.

Appendix A is a table that summarizes key information about the instruments discussed in Section II, and Appendix B consists of reprints of the actual instruments that could be published with permission. Proprietary considerations by copyright holders for some of the instruments limited our ability to publish examples of all instruments.

The assessment of clinical outcomes is not new. A tradition of scientific method has shaped psychiatric practice for a century. However, assessment is now undergoing rapid changes in instrumentation and methodology. More importantly, we foresee that outcomes assessment will have a critical role in the improvement of the quality of care, in the competition for contracts and "covered-lives," in public perception and accountability, in reimbursement, and in public policy. We hope this text will provide practitioners, clinical administrators, and appointed and elected officials with a valuable resource at this remarkable moment in the transformation of the American health care system.

Lloyd I. Sederer, M.D.
Barbara Dickey, Ph.D.

REFERENCE

1. Ellwood PM. Shattuck Lecture-Outcomes management: a technology of patient experience. *N Engl J Med* 1988;318:1549–1556.

# CONTRIBUTORS

THOMAS M. ACHENBACH, Ph.D.
*Professor of Psychiatry and Psychology*
*Department of Psychiatry*
*University of Vermont College of Medicine*
*Burlington, Vermont*

DAVID A. ADLER, M.D.
*Professor of Psychiatry*
*Tufts University School of Medicine*
*Senior Psychiatrist*
*New England Medical Center*
*Boston, Massachusetts*

C. CLIFFORD ATTKISON, Ph.D.
*Professor of Medical Psychology*
*Department of Psychiatry*
*Dean of Graduate Studies*
*University of California, San Francisco*
*    School of Medicine*
*San Francisco, California*

AARON T. BECK, M.D.
*Professor of Psychiatry*
*Center for Cognitive Therapy*
*University of Pennsylvania School of Medicine*
*Philadelphia, Pennsylvania*

JEFFREY L. BERLANT, M.D., Ph.D.
*Clinical Assistant Professor of Psychiatry*
*University of Washington School of Medicine*
*Seattle, Washington*
*Consultant, National Behavioral Health Unit*
*William M. Mercer, Inc.*
*San Francisco, California*

JOHN S. CACCIOLA, Ph.D.
*Senior Investigator*
*Treatment Research Institute-Deltametrics Inc.*
*Philadelphia, Pennsylvania*

BARBARA DICKEY, Ph.D.
*Associate Professor of Psychology*
*Department of Psychiatry*
*Harvard Medical School*
*Boston, Massachusetts*
*Director*

*Department of Mental Health Services*
*    Research*
*McLean Hospital*
*Belmont, Massachusetts*

LISA BETH DIXON, M.D.
*Assistant Professor of Psychiatry*
*Medical Director, Assertive Community*
*    Treatment Team*
*University of Maryland School of Medicine*
*Baltimore, Maryland*

JOHN P. DOCHERTY, M.D.
*Professor of Psychiatry & Vice Chairman,*
*    Department of Psychiatry*
*Cornell University Medical School*
*Associate Medical Director*
*The New York Hospital, Westchester Division*
*White Plains, New York*

ROBERT A. DORWART, M.D., M.P.H.
*Professor of Psychiatry*
*Harvard Medical School*
*Boston, Massachusetts*

ROBERT E. DRAKE, M.D., Ph.D.
*Professor of Psychiatry*
*Dartmouth Medical School*
*Lebanon, New Hampshire*

JACK DURELL, M.D.
*Professor of Psychiatry*
*University of Pennsylvania School of Medicine*
*Executive Director*
*Treatment Research Institute-Deltametrics Inc.*
*Philadelphia, Pennsylvania*

SUSAN V. EISEN, Ph.D.
*Assistant Professor of Psychology*
*Department of Psychiatry*
*Harvard Medical School*
*Boston, Massachusetts*
*Assistant Director*
*Department of Mental Health Services Research*
*McLean Hospital*
*Belmont, Massachusetts*

JAMES M. ELLISON, M.D., M.P.H.
*Assistant Clinical Professor of Psychiatry*
*Harvard Medical School*
*Lecturer on Psychiatry*
*Department of Psychiatry*
*Tufts University School of Medicine*
*Boston, Massachusetts*
*Chief, Mental Health Department*
*Harvard Community Health Plan*
*Robert H. Ebert Health Center*
*Burlington, Massachusetts*

JEAN ENDICOTT, Ph.D.
*Professor of Clinical Psychology in Psychiatry*
*Columbia University College of Physicians*
*and Surgeons*
*Chief, Department of Research Assessment*
*and Training*
*New York State Psychiatric Institute*
*New York, New York*

WILLIAM O. FAUSTMAN, Ph.D.
*Clinical Assistant Professor of Psychiatry and*
*Behavioral Sciences*
*Stanford University School of Medicine*
*Stanford, California*
*Stanford / Veterans Affairs Mental Health*
*Clinical Research Center*
*Palo Alto, California*

IAN FUREMAN, M.A.
*Senior Trainer*
*Treatment Research Institute-Deltametrics Inc.*
*Philadelphia, Pennsylvania*

GAIL M. GAMACHE, Ph.D.
*Senior Post Doctoral Research Associate*
*of Sociology*
*Social and Demographic Research Institute*
*University of Massachusetts*
*Amherst, Massachusetts*

DAVID M. GARNER, Ph.D.
*Adjunct Professor*
*Department of Psychology*
*Bowling Green State University*
*Bowling Green, Ohio*

RONALD D. GERATY, M.D.
*President*
*Continuum Behavioral Healthcare, Inc.*
*Park Ridge, New Jersey*
*Instructor in Psychiatry*
*Harvard Medical School*
*Boston, Massachusetts*

MIRIAM GIBBON, M.S.W.
*Assistant Clinical Professor of Psychiatric*
*Social Work*
*Columbia University College of Physicians*
*and Surgeons*
*Research Scientist, Biometrics Research*
*New York State Psychiatric Institute*
*New York, New York*

HOWARD H. GOLDMAN, M.D., Ph.D.
*Professor of Psychiatry*
*Director, Mental Health Policy Studies*
*University of Maryland School of Medicine*
*Baltimore, Maryland*

THOMAS K. GREENFIELD, Ph.D.
*Adjunct Assistant Professor of Psychiatry*
*University of California, San Francisco,*
*School of Medicine*
*San Francisco, California*
*Senior Scientist*
*Alcohol Research Group*
*Western Consortium for Public Health*
*Berkeley, California*

DUSAN HADZI-PAVLOVIC, M.Psychol.
*Senior Hospital Scientist*
*Division of Psychiatry*
*Prince Henry Hospital*
*Conjoint Lecturer*
*School of Psychiatry*
*University of New South Wales*
*Sydney, New South Wales, Australia*

RICHARD C. HERMANN, M.D.
*Clinical Fellow in Psychiatry*
*Harvard Medical School*
*Boston, Massachusetts*
*Resident in Adult Psychiatry*
*McLean Hospital*
*Belmont, Massachusetts*

ANN A. HOHMANN, Ph.D., M.P.H.
*Chief, Special Populations and Research*
*Methods Development Program*
*Services Research Branch*
*National Institutes of Mental Health*
*Rockville, Maryland*

ANTHONY F. LEHMAN, M.D., M.S.P.H.
*Professor of Psychiatry*
*Director, Center for Mental Health Services*
*Research University of Maryland School of*
*Medicine*
*Baltimore, Maryland*

ELIZABETH A. MCGLYNN, Ph.D.
*Health Policy Analyst*
*Social Policy Department*
*The RAND Corporation*
*Santa Monica, California*

GREGORY J. MCHUGO, Ph.D.
*Assistant Professor of Community and*
  *Family Medicine*
*Dartmouth Medical School*
*Lebanon, New Hampshire*

JOHN S. MCINTYRE, M.D.
*Clinical Professor of Psychiatry*
*University of Rochester School of Medicine*
  *and Dentistry*
*Chairman, Department of Psychiatry*
*St. Mary's Hospital*
*Rochester, New York*

A. THOMAS MCLELLAN, Ph.D.
*Professor of Psychiatry*
*University of Pennsylvania School of Medicine*
*Scientific Director*
*Treatment Research Institute-Deltametrics, Inc.*
*Philadelphia, Pennsylvania*

L. STEPHEN MILLER, Ph.D.
*Assistant Professor of Clinical Psychology*
*Department of Psychology*
*The University of Georgia*
*Athens, Georgia*

KIM T. MUESER, Ph.D.
*Associate Professor of Psychiatry*
*Dartmouth Medical School*
*Lebanon, New Hampshire*

GORDON PARKER, M.D., Ph.D.,
  F.R.A.N.Z.C.P.
*Professor of Psychiatry*
*University of New South Wales*
*Chairman, Division of Psychiatry*
*Prince of Wales and Prince Henry Hospitals*
*Sydney, New South Wales, Australia*

HAROLD A. PINCUS, M.D.
*Clinical Professor of Psychiatry*
*George Washington University*
*Deputy Medical Director*
*Director, Office of Research*
*American Psychiatric Association*
*Washington, DC*

ALAN ROSEN, M.R.C. Psych.,
  F.R.A.N.Z.C.P.
*Senior Specialist in Psychiatry*

*Northern Area Mental Health Service*
*Royal North Shore Hospital*
*Senior Lecturer in Psychiatry*
*University of Sydney*
*Sydney, New South Wales, Australia*

ROBIN L. ROSS, M.D.
*Assistant Professor of Psychiatry*
*Director of Adult Outpatient Services*
*University of Arkansas for Medical Sciences*
*Little Rock, Arkansas*

KATHRYN M. ROST, Ph.D.
*Associate Professor of Psychiatry*
*University of Arkansas for Medical Sciences*
*Associate Director*
*National Institute of Mental Health Center for*
  *Rural Mental Healthcare Research*
*Little Rock, Arkansas*

MARC SAGEMAN, M.D., Ph.D.
*Clinical Instructor*
*Hospital of The University of Pennsylvania*
*Philadelphia, Pennsylvania*

LLOYD I. SEDERER, M.D.
*Associate Professor of Psychiatry*
*Harvard Medical School*
*Boston, Massachusetts*
*Senior Vice President for Clinical Services*
*McLean Hospital*
*Belmont, Massachusetts*

SAMUEL G. SIRIS, M.D.
*Director, Adult Psychiatric Programs*
*Hillside Hospital Division*
*Long Island Jewish Medical Center*
*Glen Oaks, New York*

G. RICHARD SMITH, M.D.
*Professor and Vice Chairman*
*Department of Psychiatry and Behavioral*
  *Sciences Director*
*National Institute of Mental Health Center for*
  *Rural Mental Healthcare Research*
*University of Arkansas for Medical Sciences*
*Little Rock, Arkansas*

VIRGINIA L. SMITH
*Product Manager*
*NCS Assessments*
*Minneapolis, Minnesota*

ROBERT L. SPITZER, M.D.
*Professor of Psychiatry*
*Columbia University College of Physicians*
  *and Surgeons*

*Chief, Biometrics Research*
*New York State Psychiatric Institute*
*New York, New York*

ROBERT A. STEER, Ed.D.
*Professor*
*University of Medicine and Dentistry of New*
*   Jersey School of Osteopathic Medicine*
*Camden, New Jersey*

MELISSA J. STREETER
*Mental Health Education Coordinator*
*Mental Health Group, Neuropsychiatric*
*   Institute*
*University of California, Los Angeles*
*Los Angeles, California*

RICHARD C. TESSLER, Ph.D.
*Professor of Sociology*
*Social and Demographic Research Institute*
*University of Massachusetts*
*Amherst, Massachusetts*

HENDRIK WAGENAAR, Ph.D.
*Professor*
*Department of Public Administration*
*University of Leiden*
*Leiden, The Netherlands*

JOHN E. WARE, Ph.D.
*Research Professor of Psychiatry*
*Tufts University School of Medicine*
*Adjunct Professor of Health and Social*
*   Behavior*

*Harvard School of Public Health*
*Senior Scientist*
*The Health Institute, New England*
*   Medical Center*
*Boston, Massachusetts*

HOWARD M. WAXMAN, Ph.D.
*Director of Research and Evaluation*
*Belmont Center for Comprehensive Treatment*
*Department of Psychiatry*
*Albert Einstein Medical College*
*Philadelphia, Pennsylvania*

JOYCE C. WEST, M.P.P.
*Research Manager*
*Office of Research*
*American Psychiatric Association*
*Washington, DC*

JANET B. W. WILLIAMS, D.S.W.
*Professor of Clinical Psychiatric Social Work*
*   in Psychiatry and Neurology*
*Columbia University College of Physicians*
*   and Surgeons*
*Research Scientist, Biometrics Research*
*New York State Psychiatric Institute*
*New York, New York*

DEBORAH A. ZARIN, M.D.
*Deputy Medical Director*
*American Psychiatric Association*
*Washington, DC*

# CONTENTS

## SECTION III
## Future Directions

## SECTION IV
# Appendices

CHAPTER 1

# The Imperative of Outcomes Assessment in Psychiatry

*Lloyd I. Sederer, Barbara Dickey, Richard C. Hermann*

## THE OUTCOMES IMPERATIVE

Quality in psychiatric care is in peril. Surveys and commentaries now routinely describe a shift in the focus of patient care from clinical priorities to fiscal priorities (1–3). This transformation has been driven by the growing concern of the escalating cost of health care and by the aggressive efforts by third-party payers and utilization review organizations to manage costs by reviewing and restricting utilization of clinical services. Hospitals and health care systems are responding by reorganizing clinical services and competing for contracts to care for populations of patients. Yet efforts to provide less costly care will succeed only if careful attention is paid to both the cost and quality of psychiatric care.

A second shift in priorities, perhaps more rhetorically than realistically, is the growing demand to meet consumer needs. Although it is not entirely clear how consumer standards of quality diverge from professional standards, payers of care have used the consumer movement to raise questions about the value of psychiatric services. Regardless of the source, the pressure on clinical practice to be accountable for the outcome of care has moved outcomes assessment into the national spotlight.

In the 1990s, the quality of care initiatives are shifting from the structure and process of care to a mandate to evaluate the outcomes of care. Principally, two forces have prompted this shift. The first force predominating health care today is what Relman calls the "revolt of the payers" (4). Accurate, reliable, and quantitative assessment of the *results* of medical care must become an integral part of health care delivery if the system is to become more accountable to its payers and to the public. The second force derives from the Joint Commission on the Accreditation of Health Care Organizations (JCAHO). JCAHO accreditation increasingly is focused on continuous quality improvement that must be quantitatively demonstrated (5, 6). Quality improvement based on quantitative outcome assessment is becoming an important part of an organized system of care.

According to Donebedian, the father of quality of care research, outcome is one of three dimensions that must be measured to determine quality of care (7–9). The other two, noted above, are structure and process. Structure refers to aspects of care such as organizational design, the number and qualifications of the staff, and the facility's equipment and resources. Process refers to the services rendered to a patient during an episode of care and includes diagnostic assessments, treatments rendered, complications managed or prevented, and discharge planning. Outcomes, short term or long term, are the results of the specific procedures and treatments rendered.

Traditionally, outcome assessment has focused on the effects of discrete treatment interventions under controlled, experimental conditions (efficacy research); however, emphasis is now being placed on the assessment of patients under the naturalistic conditions in hospitals, clinics, and the community (effectiveness research). For example, in psychiatry, a controlled study of imipramine versus placebo is useful for pharmaceutical research, but health insurers would find more useful a study of the outcome of depressed patients who receive hospital level of care. The latter study would require a different methodology and new assessment instruments. Experimental trials typically are conducted with instruments that measure acute changes in symptomatology; however, outcome for patients, families, employers, and payers is not simply confined to symptomatic change. Equally important to those affected by the care rendered is the patient's capacity to function within a family, community, or work environment or to exist independently, without undue burden on the family and the social welfare system. Also important is the patient's ability to show improvement in any concurrent medical and psychiatric disorder (e.g., alcoholism and its effects on accident-induced trauma, on liver and heart disease, and on the treatment compliance of bipolar and schizophrenic patients). Finally, not only do patients seek symptomatic improvement, but they want to experience a subjective sense of health and well being.

Outcomes assessment (and its use in clinical outcomes management) is slowly developing a niche in the delivery of health care services, especially in the mental health care sector. Although the effort to integrate outcomes assessment into clinical practice is in an embryonic stage, the effort is proceeding with great urgency. The mental health care "industry," often challenged about its value and subjected to charges of inappropriate and unethical use of services, must now more than ever demonstrate its utility, effectiveness, and worth.

Outcomes assessment must become a valued aspect of the services provided by mental health institutions and the professionals who staff them. The value of outcome assessment is most manifest in its clinical utility. With the proper tools and methods, clinicians can be made more aware of patient symptomatology, risk, and functioning. Progress can be tracked, and the effectiveness of our treatment can be measured and demonstrated under naturalistic conditions. In this way, we can focus our attention on quality improvement. Continuous quality improvement (CQI), when achieved, enables clinicians to meet the needs of patients, families, and the "medical marketplace" (10). Moreover, quality improvement processes are becoming a requisite of the requests for proposals that are issued by health maintenance organizations (HMOs), managed care companies, and insurers to the provider (hospitals and clinicians) community who market their services to these buyers. They are asking providers to take CQI seriously.

Integrating outcomes assessment into clinical practice will serve several functions in addition to improving patient care. First, the development and adoption of treatment guidelines can be linked to specific outcomes. This explicit link should decrease the inappropriate substitution of less intensive treatment protocols whose appeal lies primarily in the lower charges incurred. In effect, outcomes assessment can be used to establish treatment value. Second, the integration of outcomes assessment into clinical practice can produce data to legitimize the treatment of psychiatric and substance abuse problems in the eyes of legislators contemplating changes in access to or the financing of care. Third, outcomes assessment can be seen as a marketing tool for mental health care service systems. One form of marketing, no doubt, will be the health care "report cards" envisioned by the Clinton Administration (11). If the price of care becomes less important as the principal determinant in the insurers' choice among competing health care systems, outcome data will increasingly be considered in the selection process of providers.

Finally, and perhaps most importantly, accountability through outcomes assessment offers an opportunity to regain the public trust (12). Physicians and clinicians of all disciplines currently are often held in low esteem by the consumers of medical and mental health care services. By soliciting perspectives from the patient, as well as that of the family, employer, and payer, and by focusing our concerns on improving the patient's quality of life, we can begin the process of restoring the public trust and the confidence of patients and their families.

## DOMAINS OF CLINICAL ASSESSMENT

The effectiveness of clinical services should be judged by whether there has been improvement in the patient's clinical status, feelings of well being, and functional ability. Effectiveness in these domains, although most evident in the short term (measured shortly after treatment concludes or after some shift in treatment modality), might also be assessed in the long term. Furthermore, regardless of the degree of improvement, both patient and family should be satisfied with all aspects of the care delivered. The latter includes not just the treatment provided but also activities related to the delivery of care, such as the efficiency and accuracy of the billing office or the arrangements for continuity of care.

### Clinical Outcome Assessment

The clinical assessment of outcome can be considered from two principal dimensions: symptomatic and functional. Symptomatic assessment is the collection of valid and reliable data on the presence, intensity, and duration of psychopathological symptoms. It has long played an important role in diagnosis and differential diagnosis. In prognosis, it has been used in empirical research on the efficacy of specific treatments (e.g., in randomly controlled drug studies). Symptom assessment also has been valu-able in the provision of acute psychiatric care that generally produces rapid and dramatic improvements in symptomatology. Two examples of measurable and rapid changes in symptomatology are seen in the detoxification of substance abusers and in the effects of medications on acutely agitated patients. Symptom assessment may be the best way to measure the immediate effects of a treatment.

Functional assessment is increasingly important because of the growing recognition of the economic costs of psychiatric dysfunction and disability. Employers are concerned about reestablishing productivity and patients are interested in an improvement in their capabilities (13–15). For patients, a focus on functional status, which is more directly related to their quality of life, can often be less stigmatizing than symptom-oriented assessment. An expanding appreciation of the recurrent or chronic nature of many disorders, medical as well as psychiatric, adds to the need for longer term assessment of functioning.

A patient's functional status can be assessed in multiple domains, especially interpersonal, domestic, vocational, and educational. A patient's ability for self-care, independent living, energy and zest, personal relationships, and recreational pursuits are all important aspects of functional capacity that may continue to improve in the months after symptomatic recovery. This change in functional status argues for longer term follow-up to measure any residual impairment from acute illness and to determine the gains achieved from rehabilitative interventions.

### Patient and Family Satisfaction

Satisfaction with treatment need not, but usually does, correlate with clinical outcome (16, 17). For many years, satisfaction surveys were thought to be useful public relation tools but were held in low regard by evaluators of inpatient services. Recently, the opinion of consumers of treatment has taken a more central role in the evaluation of services. The changing environment in mental health has directed attention to the needs of consumers, rather than providers, of care. Patient satisfaction is considered central to service systems when competition between plans rests, in part, on performance indicators, including patient satisfaction and patient outcomes.

Traditional patient satisfaction surveys focused primarily on hotel-type amenities (e.g., satisfaction with the food, overall cleanliness of a facility), family travel time, promptness of the service, and friendliness of the staff. Current efforts to update these surveys have led researchers in the field of patient satisfaction to place more emphasis on questions concerning the technical competence and interpersonal skills of caregivers. The latter includes questions about the extent to which patients believe they can participate in treatment planning and the staff's willingness to explain the particular benefits and limitations of different procedures or medications.

Almost every satisfaction survey asks "would you return for care or refer a relative?" A negative answer not only implies the institution now has a very unhappy patient but its contract with a managed care company or insurer may also become endangered. Some HMOs and managed care organizations require patient satisfaction to be measured and the rate of satisfaction to reach at least 90%.

Family satisfaction has greater relevance in programs that treat children or disabled adults who are under the care of their families. We are not advocating that family satisfaction be collected in place of patient satisfaction but rather that the institution in these cases has a broader constituency that must be satisfied.

Consideration of the patient or consumer perspective has become essential in the delivery of health care services. Information gained from satisfaction studies can be used to improve on treatment compliance, use of services, program design, and, in some instances, outcome (18, 19). Satisfaction studies are also useful in providing clinical and nonclinical staff with regular patient feedback (complimentary as well as critical) on their work. Satisfaction surveys are thus becoming increasingly important as an aspect of a facility's quality improvement efforts.

## ASSESSMENT INSTRUMENTS IN PSYCHIATRY

In an effort to determine which outcome instrument(s) is best for a particular situation, a plan should be developed that addresses the following questions: which patients will be included in the study? What outcomes will be most effected by the treatment? When will the outcomes be measured? Who is going to read (and use) the information provided by the outcomes study? The more specific the answer of these questions, the better the choice of outcome instrument. In research, a guiding rule is to make the measurement as precise as possible to determine the magnitude of the effect. When an instrument is not very precise, the size of the effect sought to measure will be smaller than the true size of the effectiveness of the intervention.

Collecting extensive data from large numbers of individuals is expensive and labor intensive. Therefore, most facilities have to choose between gathering a little data from all of the patients or collecting more detailed and complete data from a sample of the patients. In either case, the goal will be to define very clearly who is included and who is not included in the sample to avoid the possibility of selection bias. The justification for choosing one group rather than another will need to be explicit and understandable so that the readers of a final report will understand who was included and why. For example, when patient satisfaction surveys are left to random completion (e.g., offered on wall racks to interested consumers), a respondent bias is likely to occur. When assessment instruments are systematically applied (e.g., to every nth discharge) these biases can be minimized. Self-report measures can be used with many populations, but certain types of patients, such as those who are severely confused, disorganized, or psychomotorically retarded, may be unable to respond. The result could be a selection bias favoring the less severely ill.

As you will see in Section II of this text, the assessment instruments we have described cover well being, functioning, symptoms, satisfaction, and treatment utilization. The respondents are clinicians, patients, and their families. Almost all are intended to be used with adults, but many are written at a grade-school level and can be used by adolescents.

All of the instruments we have chosen have met acceptable standards for validity and reliability. Reliability is the accuracy and reproducability of a scale and reflects how closely a scale captures the "true" variance in scores. The higher the reliability score, the more precise the instrument. A number of approaches can be followed to test reliability, and these depend on the type of scale and its uses.

Validity depends on how well a scale measures the "outcome" construct that it purports to measure. It is more difficult to measure than reliability, especially in health care, because there is rarely a gold standard against which the scale can be compared. Most validity studies combine different approaches that accumulate evidence to support the contention that an instrument measures what it is supposed to measure. For example, construct validity may confirm that the instrument correlates highly with other measures of the same construct (e.g., diagnosis), and predictive validity may establish that the instrument effectively predicts expectable outcomes (e.g., homelessness, suicidal behavior, hospital readmission).

For facilities with limited research experience and sparse budgets for measuring outcome, other important features of an assessment instrument will include affordability and ease of administration, data entry, and analysis. The costs of assessment include the instruments themselves and the professional staff time needed for administration and analysis. Instrument

costs vary substantially; some are available through commercial concerns that charge for each copy of the instrument, others can be obtained directly from the authors at minimal cost, or some are in the public domain. Instruments require different levels of expertise for administration, ranging from those that are reliable only when administered by a clinician with specific training to those that patients can administer themselves. Staff costs can be reduced by using instruments that are self-administered, which can provide valid and reliable assessments. Like any assessment modality, however, self-report instruments can be subject to response biases. These biases can be minimized via careful design and administration (20, 21). Computer automation can further enhance simplicity of use; scanners can facilitate survey data entry; compatibility with existing hospital information systems can allow for integration of outcome data with demographic, clinical, and utilization data; and commercially available software can provide rapid data analysis and reports.

Satisfaction instruments generally do not achieve the degree of standardization that characterizes the symptom and functional instruments. Some facilities choose to tailor a satisfaction instrument to match the varied services offered and to comply with local and customary terms that describe the facility and its caregivers. A self-authored satisfaction instrument may allow for specific facility-based needs while categorizing inquiries into hotel, caregiver, treatment, and global areas. The application of computer technology, as described, will allow for automated scoring and analysis, as well as integration with other information such as clinical assessment and service utilization.

## LINKING ASSESSMENT DATA WITH PATIENT AND TREATMENT DATA

To provide a meaningful context for outcomes data, additional patient information is needed. For example, what are the demographic characteristics of the population studied? What are the clinical features of the patients receiving treatment? What are the treatments that have been provided? Each patient's utilization of clinical services, as well as aggregate information on an identified group of patients, must be recorded systematically to measure the effect on outcome. Linking clinical and satisfaction outcomes data to demographic information and service utilization will provide the database necessary to answer such fundamental questions as which demographic groups respond better or worse to treatment or which groups are more or less satisfied. We can also examine the relationship between diagnosis and clinical improvement.

## Clinical Populations

Psychiatric patients are generally quite heterogeneous. The principal *demographic characteristics* of a patient population include sex, age, race, ethnicity, language, occupation, socioeconomic status, and type of insurance coverage. The more demographic information that can be obtained, the greater the ability to identify the factors that may influence outcome.

Patient identifying information then extends to *clinical variables* that can include primary psychiatric diagnoses (both Axis I clinical syndromes and Axis II personality and developmental disorders), legal status (voluntary, involuntary, and court ordered), and substance abuse or medical comorbidity. It is also useful, when possible, to identify those patients who are disabled as a consequence of mental illness (e.g., receiving Social Security Disability Insurance), because that generally signifies severity and chronicity of illness. All of these variables have important implications for clinical outcome.

## Service Use

For psychiatric and substance abuse patients, care may be rendered at various levels of care or intensity during an episode of illness. Therefore, service use in psychiatry must be coded in such a way as to signify inpatient days, partial hospital days, acute residential days, and outpatient visits. Data storage should allow for the retrieval of a patient's treatment record at each service level during the illness episode and for an identified period of follow-up (which may be possible only if the patient remains within the same system of care).

Data may also be collected on professional services (e.g., consult psychotherapies, psychopharmacological visits), diagnostic services (e.g., psychological testing, electroencephalograms, magnetic resonance imaging), and biological treatments (e.g., pharmaceuticals, electroconvulsive therapy). Such service use can account for as much as 10–30% of facility-based costs and can be a potential predictor of outcome.

Collecting data on the use of medical services by psychiatric patients can provide a more complete understanding of a population's service utilization. Medical/surgical utilization data are also valuable in determining whether psychiatric treatment reduces costs for primary, emergency, or medical/surgical specialty care (22).

Data on the use of professional, ancillary, and hospital services are best gathered through the facility's management information system (MIS). Expanding the facility MIS for outcomes assessment can be a prohibitively costly and time-consuming effort. By downloading MIS data to a personal computer, databases can be integrated without the need to overhaul an entire system. MIS data may then be merged with clinical and satisfaction outcome data, providing a method for analyzing service use, outcomes, and satisfaction.

## OUTCOMES ASSESSMENT IN CLINICAL PRACTICE

As providers of care learn more about what treatments work for which patients under naturalistic conditions (i.e., a non-controlled patient population and nonrandomized clinical interventions), psychiatric research will shift from clinical trials to mental health services research or from efficacy to effectiveness studies. This profound change in health care research will have an equally profound effect on the way care will be provided in the future.

Every service system that exists or will emerge in the years to come must prove capable of meeting the primary goal of health care, namely, to help the patient when possible and to do no harm. Outcomes assessment offers a critically important approach to determining whether our efforts are congruent with this goal.

## REFERENCES

1. Jellinek MS, Nurcombe B. Two wrongs don't make a right: managed care, mental health, and the marketplace. JAMA 1993;270:1737–1739.
2. Schreter RF. Ten trends in managed care and their impact on the biopsychosocial model. Hosp Community Psychiatry 1993;44:325–327.
3. Foster Higgins. Survey on outcomes management. New York, 1993.
4. Relman A. Assessment and accountability—the third revolution in medical care. N Engl J Med 1988;319:1220–1222.
5. Joint Commission on Accreditation of Health Care Organizations. Chicago: The Joint Commission Guide to Quality Assurance, 1989.
6. Berwick DM. Continuous improvement as an idea in health care. N Engl J Med 1989;320:53–56.
7. Donabedian A. Explorations in quality assurance and monitoring. Ann Arbor: Health Administration Press, 1985;3.
8. Deming WE. Out of crisis [monograph]. Cambridge, MA: Massachusetts Institute of Technology, Center for Advanced Engineering Study, 1982.
9. Sederer LI. Quality, costs and contracts: administrative aspects of inpatient psychiatry. In: Sederer LI, ed. Inpatient psychiatry: diagnosis and treatment. 3rd ed. Baltimore: Williams & Wilkins, 1991;419–431.
10. Stoline A, Werner JP. The new medical marketplace. Baltimore: The Johns Hopkins University Press, 1988.
11. Bergman M. Making the grade. Hospitals and Health Networks. January 5, 1994:34–36.
12. Thier SO. Forces motivating the use of health status assessment measures in clinical settings and related clinical research. Med Care 1992; 30(Suppl):S515–S522.
13. Rice DP, Kelman S, Miller LS. The economic burden of mental illness. Hosp Community Psychiatry 1992;43:1227–1232.
14. Rupp A, Keith SJ. The costs of schizophrenia. Psychiatric Clin North Am 1993;16:413–423.
15. Greenberg PE, Stiglin LE, Finkelstein SN, et al. The economic burden of depression in 1990. J Clin Psychiatry 1993;54:405–418.
16. Eisen SV, Grob MC. Measuring discharged patients' satisfaction with care at a private psychiatric hospital. Hosp Community Psychiatry 1982;33:227–228.
17. Kalman TP. An overview of patient satisfaction with psychiatric treatment. Hosp Community Psychiatry 1983;34:48–54.
18. Linn LS, Brook RH, Clark VA, Davies AR, Fink A, Kosecoff J. Physician and patient satisfaction as factors related to the organization of internal medicine group practices. Med Care 1985;23:1171–1178.
19. Weisman CS, Nathanson CA: Professional satisfactions and client outcomes. Med Care 1985;23:1179–1192.
20. Eisen SV, Grob MC, Dill DL. Outcome measurement: tapping the patient's perspective. In: Mirin SM, Gossett JM, Grob MC, eds. Recent advances in outcome research. Washington, DC: American Psychiatric Press, 1991.
21. Dickey B, Wagenarr H, Stewart A. Using health status measures with the seriously mentally ill. Med Care (in press).
22. Strain JJ, Lyon JS, Hammer JS, et al. Cost offset from a psychiatric consultation-liaison intervention with elderly hip fracture patients. Am J Psychiatry 1991;148:1044–1049.

# CHAPTER 2

# Measuring Outcomes

*John P. Docherty, Melissa J. Streeter*

*"...when you can measure what you are speaking about, and express it in numbers, you know something about it; but when you cannot express it in numbers, your knowledge is of a meager and unsatisfactory kind. It may be the beginning of knowledge but you have scarcely, in your thoughts, advanced the state of science."*

—*Lord Kelvin*

## INTRODUCTION

The U.S. health care delivery system has undergone enormous changes in the last quarter century. Along with other areas of medicine, psychiatry must learn to cope with the extraordinary revolution that is currently changing the way Americans view health care. The nation now is demanding that mental health services be empirically based and administered with the precision of a science. A substantial attitudinal change is required to recognize the value of objective data and use it effectively.

Society is becoming increasingly intolerant of the ambiguity and the vagaries that have characterized the field of psychiatry. In fact, payers and policymakers exhibit a disturbing lack of faith in the value of mental health care. Because we have not implemented systems to effectively demonstrate the quality and utility of mental health services and have yet to approach our field with the rigor required of medicine, the necessity of these services is questioned. Payers are typically reluctant to reimburse for mental health care services, policymakers question the need to include mental health services as part of a standard benefit package, and patients doubt that they will receive the most appropriate treatment, competently delivered (1). Thus, today, virtually all of the external forces a health care organization must satisfy for its survival are now demanding that outcomes assessment, which is essential to an empirical response to these questions, be performed.

A sophisticated, comprehensive outcomes measurement system will not only allow us to effectively respond to these external forces, but such information will also provide the necessary tools to systematically improve the quality of mental health care.

Procedures are not in place to systematically monitor these variations in practice patterns, reward high quality services, or penalize low quality care. Although a substantial body of literature exists that demonstrates specific efficacy of particular treatment protocols for particular patients, few structures are available to ensure that practitioners use this information in the clinical decision-making process. Government and professional initiatives have been launched to address these problems. The Practice Guidelines of the American Psychiatric Association (2) and the extensive Depression Guidelines of the Agency for Health Care Policy Research (3) are two noteworthy examples. However, the assessment of adherence to these guidelines, the usefulness of different methods to ensure such adherence, and the impact of this adherence on patient well being is all dependent on a sophisticated and efficient system of outcomes management.

## UTILIZATION OF OUTCOMES DATA IN A HEALTH CARE INSTITUTION

Clinical outcome data can be used to achieve four main objectives: management of clinical and administrative operations, regulatory compliance, marketing, and research. The ideal outcomes management system should be designed to successfully accomplish all four of these purposes. Categorical systems may be designed to accomplish one, two, or a combination of these purposes; however, for a successful provider in the era of health care reform, the ideal outcome system should permit the accomplishment of all four goals simultaneously.

### Management of Clinical and Administrative Operations

Health care systems are expected to be responsible for the active internal management of care. Managed care companies that seek to diminish their costs and move from a "policing function" to a "facilitating function" are increasingly interested in contracting with entities that are capable of their own quantitative internal management.

How can outcomes data be used for the management of clinical operations? At its most fundamental level, monitoring outcomes data may yield information regarding a shift in the level of effectiveness of the treatment provided by the institution, which may point to the need for immediate administrative action. On a more refined level, differential changes may be noted in the effectiveness of one component of the array of services provided by the institution or of one particular patient subpopulation. Access to this data permits more precise and appropriate administrative action.

A comprehensive outcome assessment system permits the consideration of the impact of varying staffing patterns, different levels of providers, and staffing ratios on patient outcome. This critical area in the cost of mental health services may be related carefully and empirically to a patient outcome, thus providing a sound and accountable basis for managing staffing patterns and understanding the clinical and economic value of professionals of different disciplines and levels of training.

Clearly, outcomes data is essential for a meaningful system of provider profiling. Properly analyzed across providers, this data can yield information on the relative effectiveness of a specific individual; within providers, it can yield information regarding relative effectiveness of individuals with different patient subpopulations. In addition, the outcomes data may supply information on the impact of changes in treatment practices, such as greater or less adjunctive psychosocial treatment, the types of medications prescribed, and length of stay by diagnostic category. These data may have critical implications for management of both costs and payer and patient expectations.

On a slightly more complex level, data from various aspects of institutional functioning may also reveal patterns that are important in guiding administrative action. For example, the introduction of a new drug or a new physician may lead to a change in referral patterns, resulting in greater patient acuity that is accompanied by a change in the number of critical incidents. The ability to track the sequence of events that correlate with and may cause an increase in critical incidents is essential to the appropriate administrative response. Without quantitative information that is readily available and intelligibly displayed, such linkages usually are not revealed.

On the individual patient level, standardized data can be important in establishing a common language and methodology for individual patient assessment in treatment planning. With such systems, we can quantify actual progress while the patient is in treatment. Immediate data feedback allows treatment teams to determine objectively whether a particular course of treatment is yielding the expected improvement or whether a different approach is necessary.

The utilization of outcome data in clinical

and administrative operations management is a new enterprise, and time will be needed to establish the best methods for using these data. The impact of outcomes data can be significant, however, and many changes in leadership, organizational structure, and allocation of resources can be expected to follow the implementation of such a system.

## Regulatory Compliance

Some outcome assessment is required to achieve regulatory compliance, and such requirements will increase (4, 5). Attention must be paid to the specifics of these requirements as they unfold so that the proper instrumentation is selected to meet these needs. Within the framework of a comprehensive outcomes assessment and management system, however, current and future regulatory needs can and most likely will be met without substantial change in the outcome system. For example, continuing quality improvement (CQI) requirements can easily be met by the use of outcomes data on a routine basis to improve various aspects of clinical and administrative functioning. If patient satisfaction data are gathered routinely and show, for example, dissatisfaction with the admissions office, a specific project aimed at improving that score can easily be implemented without requiring new measurement or change in the hospital's routine data collection system. Additionally, a flexible system can be constructed to allow the substitution, addition, or deletion of specific items to accomplish particular CQI tasks without requiring a change in the system of assessment.

## Marketing

Perhaps the most frequent use of the mental health outcome data currently being gathered is for marketing purposes. Such data are intended to demonstrate to purchasers of care the provider's concern with the clinical status of its patients and the effort needed to assess and monitor that clinical status. This necessary and useful function of data collection allows the purchaser to develop some sense of a provider's tangible commitment to the effectiveness of its services. In addition, it provides some evidence regarding the expected effectiveness of those services.

There are significant disadvantages to developing a system that only addresses the marketing function. Although this limited system initially may seem more cost effective, it may prove to be much more expensive in the long run. Marketing systems cannot adequately provide the clinical and provider data necessary to enhance quality and ultimately to contain costs by providing the most effective treatments.

Systems that address marketing needs are characterized by discontinuous sampling rather than ongoing systematic assessment of the patient population. In addition, the data have tended to be maintained by the external agency carrying out the assessment project. Although such a structure may yield some greater sense of credibility for a purchaser of care, the most essential function of outcomes data, to provide a basis for the quantitative clinical and administrative management of the quality of care in the system (i.e., the capacity to participate in "network management"), is not supported by such a structure. For example, outcome systems that are marketing oriented will generally provide easy to read, aesthetically pleasing reports in a multicolored graphical format. This information is presented in much the same way that financial data are reported to the shareholders of a publicly held company in an annual report. Such data are clearly insufficient to support the day-to-day management of the company. Additionally, a comprehensive outcomes management system can be more flexible in producing marketing materials unique to a particular client's needs. A limited marketing system may be unable to address such special requests.

## Research

The introduction of large datasets collected from "real" populations promises to greatly enhance our research capabilities. Essentially, outcomes management systems will allow us to examine questions at every level of the mental health care system and derive pragmatic and useful information to guide key treatment, policy, and strategic planning decisions. An accessible, broad-based system of methodologically sound outcomes assessment will allow us to address important and practical clinical research questions that our present system neglects. For example, if a depressed patient fails to improve with an initial trial of a selective seratonin reuptake inhibitor (SSRI) antidepressant, what is the most effective next step? A different SSRI? A tricyclic antidepressant? Supplementation with a 5HT1A agonist? A broad program of outcomes management will allow us to rapidly and effectively address such issues.

In addition to research that addresses the efficacy of specific treatments for specific patient populations, outcomes measurement allows us to measure the effectiveness of different health care financing strategies, different clinical management systems, and different administrative policies and procedures on treatment outcome. Additionally, we can examine more objectively provider staffing models and various financial incentives to contain costs. Outcomes measurement can provide large datasets that answer such multivariate questions essential to rational health services planning.

## FEASIBILITY OF OUTCOMES MANAGEMENT

Significant advances in the technology and methodology of data collection that have greatly improved our capacity to conduct outcomes assessment as a routine part of providing medical care have occurred in the last 25 years. Specifically, great strides have been made in understanding the structure of outcome, the impact that "hidden" variables can have on the measurement of outcomes, the methodologies that support the acquisition of reliable and valid outcomes data, and the

technology that supports the efficient collection of this information.

## Structure of Outcomes

Although "outcome" is often used in a simple and global fashion, it is actually a complex construct composed of several independent dimensions. Hence, the use of outcomes in the plural form is intended to reflect the multidimensional nature of the term. Understanding the elements that comprise outcome is essential to effective conceptualization and utilization of outcomes measurement activities.

As in any area of measurement, outcomes assessment requires that the key variables be defined and operationalized. The ultimate variable for outcomes management is outcome itself. Although this may seem obvious, a precise definition of mental health outcome can be elusive. For instance, should "good outcome" for a patient with major depression be defined as a reduction in symptomatology? Improvements in interpersonal or occupational relations? An overall improvement in well being? Treatment may affect some, all, or none of these dimensions. Many clinical studies demonstrate that treatment can differentially affect one specific aspect of outcome without having a corresponding effect on any of the other outcome dimensions. For example, Strauss and Carpenter's (6) landmark work with schizophrenic patients demonstrated that commonly used outcome indicators, such as social functioning, level of symptomatology, occupational functioning, and the need for supportive resources, are only moderately correlated.

Similarly, a study of depressed women responsive to acute amitriptyline treatment (7) demonstrated that although the amitriptyline group showed a remission of neurovegetative symptomatology, little to no improvement was seen in social functioning. Conversely, although the counseling/placebo group showed improved social functioning, a relapse of depressive symptoms was experienced. The combined treatment group improved in both social functioning and depressive symptomatology, whereas the placebo group suffered continued social morbidity and a relapse of depressive symptoms. This study clearly suggests the potential for specific treatments to differentially affect certain dimensions of outcome.

Research has suggested that patient satisfaction is often independent of clinical outcome—a treatment that "works" may not necessarily leave a patient satisfied. In fact, studies have shown that staff capabilities and interpersonal skills, facility amenities, and patient expectations account for a large degree of the variance in patient satisfaction scores (8–10).

Finally, research on treatment utilization rates has demonstrated that a variety of factors, other than illness severity and treatment efficacy, affect utilization rates. Results from the RAND health insurance experiment and other studies have suggested that such variables as benefits availability, past treatment history, age, and gender affect utilization rates (11).

The relative independence of each of these outcomes measures—patient satisfaction, symptom improvement, functional improvement, and treatment utilization—highlights the multidimensional nature of outcome. A truly comprehensive and valid system should measure a broad range of outcome dimensions to accurately reflect treatment effects.

### Dimensions of Outcome

Currently, within the scientific literature for mental health care, the seven main dimensions of outcome are symptomatology (psychiatric and substance abuse), social/interpersonal functioning, work functioning, satisfaction, treatment utilization, health status/global well being, and health-related quality of life (value weighted). Chapter 3 provides a more extensive discussion of the important domains of outcomes measurement.

### Variables Affecting Outcomes Data

Three major considerations are important in the measurement of outcome: the source of the outcomes information, the timing of the outcomes assessments, and the nature of the population from which the data is derived.

*Sources of Outcome Data.* The last 20 years of clinical research has demonstrated what has been called the "Rashomon" effect: the perspectives of the patient, the provider, and the significant other groups regularly and systematically differ from one another and have a varying affect on outcomes assessment. Each of these vantage points represents a different but clinically significant aspect of the response to treatment. The patient will rate outcome according to the experienced change in subjective state, significant others will rate outcome based on change relevant to or directly affecting them, therapists will rate outcome based on the degree of change occurring as a result of the therapeutic process, employers will rate outcome based on the treatment's affect on the individual's ability to function at work, and third-party payers will rate outcome based on the intervention's success in reducing subsequent utilization of medical services (12). Thus, each of these perspectives should be assessed independently.

*Timing of Outcomes Assessment.* The timing of the evaluations has a substantial impact on the nature of the findings. For instance, it has been shown that symptomatology will regularly remit before positive changes are found in social or work functioning (13).

Outcomes measurement generally consists of three phases: baseline measurement, short-term follow-up, and long-term follow-up. The development of newer concepts, "episode of illness" and "episode of care," presents an alternative and probably a more useful framework for timing assessments of outcome. Within this framework, an episode of illness is composed of multiple episodes of care (e.g., inpatient, partial hospitalization, outpatient). The outcome system should permit assessment of each episode of care as well as regular assessments of progress through the entire episode of illness.

The baseline measures are usually collected either during the evaluation or immediately after entry into treatment for an episode of care. One constant challenge is to collect the information before treatment can exert its effects but at a point when the patient is able to participate in the process. Hence, the exact timing of the initial measurement may vary depending on the population. For instance, an intoxicated, alcoholic patient is not an appropriate candidate for complex baseline testing.

The timing of follow-up measures, however, presents a greater empirical challenge. The goal of the short-term (episode of care) follow-up is to assess the immediate effects of treatment before any additional interventions within an episode of illness. Long-term follow-up is intended to capture relapse rates, changes in resource consumption, changes in social and work functioning, and other longer term variables over the episode of illness and recovery.

Sequential measures over an extended time period are important because different treatment experiences may show very different effects depending on the time course used to evaluate them (13). Some treatments may have only long-term effects, whereas others may show an improvement on discharge followed by deterioration after discharge. Consequently, follow-up data on all dimensions are useful in determining a complete picture of the benefits gained as the result of an intervention.

Establishing a time frame for follow-up contact is a practical, initial step in setting up an outcome system. Information about the expected course of particular disorders can be helpful in selecting an appropriate time frame. For example, depression is a common diagnostic category in psychiatric facilities. For this group, follow-up assessments at discharge and about 6 months

after discharge would be sufficient to detect a patient's response to acute phase and continuation treatment (14), and a follow-up at 12 months would be sufficient to capture relapse (15, 16). Similar time frames may be appropriate for substance abuse diagnoses. However, follow-up of more than 1 year may provide valuable information for the health service planning of accountable health care systems.

In measuring patient satisfaction, which only needs to be done once, the timing is again crucial. If a mailing service is chosen, patient satisfaction questionnaires should be mailed to the patient within 4–10 days after completion of an episode of care. This timing maximizes response rates and allows the patient enough time to achieve adequate "psychological distance" from the facility to answer honestly. It is possible that questionnaires administered in the facility on discharge could lead to a positively biased response because of patient concerns regarding retaliation, anonymity, or other demand characteristics of the immediate social context (8–10).

*Patient Population Variables.* Outcomes data can only be interpreted by taking into consideration the particular population from which they are derived. In addition to clinical domains, additional background and demographics can greatly enhance the value of the data and expand the analyses that can be conducted. The recommended data to be collected are consistent with guidelines published by the National Institute of Mental Health for essential clinical management data. Such a list may be supplemented by case-mix adjustment variables relevant to the work of a specific health care system.

1. Identifying variables. Typically, three variables are required to uniquely identify a treatment episode: the medical record number, an identifying facility or program number, and an episode number.
2. Patient demographics. Variables such as age, sex, marital status, origin, and zip code are necessary to adequately de-

scribe the population of patients to whom treatment is being given.

3. Patient diagnosis. Comprehensive chart diagnoses are important and should include primary diagnosis along with all diagnoses on all axes. These diagnoses should be entered according to their Diagnostic and Statistical Manual diagnostic code because numeric data are more easily manipulated.

4. Dates of treatment. From the dates of inpatient admission and discharge, length of stay can be calculated and readmission (recidivism) can be tracked. For patients in partial hospital or intensive outpatient programs, we recommend both the dates of inclusion in the program and the number of hours per week of patient participation. These data help differentiate the patient seen 15 hours per week for 5 weeks from the patient seen 5 hours per week for 15 weeks.

5. Payer information. Data identifying the primary guarantor are obtained. The codes for these data permit the classification of patients into payer categories. Secondary guarantor information is also obtained.

6. Primary provider/attending. For inpatients, the primary care provider is usually a physician or psychologist. Each primary clinician should have a unique code that permits identification.

7. Service identifiers. Service, the most basic treatment descriptor, identifies patients by categories such as an inpatient, partial hospital, or outpatient. Other categorizations appropriate to the facility or system being evaluated can be determined.

8. Program or unit identifiers. The next level of treatment descriptor is embodied in a program and/or unit code. Sometimes both are needed to clearly identify the treatment program for a given patient. For instance, a unit number may reveal that a patient was on an adult unit and in a dual-diagnosis track or program on that unit.

9. Treatment components. Greater specificity of treatment elements can be coded and entered describing the presence of pharmacological treatment, amount and type of group therapies, vocational or other counseling, amount and type of individual therapy services, and so on.

**Methodology**

Two main bodies of research have contributed to the advances in the methodology of outcome assessment over the last quarter century. First, research such as the International Pilot Study of Schizophrenia on diagnosis and course of illness (17) led to the development of instruments for assessing outcome as well as understanding the complex structure of outcome. Studies confirm that outcome is composed of multiple dimensions such as symptoms, social and work functioning, and need for hospitalization that correlate only moderately with one another. Second, research on treatment efficacy led to an extensive development of the outcomes assessment instruments and procedures necessary to evaluate the efficacy of drug treatments and psychotherapeutic treatments.

Once decisions have been made regarding the dimensions of outcome to be measured, the appropriate providers of this information, and the timing of data collection, more specific decisions must be made in regard to procedures for collection—in other words, how the system will be operationalized.

*Instrument Characteristics.* The selection of instruments should reflect adherence to specific principles. Ideally, those instruments chosen should be comprehensive of the dimensions of interest, cost effective, easy to implement for staff and patients, adequately reliable and valid, and widely used. In addition, scales that are widely recognized and used permit comparison of results with other large databases and allow for the possibility of multisite databases at some future time.

Aside from these basic requirements, the choice of a specific instrument is largely based on convenience, personal preference, and other practical considerations, such as whether or not the instrument is in the public domain. Other specific considerations are discussed as follows.

*Self-Report Versus Interview Format.* There are pros and cons to both methodologies for collecting patient-reported data. Currently, most organizations are using self-report forms that generally are easier to administer, require less staff time, and impose less of a time constraint on the respondent. However, a backup system should be in place for individuals who have difficulty completing self-report forms because of illiteracy or other problems.

Interview forms, although requiring trained personnel to administer, have other benefits, such as fewer unanswered responses, the ability to explain certain questions, and an opportunity to maximize the utility of outcomes management as an adjunct to the therapeutic process. The interview format may be particularly useful for time-limited, in-depth studies to address a selected outcome question.

*Method of Contact.* The best method of contact is the one that works most efficiently with the target population. Mailings are relatively inexpensive; however, the typical response rate of approximately 30% is less than optimal (18). Although face-to-face administration is certainly the most desirable situation, this is both time and resource intensive and is often inconvenient for the respondents. In the case of patients who are regularly seen in an outpatient system, this may be a feasible alternative. Telephone administration is another option that is becoming increasingly more common. Research has demonstrated that telephone administration does not compromise the reliability or validity of an instrument. As technology improves, the potential for using computerized voice systems is also improving.

*Sampling.* Although we believe that outcomes data provide an invaluable clinical management tool and ideally should include every patient treated, this is not mandatory and may not be feasible. Under such circumstances, gathering data on a representative sample of patients may be preferable. However, the sample should include enough individuals of each gender, age, diagnosis, and so on to allow for meaningful analyses. Additionally, working with a sample of the population and making intensive follow-up efforts is preferable to allowing self-selection to govern the end sample. In other words, it is far better to obtain a response from 90 of 100 patients representing a scientifically valid sample than from 200 of 1,000 patients with self-selection governing the response.

A variety of reliable and valid outcomes instruments is currently available, and Section II of this book provides an excellent overview of the key instruments in the field.

## Technology

The ability to collect, analyze, and provide virtually instantaneous feedback to providers, payers, and other interested parties because of advances in the coding and integration of operating systems, the capacity of desktop computers, and other technological breakthroughs makes possible a real revolution in the usefulness of outcomes data. It is now possible to carry out data collection, storage, analysis, and reporting on a large scale, within a reasonable time frame, at feasible costs.

The three areas of technology are data collection, data storage, and data analysis. Although a comprehensive review of the technology available for each of these areas is beyond the scope of this chapter, the following sections are intended to cover the technology you may be using currently.

*Data Collection.* Today, most data are collected on paper despite the movement toward electronic medical records. Although it is true that technology can allow data entry via voice recognition, direct patient–computer interaction, and remote telecommunications, these technologies are in their early stages (19). However, optical scanning devices significantly lower the personnel time required for data entry. Depending on the speed of the instrument, the cost of an optical mark sensing device can range between $1,000 and $10,000.

A list of the elements involved in a comprehensive outcomes system was presented above. Although it may be necessary to implement new measurement systems to achieve satisfaction, symptomatology, functioning, or other clinical outcomes, new systems to collect other ancillary variables, such as demographic information, may not be needed. Because of the reporting requirements of the state health departments and of the Health Care Financing Administration, many of the data elements are already being collected. The challenge is to determine how each data element is currently collected and where this information is stored and to integrate these variables with the other outcomes elements you have chosen. It is important to store all clinical outcomes, patient satisfaction, and pertinent resource utilization data in a common database.

In constructing a system for the automation of outcomes data, you should know that a standardized electronic record format has been established for the transmission of outcomes data. This format, which has been reviewed and approved by the American Society for Testing and Materials (ASTM), was developed from standards already in existence for transmitting laboratory results and other medical information between independent computer systems. The code "HI" will identify data coded using HOI outcomes data elements codes. The HI-ASTM standards for data transmission and coding will provide the means to establish the necessary "connectivity" to permit different organizations involved in outcomes management to work together successfully. This system will also support the information exchange between health care systems, vendors of proprietary products supporting outcomes evaluations, insurers, and government agencies (20).

*Data Storage.* In the 1990s the superior hardware choice is a personal computer–based system. Mainframe vendors may attempt to convince you that data are only safe in a remote and secluded area and that no computer experience is necessary. However, mainframe systems are truly the dinosaurs of information technology and are considered "overkill" when it comes to storing outcomes data.

In addition to hardware, specific software is needed to appropriately store data. A variety of database packages now available is supported by some type of relational database management system (r-dbms) (21). It is important that a personal computer or computers used to store outcomes data use a relational database software. Each software program has different strengths and weaknesses. For instance, Microsoft makes a very user-friendly r-dbms, but it lacks the complexity and flexibility of a software called Paradox. Additionally, most experienced database managers have used Paradox, whereas Microsoft's r-dbms has only recently reached the market. Other systems such as Oracle are also available; however, many are more complicated and often require more technical support than most users truly want or need.

*Data Analysis.* A separate statistical package may be needed to actually perform the analyses. Two examples are SPSS and SAS, both of which have been widely used in the psychiatric field. Substantial advances have been made in statistical methodology and software packages that make it possible to conduct useful statistical analyses of large datasets quite inexpensively. These advances have allowed us to better analyze longitudinal data and to perform accurate and useful analyses on "faulty" datasets, such as those with large amounts of missing data.

## INTERPRETING AND REPORTING DATA

*"Data is not information. Information is data endowed with relevance and purpose."*

—*Peter F. Drucker*

A review of all of the important consider-ations relevant to interpreting data is be-yond the scope of this chapter. However, three issues should be kept in mind.

First, tests of statistical significance are critical to understanding and analyzing data. Expensive and unfair decisions may be made if this principle is overlooked. For example, one physician or hospital may ap-pear to be a much more effective health care provider than another based on both cost and outcome data. However, even though these differences may be quite large, if they are not statistically signifi-cant, they are not reliable. These data may be very unstable in that results may ap-pear very different at a second measure-ment with a larger number of patients.

Second, specific efforts should be made to take into account case-mix adjustment vari-ables that, apart from the quality of care such as severity of illness, are known to af-fect treatment utilization and outcome. Again, erroneous decisions may be reached regarding the effectiveness and value of a health care system if such "adverse selec-tion" situations reflecting skewed case mixes among different providers, programs, or systems are not considered.

Third, when using multivariable scales and dealing with diverse populations, it is important to recognize that patient changes in one subpopulation may be can-celed out by different changes in another subpopulation. These results may indicate no substantial change in the population as a whole. Therefore, the more specific infor-mation given about the type of desired and expected change, the more likely a real ef-fect will be documented. For example, out-come measures on the 36-Item Short Form Health Survey (see Chapter 8) within ho-mogeneous populations may need to be ex-amined or a predetermined subset of relevant variables may need to be used.

Once analyzed, data should be reported to the correct individuals, departments, and organizations. As discussed above, out-comes data have varied uses, and reporting requirements will differ slightly depending on the intended audience. What will not vary, however, is the fact that *the data must be presented in an accurate and meaningful manner*. The accurate, timely, relevant, and precise communication of outcomes data in health care systems re-sults in better decisions, actions, and, even-tually, quality and value (22).

A virtually limitless range of reports can be developed that include the comparison of programs, clinicians, payment sources, and age-stratified patient groups across categories of clinical outcomes; patient sat-isfaction; resource utilization; and adverse events.

It may be useful to develop focus groups with each stakeholder of the treatment process—payers, providers, patients, and managers—to determine what information they want and/or need and how they expect to use this information. Educational pro-grams may be needed to explain the mean-ing and format of reports being sent to individuals. Outcomes measurement is of no value unless it is actually used.

## CONCLUSIONS

The fact that large-scale medical out-comes databases are already in use for many illnesses proves that this work is fea-sible and useful. The Mayo Clinic has a database of over 4 million encounters and complete medical records for the residents of Olmsted County for the past 85 years. The National Cancer Institute Surveillance Epidemiology and End Results system has collected information on over a million can-cer patients. Additional databases are available for arthritis (ARAMIS), strokes (BUSTOP), renal dialysis, hypertension, and other diseases (23). Now is the oppor-tune time to put into place procedures for measuring the quality and effectiveness of mental health care.

REFERENCES

1. Mirin SM, Namerow MJ. Why study treatment outcome. Hosp Community Psychiatry 1991;42: 1007–1013.
2. Karasu TB, Kupfer DJ, Gelenberg AJ, et al.

Major depression practice guidelines. Am J Psychiatry 1993;4(Suppl):1–23.

3. Depression in primary care: detection, diagnosis, and treatment. Rockville: US Department of Health and Human Services, Public Health Service, Agency for Health Care Policy Research, 1993.

4. Transitions: from QA To CQI: an introduction to quality improvement in health care. Oakbrook Terrace: Joint Commission on Accreditation of Healthcare Organizations, 1991.

5. The transition from QA to QI: performance-based evaluation of mental health organizations. Oakbrook Terrace: Joint Commission on Accreditation of Healthcare Organizations, 1992.

6. Strauss JS, Carpenter WT. Schizophrenia New York: Plenum Press, 1981.

7. Klerman GL, DiMascio A, Weissman MM, et al. Treatment of depression by drugs and psychotherapy. Am J Psychiatry 1974;131:186–191.

8. Hall MC, Elliott KM, Stiles GW. Hospital patient satisfaction: correlates, dimensionality, and determinants. J Hosp Marketing 1992; 7:77–90.

9. Hsieh MO, Kagle JD. Understanding patient satisfaction and dissatisfaction with health care. Health Soc Work 1991;16:281–90.

10. Elbeck M, Fecteau G. Improving the validity of measures of patient satisfaction with psychiatric care and treatment. Hosp Community Psychiatry 1990;41:998–1001.

11. Keeler EB, Manning WG, Wells KB. The demand for episodes of mental health services. J Health Economics 1988;7:369–392.

12. Mintz J, Auerbach AH, Luborsky L, et al. Patient's, therapist's and observers' views of psychotherapy: a "Rashomon" experience or reasonable consensus? Br J Med Psychol 1979; 46:83–89.

13. Mintz J, Mintz LI, Arruda MJ, Hwang SS. Treatments of depression and the functional capacity to work. Arch Gen Psychiatry 1993; 49:761–768.

14. Keller, MB, Lavori PW, Mueller TI, et al. Time to recovery, chronicity, and levels of psychopathology in major depression: a 5-year prospective follow-up of 431 subjects. Arch Gen Psychiatry 1992;49:809–816.

15. Shea MT, Elkin I, Imber SD, et al. Course of depressive symptoms over follow-up: findings from the National Institute of Mental Health treatment of depression collaborative research program. Arch Gen Psychiatry 1993;49:782–787.

16. Frank E, Kupfer DJ, Perel JM, et al. Three year outcomes for maintenance therapies in recurrent depression. Arch Gen Psychiatry 1990; 47:1093–1099.

17. World Health Organization. The international pilot study of schizophrenia. Geneva: WHO Press, 1973;1.

18. Steiber S. Measuring and managing patient satisfaction. Chicago: American Hospital Publications, 1990.

19. Ball MJ, Douglas JV, O'Desky RI, Albright JW, eds. Health care information management systems: a practical guide. New York: Springer-Verlag, 1991.

20. McWilliam C, Paradise Y, Ward R. Outcomes management at Henry Ford health systems center for clinical effectiveness: current reality or future vision. Group Pract J 1994;43:49–56.

21. Fain E. Today's or tomorrow's computer systems? Behav Healthcare Tomorrow 1994; 3:25–31.

22. Davies AR, Doyle MA, Lansky D, et al. Outcomes assessment in clinical settings: a consensus statement on principles and best practices in project management. Joint Comm J Qual Improv 1994;20:6–16.

23. Ellwood P. Shattuck Lecture-Outcomes management: a technology of patient experience. N Engl J Med 1998;318:1549–1556.

CHAPTER 3

# Domains of Study and Methodological Challenges

*Elizabeth A. McGlynn*

Outcomes, in the context of this chapter, refer to health outcomes. Therefore, one must consider what definition of health is being used. The World Health Organization (1) defines health as "a state of complete physical, mental, and social well-being and not merely the absence of disease or infirmity." This definition is comprehensive and implies that outcome domains should include both positive (well being) and negative (disease status) dimensions. The specific outcomes of interest further depend on the perspective being considered; because different individuals and groups tend to value those outcomes most salient to them, the domains of outcomes assessment will necessarily differ. Some of the most familiar perspectives and their primary domains of interest are summarized in Figure 3.1. To obtain perspectives from each of the key participants, a variety of assessment activities is needed. Moreover, the conclusions may differ in determining whether outcomes are positive or negative, depending on the perspective assessed.

Outcomes must be viewed as the result of a particular process. The term outcomes

itself implies a longitudinal perspective—an observation of an occurrence between two points in time. Epidemiology, for example, examines outcomes that result from the natural course of a disorder (i.e., without treatment). These outcomes generally represent the baseline against which treatment is assessed. Studies of the efficacy of preventive interventions consider whether modifying certain risk factors (while controlling for those risk factors that are not modifiable) is associated with improved outcomes. Treatment efficacy considers whether outcomes are improved as a result of a specific intervention, holding constant the risk profile of the patient.

In determining the optimal time frame for outcome assessments, the expected rate of change in outcomes for the intervention being evaluated and the anticipated attribution of outcomes should be considered. Both short-term and long-term outcomes are important. Short-term outcomes might refer to the immediate effect of a treatment intervention (e.g., response to a new antipsychotic medication), whereas long-term outcomes might refer to an assessment of whether results are maintained after intensive treatment interventions cease (e.g., several months after a behavioral skills training course has been completed). The more time that passes between the assessment and the intervention being studied, the greater the chance that intervening factors will influence the observed outcomes, thus diminishing the ability to attribute results to the

| Perspective | Primary Domain |
|---|---|
| Physicians | Clinical status |
| Clients | Functioning in everyday life |
| Families | Impact on family |
| Purchasers | Cost of care |
| Society | Allocation of scarce resources |
| Researchers | What is measurable |

**Figure 3.1.** Perspectives and their Primary Domains

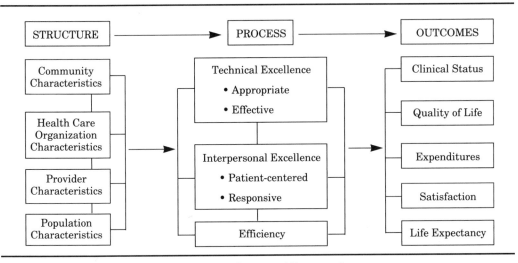

**Figure 3.2.** Conceptual Framework

intervention. On the other hand, assessments that occur too quickly may prevent an observation of the real benefits of an intervention. For example, many antipsychotic medications may take 6 weeks or more to affect symptoms; assessments done within 2 weeks of starting treatment may give a biased view of the efficacy or effectiveness of treatment. Outcomes also occur in a context. The framework provided by Donabedian (2) for studying the quality of care illustrates a way to conceptualize the context in which outcomes are observed (Fig. 3.2). The delivery of care and the system itself (technical and interpersonal excellence) should be considered if we are to understand observed variations in outcomes. Some parts of the context are more important for certain outcome domains. For example, technical excellence (i.e., care that is appropriate and effective) is likely to be most predictive of clinical status, whereas interpersonal excellence (i.e., patient centered, responsive) is more likely to be predictive of satisfaction and quality of life.

## OUTCOMES ASSESSMENT

Outcomes may be assessed at different levels, and the technology for making these assessments is determined by the way in which the information will be used (Fig. 3.3).

In clinical trials, the efficacy of certain interventions may be established. Efficacy refers to outcomes for specific groups of patients (generally without comorbidities or other complicating factors) treated in strictly controlled settings by highly qualified practitioners.

Effectiveness refers to outcomes for real patients treated in common practice settings by average practitioners. The benchmark used for effectiveness studies is the result from efficacy studies.

Quality assessment, which is a focal point of health reform, evaluates the rea-

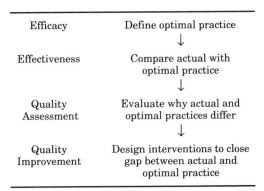

**Figure 3.3.** Different Levels of Outcomes Assessment

sons why actual practice may fail to achieve the results observed in clinical trials (i.e., assessment of the gap between efficacy and effectiveness). Two key differences between clinical trials and actual practice are the quality of the care delivered by health professionals and the case mix of patients treated. A quality assessment, for example, might show that patients with depression who do not achieve the symptom control expected from their antidepressants are receiving suboptimal doses. Alternatively, a certain medication may not seem to work as well in patients with certain comorbid disorders—a group that might not have been studied during a clinical trial. In short, quality assessment offers a mechanism for exploring whether the gap between optimal and actual results can be narrowed by improving the delivery of care or whether there are real limitations on the outcomes that can be achieved in patients whose profiles differ from those enrolled in trials.

Quality improvement activities are designed to close the gaps between best practices and actual practice. For example, a quality-improvement team might provide a continuing education conference for psychiatrists on dosing strategies for antidepressant medication and follow-up with feedback to individual physicians about their prescribing patterns. Many quality problems have been shown to result from problems in the system (e.g., laboratory results are not sent to the physician in a timely manner). Other activities designed to improve the delivery of health care depend on the ability to change ingrained behavior.

## Dimensions of Effectiveness

Effectiveness studies seek to answer the question does medical care make a difference? In an era of constrained resources, providing the effectiveness of interventions may be a critical step for organizations making coverage decisions. To answer this question, two different dimensions of analysis can be addressed. The first dimension of analysis is population

based. For example, the impact of an intervention on life expectancy, mortality rates, and morbidity of a specific population would be measured. The key challenge is to determine the component of observed differential outcomes that results from different interventions as opposed to social and environmental factors. The second dimension is the effectiveness of delivering a specific intervention—can we do a better job of providing the particular intervention. The field of quality improvement is based on this analysis. These two dimensions of inquiry, although related, can produce quite different answers. It is possible to provide an intervention that is very effective when administered properly, but providers may not always deliver that intervention with highly technical or interpersonal excellence.

Examples of efficacious interventions that are not effectively implemented include a variety of preventive services (e.g., mammography, childhood immunizations, pap smears), surgical interventions (e.g., bypass surgery performed so poorly that the risk of mortality is substantially increased), and medical interventions (e.g., antibiotics prescribed for too short a course). Certainly, in many of these cases, an element of patient adherence factors into the effectiveness of the intervention, but the interpersonal excellence with which treatment recommendations are given to patients may substantially influence adherence and, in turn, outcomes.

## Levels of Analysis

The levels of analysis that might be considered include state, community, health plan, facility, health care providers, or the individual patient. Health reform performance domains focus primarily on health plans, facilities, and providers. The ability to draw conclusions depends on the number of observations from any of these groups and the expected distribution of individuals across different outcomes. In a study of outcomes from a disease with low prevalence in a popula-

| Outcome Domain | Data Source | | |
| --- | --- | --- | --- |
| | Claims/Administrative | Clinical | Survey |
| Clinical status | | x | |
| Functional status | | x | x |
| Quality of life | | | x |
| Adverse events | x | x | |
| Satisfaction with care | | | x |
| Expenditures | x | | |

**Figure 3.4.**  Best Sources of Data by Outcome Domain

tion or with relatively rare bad outcomes, large sample sizes may be required to draw conclusions about the importance of any difference observed by providers or health plans.

For example, to conclude that a two percentage point difference in the rate of low birthweight births (prevalence of 1%) between two health plans was statistically significant, a sample of 1,800 births per plan would be needed. For small plans, this sample may be more births than occur in a year; in addition, it is unlikely that this outcome measure could be used to make comparisons among physicians. Other diseases may occur too infrequently in the population to be included in an evaluation of health plan quality (e.g., schizophrenia in a private health plan).

## Sources of Data

Another major consideration is the reliance on data sources to obtain information on outcomes (Fig. 3.4). Each potential source of data has strengths and limitations that should be considered in designing a data collection strategy. For example, the medical record may be a good source of data on technical aspects of care, critical test results, and inpatient processes of care. However, it may be a relatively poor source of information on interpersonal aspects of care, normal history findings (e.g., patient is not a smoker), and outpatient processes of care. Patient or enrollee surveys can be good data sources for symptoms, functioning, and in-

terpersonal aspects of care but may not be useful for obtaining clinical findings or specific technical processes. Administrative data may be useful for examining patterns of visits and test but may not include details about the content of visits or the test results. All of these data sources potentially can be used for outcomes studies, but it is important to consider which outcomes are of interest and whether the data source is adequate for obtaining information on those outcomes.

Many general data collection issues arise when considering study designs and data system development. First, will the outcomes data include only those who use care or the entire population? This question is important if access will be a problem, and observations about outcomes will be biased if only users of care are examined. Second, will the data include all individuals or a sample? Everyone in the population does not need to be included. For cost and efficiency concerns, it may make more sense to draw a random sample that is representative of the entire group being studied. Third, will data be collected at a single point in time or at multiple points? As mentioned earlier, outcomes implies a longitudinal design, suggesting that data collection at a minimum of two points in time is required. Fourth, if collecting data over time, will the same samples be included or will a new sample be drawn each time? Collecting information on the same individuals over time is the only way to obtain truly longitudinal data; the other strategy is a series of cross-sectional analyses that might not capture other sources of variation occurring in the observed population.

## Criteria for Selecting National Performance Measures

The criteria for selecting national quality performance measures, outlined in President Clinton's health plan initiative, are standards for selecting study conditions. These conditions include the following:

- Aspects of care (high prevalence, significant morbidity or mortality, high cost, acknowledged public health objectives) that are most important;
- Representative services that can be reliably and validly measured;
- Performance of services that have the widest variation;
- Processes of care that have validated outcomes measures;
- Outcomes that have been attributed to health care interventions and where risk adjustment methods exist.

A number of mental health care conditions meet the first criterion: affective disorder is very prevalent, dementia imposes significant morbidity, suicidality results in premature mortality, schizophrenia is costly, and substance abuse is included in the public health objectives.

Some common outcomes domains used to evaluate mental health care include mortality (preventable, premature), complications (e.g., side effects), readmission or relapse, psychiatric symptoms, physical symptoms (e.g., untreated medical comorbidity), and functional status. Also, rates of incarceration in a community could be indicative of an outcome that suggests system failure—entry of those with mental illness in the jail system rather than the mental health system.

In evaluating the usefulness of any particular measure, a variety of criteria are commonly used: reliability and validity, mode of administration, and degree of sensitivity to health outcome changes. Other factors to consider are the relative burden placed on the respondent, the level of training required by those who are collecting the data, and the ease with which scores can be interpreted. Implementing the results of outcomes studies should determine the scientific rigor required of the measurement tools. Basically, the more information available potentially affecting the behavior of individuals, the greater the responsibility for ensuring that the tools of assessment are producing real information.

## CONCLUSIONS

A variety of research tools exists to assess the outcome domains discussed in this chapter. Although researchers are likely to continue developing new tools and refining existing ones, the newest area of investigation is the use of outcome and other measures to monitor system performance. In this application, short form measures that can be administered easily by nonclinical lay persons or that can be self-administered by respondents are perhaps the most useful tools. However, care must be taken in developing short form measures to evaluate whether they produce reliable and valid information. As outcomes measurement moves from research to practice settings, a reduction in the scientific rigor for measurement and analyses may be seen; consequently, the accuracy of the information is decreased substantially and the confidence in drawing conclusions is lessened. Maintaining rigorous standards during implementation of these new applications is critical.

Although the interest in using outcomes measurement for a variety of purposes is considerable, collecting information about the factors that contribute to the outcomes is important. This includes both the actuarial process of care (i.e., what is done by the health services system for an individual) and the external factors that might influence outcomes (e.g., individual behaviors, socioeconomic status, comorbid medical conditions). Accounting for these external factors will contribute to clarifying where the best opportunities for improving outcomes exist—enhancing the skills of health professionals delivering care or working with patients to increase adherence to recommended treatment strategies.

REFERENCES

1. World Health Organization. Constitution. In: Basic documents. Geneva, Switzerland: World Health Organization, 1948.
2. Donabedian A. Evaluating the quality of medical care. Milbank Q 1966;44:166–203.

CHAPTER 4

# USING OUTCOMES ASSESSMENT FOR QUALITY IMPROVEMENT

*Howard M. Waxman*

## INTRODUCTION

Recently, I described the initial development of a hospital outcome evaluation program (1) based at the Belmont Center for Comprehensive Treatment, a private non-profit psychiatric facility located in Philadelphia. This program, conducted by a small number of staff in the hospital's research department, was designed as a cost-effective model applicable to the special needs of any institution. Our experience with the program indicates that the model deserves serious examination and possible replication as a practical means to effect positive changes in health care networks. The model, which allows for continuous review and improvement in treatment outcomes and other measures of quality, has greater potential than the simple demonstration of outcome results. Our program continues to test the limits of this approach to improve the operation of our services and deliver a better health care product.

We believe that local ownership of the data collection and reporting procedures enhances the quality improvement process. Clinicians take more responsibility for an outcome process that has not been imposed on them. Also, we find that the quality of the information obtained from the interaction between patient and therapist is less likely to be degraded. Our outcome program has served as the basis for a dynamic interplay between the quality-improvement committees and the research department. By incorporating new data and new ideas, the program has created a common groundwork that fosters communication between clinical and research staff in our hospital, between our hospital and managed care companies, and among other hospitals. We have found that outcome assessment can be conducted without sacrificing the patient's right to privacy and without placing an undue burden on the operation of the clinical programs. In this chapter, I review and update the development of the system currently in operation at our hospital and encourage the development of similar programs in other institutions.

## DEVELOPING AN OUTCOMES INFRA-STRUCTURE

### Choosing Instruments for Assessment

An outcome program requires carefully chosen assessment tools. Each instrument has its own unique characteristics and each is specially suited to certain conditions; no single data collection instrument is acceptable for every clinical situation. It often takes time to fully appreciate the characteristics and limitation of each instrument. We selected instruments that were supported by significant investigational literature. For our inpatient programs, we use begin by using the Client Satisfaction Questionnaire (CSQ-8) (2), the Brief Symptom Inventory (BSI) (3), and the MOS 36-Item Short Form Health Survey (SF-36) (4). These instruments provide global assessments of three constructs: client satisfaction, symptom severity, and health status and functioning. They are relatively easy to administer and provide a good orientation to outcome evaluation for clinical staff. More detailed information on these instruments can be found in Section II.

Comparison of BSI scores at admission and discharge yields one measure of "improvement" after inpatient treatment. The CSQ-8 scores collected at discharge indicate satisfaction levels. Our complete satisfaction questionnaire also provides space for written comments and answers to 30 other questions that we developed for the project. These additional items ask more specific questions about Belmont's clinical services. The SF-36 has been used at admission and is just beginning to be used during follow-up assessment. We are also now just beginning to collect data from our outpatient, partial, and satellite programs.

## Using Computer Technology

Our preferences for hardware and software requirements are based on personal experience. We use a National Computer Systems (NCS) mark sense reader that automatically scans documents and enters the data into a database. This technology represents an initial investment and requires training, yet it saves considerable time and expense in what would otherwise be an extraordinary job of data entry in an organization that sees over 2,000 inpatients a year and has over 35,000 outpatient contacts. Using the scanner, we are able to gather and enter information on all consenting patients at multiple points without employing a small legion of data entry clerks. We use IBM-compatible computers, which are compatible with our software and the NCS scanner. Our choice of software is SPSS for Windows, a well-known statistical software package that can be used to analyze data in the outcome database. Expert advice is recommended if sufficient graduate training and postgraduate experience is lacking in this area.

The database, which is the center of the entire outcome evaluation network, now has some information on over 10,000 patients and is growing rapidly. This includes administrative and admitting data on all 10,000 ptients and client satisfaction data on 4,500 patients, admission BSI and SF-36 data on 1,150 patients, and complete admission and discharge BSI data on 720 patients. These different numbers result from the staggered phase-in of the program with client satisfaction data collected since July 1994 and BSI and SF-36 data collected since February 1994. It also reflects different compliance levels for the different questionnaires.

The database has proven invaluable for a wide variety of purposes, including quality improvement studies, and new variables can be added to the database for special purposes. Multiple files can be merged by accessing special coded numbers that identify each patient and each patient contact. This system promotes the safeguarding of confidentiality by separating patient files containing personal information from the remaining data. In the research department, this information is combined to create a complete database.

Our program gathers information directly from the patients who were asked to complete the rating scales (sometimes with assistance) at different points in the treatment process. The program is organized so that one staff member from each unit or program has the oversight responsibility for data collection. The staff member, typically a nurse case manager, ensures that patients are given the rating scales, that they have the necessary help to complete them, and that the scales are returned to the research department. Thus, the clinical staff guarantees the quality and integrity of the data-collection process, provides essential information to the research department concerning the quantity and quality of the information, and assists in the interpretation of the data. In our hospital, staff meetings are held regularly as part of an informal outcome's task force. In these meetings, discussions center on compliance with data-collection procedures, instructions for proper interviewing skills, and results obtained.

## THE QUALITY-IMPROVEMENT PROCESS

Our results, which are reported to the hospital's quality-improvement committees, take several forms. The most visible form is the Belmont Hospital Report Card, a quarterly review of our quality indicators, including clinical outcomes. The report card is produced by the research department using the statistical and graphics capabilities of the SPSS-Windows software and is formally presented to the hospital's utilization review committee, chaired by the medical director. The report card is also presented to the quality management committee, the oversight quality committee for the hospital. The report card displays summary statistics and trends in tabular and graphic form. Thus far, trends have been presented for the following indicators: client satisfaction, symptom improvement, functional status, recidivism, discharge status, and length of stay. The aggregate results are presented for the entire institution, and separate results are reported for each of the units. In addition, tables are created to show the proportion of patients on each unit who are satisfied with aspects of the treatment services as defined by our hospital questionnaire.

The actions of the quality-improvement committees can be classified as *organizational, informational,* and *preventive.* Organizational actions consider the types of information presented at the meetings and the format in which they are displayed. Informational actions request *focused studies* from the database, from medical records, or from other sources. Preventive actions are changes in the process of the clinical programs. At this point in our program, most of the actions have been organizational and informational. The additional database analyses that have frequently been requested become internal quality improvement studies that use descriptive and inferential statistics to further analyze database information for preventable sources of poor performance. Reports of these research projects, including results,

discussions, and conclusions, are presented to the committees. Thus far, reports have been completed on client satisfaction, recidivism, and discharge status.

More recently, the database requests have been to identify medical record numbers for individuals in poor performance groups. For client satisfaction, a poor performance group is identified by dissatisfaction with services (score of 20 or less on the CSQ-8). For recidivism, readmissions within 30 days is our current target group. For discharge status, individuals with AWOL (away without official leave) or AMA (against medical advice) discharge are selected for special study. Finally, for treatment response, our quality committee initially has selected for study those individuals who do not show improvement in using BSI scores from admission to discharge. Chart reviews of specific patients are sometimes conducted as a quality improvement activity during the committee meetings. In specific instances, independent investigations of problem cases have been conducted by staff members.

## SOME PRELIMINARY FINDINGS IN MEASURING CLIENT SATISFACTION

Figure 4.1 shows the distribution of CSQ-8 scores from our inpatient units, based on results from the first sample of 3,500 patients to complete the form. The results are obviously skewed toward high satisfaction levels. Our response has been to ignore patients who score in the high satisfaction range and address our quality-improvement activities to those who score in the low range scores from 8 to 20 (2). About 8% of the patients fall into this category. Figure 4.2 shows trends in client satisfaction data that can be presented in the hospital report card; indicates the percentage of patients each month whose CSQ-8 results show low, medium, or high satisfaction with services; and shows the stability of the measure and how it can be used to form a baseline. Similar graphs are created for different units and different segments of the patient population (i.e., sex, age, race).

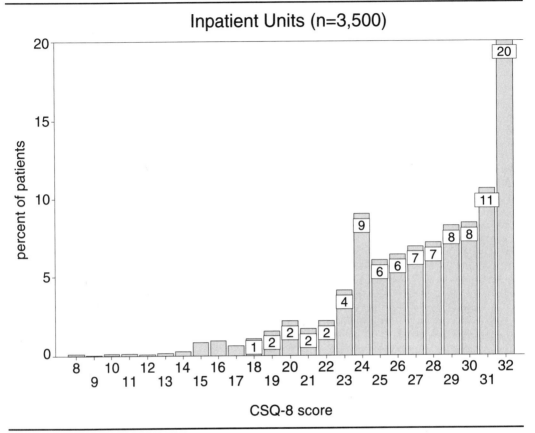

**Figure 4.1.** Distribution of CSQ-8 Scores

Table 4.1 displays correlation coefficients for the individual CSQ-8 items obtained on the same group of 3,500 patients. High correlations can be seen between each of the individual items and between each of these items and the total score.

One of our first focused database studies examined correlates of poor client satisfaction. Substantive analyses were possible because the database contained client satisfaction data on several thousand individuals. Client satisfaction was examined as a function of such variables as length of stay, race, age, sex, diagnosis, unit, and admission status. Age was the only variable found to be associated with client satisfaction scores, with the youngest and oldest age groups showing somewhat lower satisfaction levels. A separate pilot project relating symptom improvement to client satisfaction, however, yielded statistically significant and perhaps clinically important data.

Table 4.2 shows results from a sample of 183 patients grouped according to their level of treatment response. High treatment respondents were defined as those who showed a greater than 40% reduction in BSI total scores (nontransformed Global Severity Index scores). Table 4.2 also divides patients into low (8–20), medium (21–26), and high (27–32) satisfaction levels (2). We found that 21 of 22 of our most dissatisfied respondents were in the group showing poor treatment response. Of the 82 respondents who showed high treatment response, *only 1* expressed dissatisfaction with treatment. These results were

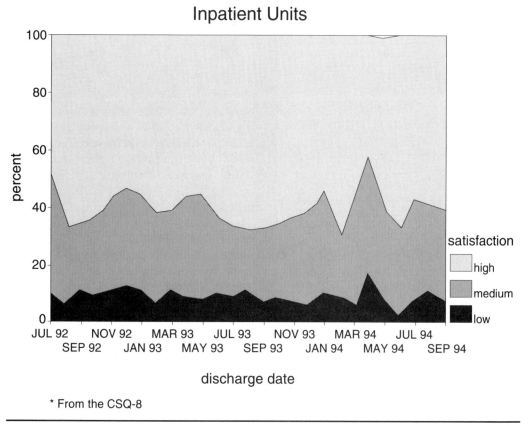

**Figure 4.2.** Trends in Client Satisfaction*

**Table 4.1. Correlation Coefficients of Individual CSQ-8 Items**[a]

|  | CSQ1 | CSQ2 | CSQ3 | CSQ4 | CSQ5 | CSQ6 | CSQ7 | CSQ8 | CSQ Total |
|---|---|---|---|---|---|---|---|---|---|
| CSQ1 | 1.00 | 0.85 | 0.79 | 0.83 | 0.80 | 0.83 | 0.82 | 0.80 | 0.73 |
| CSQ2 | 0.85 | 1.00 | 0.83 | 0.85 | 0.83 | 0.85 | 0.83 | 0.82 | 0.78 |
| CSQ3 | 0.79 | 0.83 | 1.00 | 0.81 | 0.79 | 0.84 | 0.80 | 0.79 | 0.73 |
| CSQ4 | 0.83 | 0.85 | 0.81 | 1.00 | 0.82 | 0.84 | 0.82 | 0.87 | 0.77 |
| CSQ5 | 0.80 | 0.83 | 0.79 | 0.82 | 1.00 | 0.82 | 0.82 | 0.81 | 0.75 |
| CSQ6 | 0.83 | 0.85 | 0.84 | 0.84 | 0.82 | 1.00 | 0.85 | 0.83 | 0.76 |
| CSQ7 | 0.82 | 0.83 | 0.80 | 0.82 | 0.82 | 0.85 | 1.00 | 0.82 | 0.77 |
| CSQ8 | 0.80 | 0.82 | 0.79 | 0.87 | 0.81 | 0.83 | 0.82 | 1.00 | 0.76 |

CSQ1    How would you rate the quality of service you received?
CSQ2    Did you get the kind of service you wanted?
CSQ3    To what extent has our program met your needs?
CSQ4    If a friend were in need of similar help, would you recommend our program to him/her?
CSQ5    How satisfied are you with the amount of help you received?
CSQ6    Have the services you received helped you to deal more effectively with your problems?
CSQ7    In an overall, general sense, how satisfied are you with the service you received?
CSQ8    If you were to seek help again, would you come back to our program?

[a]n = 3,500

**Table 4.2. Relationship of Client Satisfaction to Treatment Response**[a]

| | | Symptom Reduction | | |
|---|---|---|---|---|
| | | Low | High | n |
| Client Satisfaction | Low | 21 (20.8) | 1 (1.2) | 22 |
| | Medium | 33 (32.7) | 23 (28.0) | 56 |
| | High | 47 (46.5) | 58 (70.7) | 105 |
| | n = | 101 | 82 | |

[a]n = 183

interesting vis-a-vis the literature, which has been equivocal on the relationship between client satisfaction and treatment response (5–10). One factor that may have contributed to our finding is that both the client satisfaction and the "post-"BSI data were collected at discharge. Future investigations could determine whether this temporal contiguity may, in some way, be an important factor in the significant association of these two measures. When patients feel relief from symptoms, they may attribute their improvement to their surroundings—the hospital and staff.

As mentioned above, we have conducted similar studies of other outcome indicators, including recidivism and discharge status. As with the study of client satisfaction, these studies use variables in the database to understand as best we can how the hospital operates and looks for potential avenues to enhance our performance. Future plans call for an examination of correlates of poor treatment response using the BSI and SF-36 data.

## ASSESSING OUR OUTCOME PROGRAM

Our outcome program combines the use of computer hardware and software with rating scales scientifically proven to reflect subjective reports of well being. The system, which is only as good as the information it is given, must constantly question the validity and reliability of that information. What are the patients really telling us? Is the infor-

mation worthwhile? Are they telling us what they think and feel or are they telling us what they think we want to know?

We believe that an inhouse outcome data collection system creates an environment that is especially conducive to periodic checks on reliability and validity. We constantly question our own choices of rating scales and data collection procedures based on concerns that arise during assessment. For example, we observed some patients leaving the hospital prematurely against medical advice (AMA) and others refusing to fill out the questionnaires. Thus, although we were getting a compliance rate of between 60% and 70% of those patients that were discharged normally, we were still missing the others, and thus, were not obtaining any information from those that left AMA. We were concerned that our client satisfaction measurement process might be missing those persons who were most dissatisfied. Although our satisfaction results reflected favorably on the hospital, we knew that they were not satisfactory for internal quality review. We found a partial answer by examining our own database; some of the patients who either refused to fill out the forms or who left AMA were later readmitted for more treatment. Our examination of the satisfaction ratings on those patients revealed that they were not substantially different from those that were completed by patients after a normal discharge. Although we were unable to sample those patients who did not return, these results gave us somewhat greater confidence in the reliability of our data collection process.

Another concern was that many of our patients, especially those functioning at a lower level, might not be able to understand the satisfaction questionnaire. Fortunately, we collect written comments from the patients in addition to using the standard rating scales for satisfaction. Using a random sample of 70 patients, we asked a rater to compare a patient's written comments with his/her answers on the rating scale; thus, we were able to obtain another check on the validity of our own data. We discovered an extremely high correspondence between the written comments and the results of the rating scales. Ninety-eight percent of patients with high satisfaction scores also gave favorable written comments, and 88% of those with low satisfaction scores gave negative written comments. Although these studies answer some concerns about the use of satisfaction rating forms, we continue to think of new ways to ensure their reliability and validity. The most important consideration is to determine accurately how each patient feels and thinks. Without this data as a basis, an outcome system is limited, no matter how sophisticated the technology or how large the database.

We have found that the results of rating scales and other measures of quality, such as discharge status and recidivism, must be carefully evaluated in the context of the clinical program and not simply taken at face value. For example, dissatisfaction with family therapy expressed by adolescents may say less about the program than it says about the problems these adolescents have coping with feelings aroused by the presence of family members. In a program dealing with eating disorders, low levels of symptom improvement in some patients may not reflect poor treatment response but may actually reveal the successful elicitation of trapped feelings of anger that may be related to the patient's condition. On the other hand, high satisfaction with inpatient treatment services does not necessarily imply satisfaction with a short length of stay that may have been mandated by a managed care company. Our experience in obtaining and interpreting data has made us realize the importance of thoroughly considering all data results before drawing any conclusions.

## FUTURE DIRECTIONS IN OUTCOME ASSESSMENT AND QUALITY IMPROVEMENT

The Belmont program has been operating for approximately 3 years. Our current plans call for a continued "roll-out" of the program to encompass greater numbers of outpatient, partial hospitalization, and satellite programs. We will also begin to use assessment instruments that more specifically measure the needs of each patient population. The CSQ-8, the SF-36, and the BSI are broad general purpose outcome measures. We will continue to examine the appropriateness of these instruments and substitute others if necessary. We must also work with the staff from each program to identify more precise measuring instruments for each patient population. To accomplish this task, we have asked the clinical leaders of the hospital to more clearly define the philosophy for each treatment program, including measurable treatment goals. The hospital is also working toward the development of more formal treatment guidelines. Once these goals are defined, different outcome assessment instruments may be chosen to supplement those we already use. In addition, we will develop questionnaires that contain items identifying key areas for clinical management on the basis of treatment guidelines and clinical pathways. Thus, new data on compliance with the treatment process will be developed in conjunction with additional outcome variables, thereby creating more clearly defined programs that integrate treatment process with outcome evaluation data.

We hope that outcome measures will help clinical management by providing vital information on the operation of the treatment programs. This relationship must be reinforced continuously so that each part plays its role in the process. We also draw a distinction between executive decisions that are made in regard to a program's operation and management decisions that affect the fine tuning of a program through the continuous quality-improvement process. At a time of historic changes in the delivery of mental health services, both types of decision processes are critical, and outcome data can be used to support each of these decision processes.

A hospital-based outcome program promises to promote the merger of process measures with outcome measures in quality improvement. The improvement of clinical outcomes also can be achieved by using treatment guidelines and clinical pathways and/or well-defined treatment protocols. With clearly defined treatments, compliance with treatment protocols can be measured. Another task for the quality-improvement committee would be to assess the outcome results against the compliance data. If clinical outcomes are poorer than expected, it becomes necessary to check and improve compliance with the guidelines. If this is accomplished and outcomes are still not satisfactory, it may be time to reexamine and modify the guidelines, lower the expectations for treatment response, or abolish the program.

Improvements gained from an outcome program should reflect the refinement of clinical management practices rather than the development of new treatments. The development of new treatments is generally accomplished by experimental methods where variables are more controlled and greater correlations between treatment and outcome variables are achieved. The quality-improvement model outlined here uses correlational analyses to identify predictors of quality. Changes are seen against an ongoing baseline. There are obvious methodological limitations to the use of correlational analyses and assessments against baseline without proper control or comparison groups. Yet the quality-improvement model is better suited to practice settings where random assignment to treatment and nontreatment control groups might be viewed as improperly denying treatment. The techniques of large-scale data analyses from inhouse databases can be very powerful. We caution against acting spuriously on results of these analyses without careful consideration of the influence

of confounding variables and other artifacts such as regression to the mean. Trained statisticians and methodologists as staff or consultants are necessary to prevent against the improper use of outcome data that could lead to erroneous conclusions and reductions in the quality of care.

In our program, we have only begun to explore those quality-improvement activities that could incorporate outcome assessment data. In addition to the possibilities outlined in this chapter, many more activities could be undertaken. These include the use of inservice training and lectures to further educate staff in the latest treatment advances, collaboration in national research programs, and participation in pharmaceutical clinical trials to test the effectiveness and safety of new and promising pharmacological agents. New program development can be based on pilot programs tested with the technology of outcome data assessment. Based on reviews of internal outcomes data and published outcomes literature, vigorous discussions by quality-improvement committees can result in the development of new activities

## CONCLUSION

This chapter is written for those who wish to begin the development of an outcome program at their institution. It describes, in some detail, the development of the program that is now in active use in a 147-bed psychiatric facility. The program gathers information about client satisfaction, symptom improvement, and quality of health and life using three standardized rating scales that are found in Section II of this book. Our data derives from self-administered forms that are scanned by a machine and directly entered into a computer database. The database is used to analyze the information and generate reports that are presented to the hospital's quality-improvement committees. The information gathered becomes part of the indicators of hospital quality. Standards are established for acceptable performance and actions are taken to improve performance in areas considered problematic by clinical staff. The program provides continuous monitoring through comparison of new data to the established baseline.

In the future, one of the primary goals of our outcomes assessment team will be to improve our performance on clinical outcome indicators. The quality-improvement process must take into account those indicators that show the greatest amount of change and determine the best methods for interpreting and applying this data. In this regard, the role of an experienced data analyst is essential to any successful outcomes assessment program.

*Acknowledgments.* Appreciation is expressed to William Dubin, M.D., for his unfailing support and guidance in all phases of this project; to Cathy Jaeger, R.N., and the Nursing Department at Belmont for considerable assistance with data collection and excellent advice; and to Ruth Pessah for her excellent assistance with office management and coordination. All work has been supported by funds from the Albert Einstein Healthcare Network.

REFERENCES

1. Waxman HM. An inexpensive hospital based program for outcome evaluation. Hosp Community Psychiatry 1994;45:160–162.
2. Larsen DL, Attkisson CC, Hargreaves WA, Nguyen TD. Assessment of client/patient satisfaction: development of a general scale. Eval Prog Planning 1979;2:197–202.
3. Derogatis LR, Melisaratos N. The brief symptom inventory: an introductory report. Psychol Med 1993;13:595–605.
4. Ware JE, Sherbourne CD. The MOS 36-item short-form health survey (SF-36). Med Care 1992;30:473–483.
5. Carmel S. Satisfaction with hospitalization: a comparative analysis of three types of services. Soc Sci Med 1985;21:1243–1249.
6. Drake RE, Wallach MA. Mental patients' attitudes toward hospitalization: a neglected aspect of hospital tenure. Am J Psychiatry 1988;145:29–34.
7. Fleming GV. Hospital structure and consumer satisfaction. Health Serv Res 1981;16:43–63.
8. Nguyen TD, Attkisson CC, Stegner BL. Assessment of patient satisfaction: development and refinement of a service evaluation questionnaire. Eval Prog Planning 1983;6:299–313.
9. Roback H, Snyder WV. A comparison of hospitalized mental patients' adjustment with their attitudes toward psychiatric hospitalization. J Clin Psychol 1965;21:228–230.
10. Weinstein RM. Patient attitudes toward hospitalization: a review of quantitative research. J Health Soc Behav 1979;20:237–258.

# CHAPTER 5

# Outcome Evaluation in Psychiatric and Substance Abuse Treatments
## Concepts, Rationale, and Methods

*A. Thomas McLellan, Jack Durell*

## INTRODUCTION

Our society has become increasingly concerned about the dramatic rise in the costs of treating substance dependence and mental illness, particularly in terms of lost productivity, social disorder, and health care utilization (1, 2). Although the public demands more availability of services and greater financial support, policy makers, providers, and payers question the efficacy and value of mental health care (3).

In response to these concerns, we have seen a growing demand to evaluate and demonstrate the quality of and the need for mental health services. Because the past decade has significantly advanced the standardization of diagnoses and the reliable measurement of symptoms and functional status, the outcome of mental health and substance dependence treatment programs now can be evaluated validly in naturalistic treatment settings (4).

In our opinion, attendance at national provider meetings and a review of the scientific literature indicate, despite well-intentioned efforts, frequent misapplications of evaluation designs and the use of poorly conceptualized evaluation procedures. These procedures not only fail to provide useful information but may yield inaccurate findings that could damage the developing field of outcomes assessment. For these reasons, we offer various conceptual and methodological principles that we believe are associated with appropriate, and more successful, outcome evaluation efforts.

We discuss treatment expectations and outcome evaluation methods for both substance dependence and mental health within a common framework. Major differences do exist among patient subgroups within and between each of these two diagnostic categories (e.g., methadone-maintained opiate dependent versus prescription benzodiazepine abusers, chronic schizophrenics versus agoraphobics). At the same time, these disorders often occur simultaneously, especially among treated samples. Many mental health care facilities offer identical services for the care and treatment of both disorders, often in the same settings and by the same practitioners. In evaluating treatment of these disorders, we believe that the goals and procedures used share more conceptual and procedural similarities than differences.

First, we discuss the reasonable expectations of psychiatric and substance abuse treatments that we believe form the basis for evaluation criteria. In addition to symptom reduction, we consider general rehabilitation goals such as functional improvement and decreased utilization of health and social services to be important in determining the value of these treatments.

Next, we examine the differences in forms of treatment and goals between inpatient and outpatient care. Because each plays a different role in achieving patient rehabilitation, we do not believe outcomes should be evaluated using the same criteria or the same points in time.

Finally, we build on these conceptual issues and provide a brief, practical description of the five cardinal features that, in our view, characterize successful outcome evaluations:

1. Patient sampling should take place at admission and on completion of treatment.
2. Outcome status and change should both be measured.
3. Medical and functional status should be measured as well as primary symptoms associated with psychiatric illness and substance abuse.
4. Standardized measures appropriate to patient samples should be used.
5. Evaluations should include follow-up rates of at least 70% to ensure valid results.

We believe these features are commonly neglected or improperly applied in poorly designed studies, and we hope to offer practical guidelines to those facilities planning to undertake evaluation studies.

## REASONABLE EXPECTATIONS AND GOALS FOR EFFECTIVE TREATMENT

A major issue to be considered before an evaluation of either substance dependence or mental health treatment is a clear expectation of treatment effectiveness. If these treatments "work" perfectly, what should they accomplish? This issue is not merely academic or philosophical because it forms the basis for determining the form of treatment, including appropriate goals, patient placement criteria, and staffing patterns and treatment duration. It is the criteria against which we measure effectiveness.

Patient expectations must be considered first. Although there are exceptions, generally most patients entering treatment want relief from the primary symptoms that led to their seeking treatment regardless of the cause. Typically these symptoms are problematic in their own right but also prevent the patient from functioning personally,

socially, and occupationally. From the patient's perspective, at least two desired outcomes of medical care generally are expected: relief from the primary symptoms and restoration of unimpaired or improved functional status. If the primary symptoms are the only impediments, the relief of these symptoms will permit both patient expectations to be fulfilled. However, the mere reduction of symptoms does not always guarantee other patient goals, and treatment cannot be considered truly effective unless both expectations are attained.

These expanded ideas regarding the general rehabilitative expectations of substance dependence and psychiatric treatment are consistent with the outcomes of general medical care. In their work, Stewart and Ware (5) state:

> Since the 1970s, however, the emphasis in America on what patient outcomes to measure to determine health status has been shifting. The focus on the outcomes of medical care is now shifting to the assessment of functioning, or the ability of the patients to perform the daily activities of their lives, how they feel, and their own personal evaluation of their health in general. (p. 51)

Major differences can be seen in outcomes for physical and mental health treatments, but as the authors suggest, generic functional indicators appear to be relevant to both.

Other groups can be directly or indirectly affected by the problems of the patient, and they may have legitimate expectations of their own. For example, employers want their employee returned to functional effectiveness after treatment and want to be able to assure other employees that they need not fear injurious behavior from the instability associated with psychiatric illness and/or substance abuse. Family, neighbors, and law enforcement officials want an end to worries, embarrassments, and social disruptions. Finally, providers and third-party payers expect effective treatment to result in decreased utilization rates, thereby offsetting costs.

The expectations of the patients and other affected groups extend beyond the goal of reducing the primary symptoms that resulted in the initiation of treatment. We believe these expectations are generally reasonable goals for most psychiatric and substance dependence treatments and performance on these expectations can and should be measured as part of a meaningful outcome evaluation.

Our position does not assume that all patients will achieve full satisfaction of their expectations or that any single part of a multifaceted intervention will, by itself, effect the total outcome. Although the overall goals of comprehensive care should be based on the above expectations, particular treatment approaches and health care settings are designed to address only a subset of these expectations. The achievement of the full range of expectations requires an integration and coordination of the separate parts of the treatment program.

In setting up an outcome system, any single treatment program should be evaluated against the specific expectations and treatment goals appropriate for that particular segment of treatment. In addition to sharing responsibility for achieving the full set of goals listed above, it is important to measure the integration of each treatment into the larger network of care. For example, a patient needing hip replacement surgery typically presents with symptoms that include pain and restricted motion. Although the patient's immediate goal may be the relief from pain and the continued degradation of the joint, the ultimate expectation of the patient and others affected by the problem would be the return to relatively unrestricted, painless ambulation.

This ultimate goal cannot be achieved by even the most successful surgery without significant and ongoing rehabilitation therapy. The surgical and rehabilitation specialties must work together to help the patient realize full satisfaction. The concept of individual responsibility for achiev-ing specific goals, combined with the shared responsibility for integrating separate goals, forms the basis for the divided evaluation strategy described below.

## DIFFERENCES BETWEEN OUTPATIENT AND INPATIENT TREATMENT

In establishing a framework for outcomes assessment, important consideration should be given to the differences in variables affecting outcomes in inpatient and outpatient care. These treatments should not be evaluated on the same goals.

### Goals of Inpatient Treatment Programs

Since the advent of managed care strategies in the United States, inpatient care has been considered "acute" or "short-term" care treatment in both substance abuse and mental health settings. Except in certain catastrophic cases requiring chronic care in a psychiatric hospital or ongoing treatment in drug abuse centers, most inpatient care today is restricted to less than 2 weeks (6). Admission to inpatient treatment programs is limited to those patients with severe, comorbid medical problems; psychiatric and/or substance dependence symptoms that cannot be controlled in an outpatient setting; and severe social instability. The goals of these brief, acute inpatient settings follow from the admission criteria and encompass the medical and psychological stabilization of the patient and the development of an effective discharge plan that *includes continued outpatient care.* The goal of acute inpatient treatment is not rehabilitation but removal of the barriers to outpatient care that, in turn, will allow for the overall goal of rehabilitation. Specifically, inpatient treatment expectations include the amelioration and stabilization of all of the symptoms that were "out of control" even with outpatient care and thus were responsible for the inpatient admission. The inpatient program, if properly designed, should provide active referral and engagement of discharged patients into outpatient care and should not be expected to cure or eliminate the problems associated with the inpatient care episode alone.

## Outcome Evaluation of Inpatient Treatment

Outcome evaluation should take place within 2 weeks to 1 month after discharge. Generally, inpatient care can be considered successful if, shortly after discharge, the patient has experienced adequate symptom reduction to permit continuing care on an outpatient basis and has entered an appropriate outpatient program (i.e., based on level of service intensity needed). Effectiveness evaluated solely at the time of discharge only permits an assessment of primary symptom reduction. Although this goal is important, under this criteria only a minimum level of performance would be achieved by most contemporary inpatient substance abuse and psychiatric programs. An adequate assessment of the additional goals of integrating the patient into an appropriate level of outpatient care and achieving ultimate rehabilitation cannot be evaluated at discharge. In addition, evaluation at discharge does not indicate whether the symptomatic improvements will endure the stresses of daily life outside a hospital setting.

In contrast, inpatient care evaluated beyond 1 month will miss the opportunity to measure the patient's integration into continued outpatient care. If a patient has entered into ongoing outpatient treatment, any favorable results detected in an evaluation beyond 1 month may be due to the direct effects of the outpatient care itself and cannot be appropriately attributed to the inpatient component of care.

## Goals of Outpatient Treatment Programs

The levels and approaches of mental health care for outpatients vary in intensity and scope depending on the myriad of medical, psychiatric, substance abuse, and other psychosocial problems presented by the patient populations. By necessity, our discussion is limited to outpatient care designed for sufficiently dysfunctional patients who have received inpatient care. The essential goal of outpatient treatment is to maintain the changes initiated in the acute care setting and to prevent a relapse to hospitalization or to another restrictive form of treatment. Typically, relapse is prevented in both substance dependence and general psychiatric settings through proactive assessment and treatment of problems likely to promote the return of serious primary symptomology. Patients are required to make behavioral changes designed to minimize stress, promote adaptive behavior, and avoid situations that may result in relapse.

Varied and ongoing problems in a patient's life could lead to symptom recurrence after treatment. Although these "psychosocial" problems may not have been related to the original etiology of the psychiatric or substance abuse problems under treatment, they may be intimately related to relapse after treatment. Difficulties that need to be addressed in ongoing rehabilitation treatment, and the behavioral changes necessary to offset them, can require protracted treatment to develop and implement appropriate interventions designed to address these risks to symptom exacerbation and relapse.

## Outcome Evaluation of Outpatient Treatment

Given the potential range of assessments and behavioral interventions needed to sustain protection from symptom exacerbation, the most appropriate time to evaluate the goals of severely ill outpatients would be no earlier than *3 months and possibly not before 12 months*. A review of patients receiving treatment for substance abuse over a 1-year period indicates that 60–80% of the cases suffering ultimate relapse do so within 3–4 months (7). Outpatient care can be considered successful at a 3-, 6-, or 12-month follow-up point, regardless of whether outpatient care is ongoing, if the patient has not required inpatient care, and no increase has been seen in the severity of problems that could promote relapse. In addition, consideration should be given to measuring the success of more subjective goals, such as patient satisfaction and sense of well being, which we address later.

## THE DESIGN AND IMPLEMENTATION OF OUTCOME EVALUATIONS

### Clinical Trails Versus Outcome Evaluation

In the most rigorous measurement of treatment efficacy, controlled clinical trials, a random sample of patients receiving treatment is compared with those who do not receive treatment. Similarly, in assessing outcomes between patients treated in program X with those treated in program Y, randomly selected samples of an appropriate patient population, randomly assigned to both programs, would have to be compared. Even under rigorous measurement conditions, outcome data from a single program will have limited interpretability unless comparisons can be made to a larger reference group. Without comparison data, even clear evidence of significant benefits to a large population of treated patients may simply reflect outcomes that may have been seen with *any* or *no* treatment. Similarly, a low improvement rate may not necessarily indicate ineffective treatment but only a poor prognosis among the sample treated. In evaluation research, various comparisons produce different types of feedback.

### Historical Controls

Randomly selected samples of discharged patients from the same program can be studied over several years, and the results can be measured using the same standardized techniques. Comparison data obtained from these longitudinal studies would measure the differences in patient outcome over time, assuming no change in admission severity of the patients.

### Severity-Adjusted Comparisons

A better approach would be to measure the severity of the patients' problems when treatment starts, assessing the previous 2 weeks or month and again at follow-up and repeating this practice over the course of several years. Measuring the severity of admission problems provides outcome data similar to that provided under historical control procedures and also permits three additional analyses: determination of "improvement" from admission to follow-up as well as the status of the patient at discharge; comparison of admission severity over time; and comparison of the outcomes of patient subgroups over years matched for admission severity, diagnoses, or both.

### Database Comparisons

Collecting additional admission information provides severity-adjusted comparisons of program effectiveness over time. However, when the only data available are unique to one program, we cannot determine whether the treatment provided in that program is better or worse than treatment provided in another program for a comparable set of patients. This is the case even when the data are repeated over time and are taken from different patient samples. Therefore, a better result could be achieved by using well-validated instruments that have been widely used in similar evaluations of other treatment programs and patient samples, thereby providing a database of *comparative* treatment outcomes.

Our study of the comparative effectiveness of two forms of treatment of substance-dependent patients shows methods for using these various assessment options in practice and the benefits obtained from these procedures (8). For example, in the treatment of psychiatrically complicated substances abusers, staff from program A determined that the improvement rates and outcomes after 6 months of care were poor (worse than expected). To evaluate this observation, the program sampled a group of these patients at admission and followed them through treatment for 6 months. Results showed that improvement on many functional domains (e.g., employment, crime, drug use) was minimal, and outcome status at the 6-month point did not come close to expectations. To verify this result, program A resampled again the following year and found that the improvement rate and the outcome status were even worse. On examination, severity of symptoms at admission was shown to be significantly higher in the second group of patients. This additional data seemed to indicate that treatment effectiveness at least was not getting worse.

Despite these findings, because outcomes did not approach expectations and improvements were found in patients with less severe symptoms, the staff from program A concluded that their treatment program was ineffective with psychiatrically ill substance-dependent patients. The most responsible solution was to refer the patients to program B, which was 50 miles away.

Before making this policy change, a third evaluation was undertaken actually comparing the performance of two samples of patients at both programs (matched on the same, well-validated measures of problem severity at admission). Results again indicated only modest improvement rates for the patients in program A. However, matched samples of patients referred to program B actually showed *negative change and even worse outcome status* after comparable treatment. Because program A used the same measurement instruments and evaluation procedures, results indicated treatment effectiveness for patients with approximately the same admission severity when compared with the available alternative type of treatment.

The nature of the evaluation design, the selection of the patient sample, and the choice of outcome measures and evaluation intervals all profoundly affect outcomes assessment. In the next section, we propose methods of evaluation designed to capture those essential features that permit meaningful interpretation of results using practical, nonintrusive, economical procedures.

## PROCEDURES FOR OUTCOME EVALUATIONS

### Measuring Outcome at Admission and at Completion of Treatment

Outcome evaluations can be an invaluable management tool, but perhaps the most important question for the purchaser of treatment would be what are the likely outcomes for patients referred to your program?

The best response to this question would be to evaluate patients at admission when the program accepts responsibility for treatment. For "intent to treat evaluations," patient samples should be randomly selected at this time and followed throughout the course of treatment. This technique is designed for all patients admitted to a program and outcomes should be assessed regardless of whether the patient completes the program.

"Treatment maximization evaluations" measure outcomes of patients discharged after completion of the full course of treatment and estimate the effects of treatment when the full "dose" and regimen have been provided. However, the results may be misleading because the sample of those completing treatment may represent a minority of the more motivated or least severely affected patients. Either of these biases would lead to a higher likelihood of completion or a better prognosis. Data from this type of study is pertinent only when the large majority of admitted patients is certain to complete the full course of treatment.

Obviously, with individual evaluation designs, estimates of effectiveness vary. For example, in evaluating treatment effectiveness for patients with tuberculosis, comparisons can be made between a sample of patients who enter treatment with those who complete the full course of therapy. Results may indicate that only 50% of the patients may complete the full course of treatment. At the same time, 100% of those patients who do receive the full doses of isoniazid become symptom free. This illustrates the traditional differentiation between efficacy—the results of an intervention applied under optimal circumstances—and effectiveness—the results of an intervention in a standard population under real-world conditions.

In our opinion, the "intent to treat" design is easy to implement, yields valuable data, and, given appropriate sample sizes, permits treatment evaluation in those patients who do not complete the full course of treatment.

Ideally, outcomes data should include every patient treated; however, this is not always required. Gathering data on a representative sample of 50 to 100 patients may be preferable and may provide as much useful information as a larger group, depending on the sensitivity of the outcome measure and the statistical power of the design (9). Consecutive admissions typically produce a representative sample in a rapid and efficient manner. Over the past few decades, researchers and statisticians have perfected sampling techniques that provide the most efficient and scientifically valid methods for estimating treatment efficacy and effectiveness. Following *all* patients who enter a treatment program is extremely expensive and time consuming. Close monitoring is required to assure that the scientific validity of the measurement is not eroded by the length of time involved and inevitable changes in staff and clinical procedures commonly seen over extended periods of time. A careful study of a smaller, randomly selected patient sample provides as much information as would continuous evaluations.

## Measuring Outcome Status and Change

In these areas of measurement, outcomes assessment must take into account variables such as socioeconomic status, functional status, severity of symptoms,

and time of evaluations. For example, in a program designed to treat chronic, lower socioeconomic strata schizophrenics, the change in symptomatic status from admission to follow-up might show significant and clinically important levels of improvement. At the same time, if we look at a patient's functional status or outcome at a posttreatment evaluation, we might see very low absolute levels of function. Conversely, a program designed to manage general anxiety disorders or alcohol abuse among working, insured, middle class patients may show only modest improvements in symptomology from admission to posttreatment evaluations but good functional status, acceptably low levels of health care utilization, and other favorable outcome status measures largely because of the good pretreatment starting points.

Outcome evaluations often measure follow-up status as well as general, historical indicators (e.g., medical, social, and family role) of the patient's functional status at admission. These case-mix adjustment variables are used to mathematically equate the outcome status of the target group with the expected outcomes for groups with comparable levels of pretreatment impairment. Decisions regarding effectiveness may be made erroneously if these variables are not considered. This statistical adjustment offers little direct information about the improvement of an individual patient's condition. From a clinical and practical perspective, the measurement of several target aspects of a patient's functional status for comparable periods of time before the start of treatment and before each evaluation point is worthwhile. For example, if reduction of depression symptoms is a target goal, a standard measure of depression can be collected easily and validly from the patient (reporting the past week or month) at admission, again at discharge, and at subsequent follow-up points. This procedure measures both outcome status and symptomatic change.

## Measuring Social Function, General Medical Status, and Target Symptoms

The expectations often placed on treatments for substance dependence and psychiatric illness and the influence of a wide range of variables on relapse indicate the importance of evaluating all functional areas along with target symptoms presented at treatment admission. In practice, the same methodology required to measure improvement and outcome status in the target problem areas also permit measurement of improvement and outcome status in the areas of employment and self-support, family and social relations, and utilization of medical and social services.

**Suggested Measurement Domains for Evaluating Treatment Effectiveness.** The adoption of broad rehabilitation expectations is reasonable and useful when evaluating the outcomes of substance dependence or psychiatric treatments, taking into consideration both patient and societal goals. We suggest four independent outcome domains important to measurement: reduction of primary symptoms (psychiatric and/or alcohol and drug abuse); improvement in health, personal, and social function; cost of care; and reduction in public health and safety threats.

In our view, the first two domains are consistent with the primary and secondary measures of effectiveness typically used for evaluation by the Food and Drug Administration in controlled clinical trials (10) and conform to accepted methods used by other health care services (5). The third domain, cost, is a major consideration in the provision of all health and social services and in the overall value of a treatment. The last outcome dimension, which acknowledges the significant concerns associated with addiction, is more specific to the treatment of substance abuse. We discuss each domain and appropriate measurement.

Reduction in primary symptoms is the most important goal of psychiatric treatment and can be measured objectively by independent evaluators. For substance abuse, measurements can be obtained by urinalysis for drug screening or by breathalyzer readings of blood alcohol levels. Under appropriate conditions, when confidential information is collected by independent evaluators without penalty for accurate reporting, research has shown that self-reports of alcohol and drug abuse can be reliable, accurate, and sensitive measures of this primary dimension of effectiveness.

From a societal perspective, improvement in a patient's functional status is important to symptom reduction, which, in turn, results in cost savings. In addition, these improvements are related to maintaining gains in the primary outcome area of substance use. Specific instruments have been developed (11) to measure improvements in functional status. For example, inventories of general health and psychological symptoms and measures of family function, employment history, and earnings can be reliable and valid when collected directly from the patient through confidential self-reports, clinical evaluations, or employment records.

From the provider's perspective, basic costs of care should be measured by reviewing patient insurance and billing records. Instruments for measuring direct costs also should take into account charges to the patient as well as such additional costs as out-of-pocket expenses, lost time from work, and transportation to and from treatment. Although these basic elements of costs can be measured with relative ease and can provide a reasonable approximation of the major components of all costs for comparison purposes, they do not provide a comprehensive record of all costs. Measuring such indirect costs as overhead or capital expenditures is beyond the scope of this discussion.

Perceived threats to public health and safety from patients with substance abuse disorders come from behaviors associated with the spread of infectious diseases or, in the case of psychiatric illness, commission of criminal acts. Because of the importance of these societal fears, we have set up a special criterion domain to evaluate treatment effectiveness. Specifically, activities such as sharing needles, having unprotected sex, and exchanging sex for drugs are serious behaviors linked to addiction that pose significant threats to society. Confidential self-reporting techniques can be used to accurately measure these behaviors. Objective measures of the acquisition of infectious diseases, such as the acquired immunodeficency syndrome, can be obtained by laboratory tests in a target sample of patients but do not reflect the spread of these diseases to other members of society through patient contact.

Crimes committed under the influence of alcohol or drugs are major threats to public safety. Techniques for measuring these activities include confidential self-reports through interviews and questionnaires. Objective measures of the results of these acts can be obtained from public arrest and conviction records, but these measures typically underestimate the extent of the criminal and dangerous behaviors actually performed.

Recent evaluations have focused on two important variables of outcome assessment from a consumer perspective: duration of treatment and patient satisfaction after treatment. Treatment retention is a reasonable assessment of a program's success in convincing a patient to pursue a specified rehabilitation course. Patient satisfaction is a good indicator of a program's ability to reduce primary symptoms and to provide additional help. Each measure provides useful information; however, neither offers a direct assessment of the primary goals of treatment, either psychiatric or substance dependence, in either inpatient or outpatient settings. Variables such as family and employer pressures can be as responsible for treatment retention as the direct efforts of the treatment program itself. Similarly, factors such as accessibility

of service, quality of staff, and physical attributes of a particular facility can be as important in eliciting patient satisfaction as the program's effectiveness in achieving the target goals. We do not argue against the use of these measures but point out that they are not substitutions for direct and valid measures of symptom reduction and functional status.

## Using Standardized Measures in Outcome Evaluation

To obtain reliable and valid measurements for the target populations under study, well-standardized instruments must be used. Two important reasons for this approach include using statistics to maximize reliability and sensitivity of the measures taken and establishing comparison conditions.

The overall validity of the conclusions reached is a joint function of the measure's reliability (the extent to which it is reproducible) and sensitivity (the extent to which true changes in functional status can be detected). For example, in treating depression, using a proven instrument, along with other program developed measures, will ensure that the evaluation detects true change in the symptoms of the patient population. Standardization will assist in determining the size and composition of the patient sample to be recruited for the outcome evaluation (9). In addition, a standard measure offers a method against which any new measure of depression can be validated.

Using standardized measures permits comparison conditions. Results obtained from a single evaluation can be measured against results from a larger database of comparable patient samples and treatment conditions. This factor is extremely important in those evaluation designs that lack an untreated control group or local comparison groups. Without comparisons, outcome data collected from a single treatment or program cannot be interpreted scientifically.

## Using Follow-Up Contact Rates for Valid Results

Many outcome evaluations fail to represent adequately the patient sample at an appropriate point after the termination of treatment. Earlier, we noted the importance of representing the "average" patient entering treatment using random or consecutive sampling techniques. However, if the follow-up rate for this representative sample is only 50–60%, the contact group may not be representative of the original sample or, in turn, the larger population. A 50% contact rate may represent only the most improved and most functional group from the original sample. Conversely, depending on the techniques used to recontact the patients, this group may be the most impaired or least functional. In either case, the effectiveness of the treatment program for the average patient cannot be assessed properly if the results are retrieved from a nonrepresentative subgroup.

Thus, we can conclude that posttreatment contact rates of 85% or higher are desirable to minimize sampling bias. Rates below 70% are likely to misrepresent the sample and should be regarded with caution. In fact, in compliance with the Food and Drug Administration, studies offering evaluation information on a new drug must include at least a 70% follow-up rate (10).

Many program administrators have produced posttreatment data on a standardized outcome measure from a large patient group collected at a posttreatment evaluation point. Unfortunately, these data often are derived from patients completing treatment programs and may represent only 50% or less of those completers responding to the follow-up. In our opinion, *this data is not interpretable.* Because the percentage of admitted patients actually completing the program is not indicated (and may range from 10% to 90%), this evaluation design produces limited information under the best of circumstances. More problematic, these data may not represent adequately the treatment effectiveness for program completers, despite the often large absolute number of cases. The results represent only a small, biased percentage of those completers, usually the most motivated cases. In short, the time, energy, and money invested in the efforts to obtain a true evaluation may be wasted.

In practice, we consider follow-up contact to be the most difficult, most expensive, but most important aspect of an outcome evaluation. To ensure the success of follow-up contact, effective techniques should be initiated at treatment admission when the patient is evaluated, is assured of confidentiality, and is asked to provide contacts at the designated follow-up point (5). These references should be checked for accuracy during the course of treatment, and the patient should be reminded of the pending follow-up contact at the time of discharge. When financial incentives and a private telephone line for receiving collect calls are added to these techniques, follow-up contact rates of 85% or higher can be achieved (12, 13).

## CONCLUSIONS

Psychiatric and substance abuse treatments can be evaluated scientifically. Public concerns, financial expenditures, and the availability of measures and procedures for producing valid and nonintrusive information demand that we implement systems to effectively demonstrate the rationale for and quality of mental health care. The results of our studies should encourage the efforts of others to assess treatment outcome among psychiatric and substance abuse patients. Realistic treatment expectations and the utilization of appropriate evaluation designs and measurement techniques are important factors in outcomes assessment. When appropriate designs are applied in a rigorous manner, the results offer heartening indications that many forms of treatment can be effective in reducing target symptoms and achieving rehabilitation (14–17). At the same time, not all treatments are effective by any standard; some are better than others and the cost effectiveness among treatments varies greatly (4, 18).

Evaluation methods are still evolving and require better techniques for measuring the patient, the program setting, and the services provided. Further research efforts will accomplish this goal, but in the interim, existing treatments can and must be evaluated using appropriate and available scientific procedures.

## REFERENCES

1. National Institute on Drug Abuse. See how drug abuse takes the profit out of business. Washington, DC: Department of Health and Human Services, U.S. Government Printing Office, 1991.
2. Merrill J. The cost of substance abuse to America's health care system. Report 1. Medicaid hospital costs. New York: Columbia University, Center on Addiction and Substance Abuse, 1993.
3. Saxe L, Dougherty D, Esty K, Fine M. The effectiveness and costs of alcoholism treatment [case study 22]. Washington, DC: Office of Technology Assessment, 1983.
4. McLellan AT, Grissom G, Alterman AI, Brill P, O'Brien CP. Substance abuse treatment in the private setting: are some programs more effective than others? J Subst Abuse Treat 1993;10:243–254.
5. Stewart AL, Ware JE. The medical outcomes study. Santa Monica: The Rand Corporation, 1989.
6. McClure W. Health care reform: the buy right strategy. National Education Association, Retirement and Benefits Forum, October 20, 1990.
7. McLellan AT, Metzger D, Alterman AI, Cornish J, Urschel H. How effective is substance abuse treatment—compared to what? In: O'Brien CP, Jaffe J, eds. Advances in understanding the addictive states. New York: Raven Press, 1992.
8. McLellan AT, Griffith J, Childress AR, Woody GE. The psychiatrically severe drug abuse patient: methadone maintenance or therapeutic community. Am J Drug Alcohol Abuse 1984;10:77–95.
9. Kraemer HC, Thiemann S. How many subjects? Statistical power analyses in research. Newbury Park: Sage Publications Inc., 1987.
10. Food and Drug Administration. Compliance policy guidelines. Associate Commission for Regulatory Affairs 1980;21 CFR 310.
11. McLellan AT, Luborsky L, O'Brien CP, Woody GE. An improved evaluation instrument for substance abuse patients: the Addiction Severity Index. J Nerv Ment Dis 1980;168:26–33.
12. Alterman AI, Droba M, McLellan AT. Response to day hospital treatment by patients with cocaine and alcohol dependence. Hosp Community Psychiatry 1992;43:930–932.
13. McLellan AT, Luborsky L, Woody GE, O'Brien CP, Druley KA. Increased effectiveness of substance abuse treatment: a prospective study of patient-treatment "matching." J Nerv Ment Dis 1983;171:597–605.
14. Miller WR, Hester RK. The effectiveness of alcoholism treatment methods: what research reveals. In: Miller WR, Heather N, eds. Treating addictive behaviors: process of change. New York: Plenum Publishing Corp., 1986.
15. Moos RH. Evaluating treatment environments. New York: John Wiley & Sons Inc., 1974.
16. Shea MT, Elkin I, Imber SD, et al. Course of depressive symptoms over follow-up: findings from the NIMH treatment of depression collaborative research program. Arch Gen Psychiatry 1992;49:782–787.
17. Reynolds CF, Frank D, Perel JM, et al. Combined pharmacotherapy and psychotherapy in the acute and continuation treatment of elderly patients with recurrent major depression. Am J Psychiatry 1992;149:1687–1692.
18. McLellan AT, Grosman DS, Blaine JD, Haverkos HW. Acupuncture treatment for drug abuse: a technical review. J Subst Abuse Treat 1993;10:569–576.

# CHAPTER 6

# Outcomes Management Strategies in Mental Health
## *Application and Implications for Clinical Practice*

*Robert A. Dorwart, GAP Psychopathology Committee[a]*

## INTRODUCTION

We discuss in this chapter outcomes management strategies in clinical practice, with an emphasis on their application and implications. We present a case study that deals with the management of clinical problems by integrating traditional clinical evaluation with outcomes-oriented thinking. Using typical outcomes management techniques, we describe the case in detail, allowing the reader to understand the nature of the clinical problem (and to permit consideration of alternative treatment strategies), to grasp the context of a typical outcomes management program within a managed care system, and to understand how the use of outcomes management systems can improve the quality of care and the cost-effectiveness of treatments.

## CASE STUDY

Dr. Donna Smith, a psychiatrist and a member of a preferred provider organization (PPO), has been contacted by a PPO case manager requesting information about an outpatient she is treating. The case must be reviewed because the PPO requires authorization for further treatment.

### Patient Information

The patient, Max Fine, is a 50-year-old accountant diagnosed with major depres-

sion. When first seen, he was unable to work, and this lack of occupational functioning was compounded by the fact that the busy season for tax preparation was fast approaching. His symptoms and level of impairment were moderate to severe. After treating Mr. Fine, Dr. Smith's evaluations indicated that his symptoms were largely resolved. Although he reported feeling a bit better, Mr. Fine was still unable to work. Dr. Smith examined Mr. Fine weekly for 6 weeks to assess pharmacotherapy and to provide cognitive behavioral psychotherapy. Mr. Fine's employer requested an estimated time for his return to work.

### Treatment Plan and Outcome Considerations

Mr. Fine's insurance plan required patients to see doctors affiliated with a PPO that used a review/outcomes management system. Dr. Smith described her treatment plan to the case manager and indicated that she was requesting continued visits for further treatment, predicated on data demonstrating the efficacy of pharmacotherapy and cognitive behavioral therapy for treating moderately severe depression. She explained that Mr. Fine did not improve as quickly as all those involved in his case had hoped. All concerned questioned why this usually efficacious treatment strategy had not been fully successful. In Mr. Fine's case, why did symptoms lessen while no improvement was seen in functioning?

As they discussed the case, Dr. Smith and the case manager addressed the fol-

[a]David A. Adler, M.D.; Jeff L. Berlant, M.D., Ph.D.; Lisa Beth Dixon, M.D.; John P. Docherty, M.D.; James M. Ellison, M.D., M.P.H.; Howard H. Goldman, M.D., Ph.D.; Marc Sageman, M.D., Ph.D.; and Samuel G. Siris, M.D.

lowing questions that highlighted the concepts integral to a successful outcomes management strategy: Was the diagnosis correct? Should Mr. Fine continue in cognitive behavioral therapy? Was he taking his medication? Was imipramine, as currently prescribed, the best form of pharmacotherapy? Would prescribing a selective serotonin reuptake inhibitor (SSRI) be a better option? Would the increased cost of an SSRI result in greater value, through greater compliance (if that was a problem) and better effect? Would the added benefit to his employer of an earlier return to work warrant the cost of intensified treatment (cost-benefit)?

Current changes in health care financing have challenged psychiatrists like Dr. Smith to consider outcomes in a more developed, systematic manner that is open to professional and public scrutiny. Policy planners, the managed care industry, third-party payers, and the federal government continue to demand answers to the questions, "What are we paying for?" and "Do our treatments work?" (1). This chapter attempts to define and clarify outcomes assessment and to encourage its use by mental health and substance abuse professionals.

## Outcomes Definitions

As with Mr. Fine's treatment, outcomes are divided into clinical and functional categories: clinical outcomes describe the psychiatric and physiological signs and symptoms of disease or disorders and functional outcomes describe levels of social role performance (2). Stewart and Ware (3) discuss the ways in which health status can affect the quality of life by dividing outcomes into five distinct dimensions:

1. *Physical health*, which refers to "the performance of or ability to perform daily self-care activities";
2. *Mental health,* which addresses the realms of behavioral dysfunction, symptoms of psychological distress or well being, and cognitive functioning;

3. *Social functioning,* which encompasses social contacts and resources;
4. *Role functioning,* which refers to "the performance of or capacity to perform usual role activities";
5. *General health perception,* which rates the self-perceptions of individuals about their global level of well being, energy, and vitality.

This approach illustrates the shift from a reliance on the provider perspective of assessing signs and symptoms of disease to the patient perspective of assessing functioning and well being. The interest in outcomes has also encouraged the evaluation of medical services or procedures within frameworks that the mental health field has long recognized as important, such as the status of social and role functions, emotional health, cognitive function, and satisfaction with life (4, 5).

## Process of Outcomes Assessment

**Measurement.** Measurement refers to the use of time intervals to determine a change in condition. Dr. Smith has been engaging in informal measurement of outcomes, using global ratings to assess Mr. Fine's progress based on his reports of symptoms at particular points in time. Because she has gathered information in multiple domains, she is aware that he is doing better in some respects than in others. In organized systems, uniform measures of symptoms and functioning might be used to promote comparability and accountability.

**Monitoring.** Monitoring refers to the use of periodic assessment of treatment outcomes to permit inferences about what has produced change. Dr. Smith has been tracking the progress of Mr. Fine at regular intervals during each weekly visit. By repeated measurement of clinical symptoms and functioning, Dr. Smith has become aware of the divergence in improvement between the two domains.

**Management.** Management refers to the use of monitoring information in the management of patients to improve both the clinical and administrative processes for delivering care. Dr. Smith's PPO has been collecting information on the outcomes of several conditions that she treats. The PPO staff have provided her with a profile comparing the response rates of her patients diagnosed with depression and treated with imipramine to the response rates of those treated by other psychiatrists in the PPO. The crude data indicate that her patients' functional improvement lagged behind their symptomatic improvement. Although this is true of other physicians' patients as well, Dr. Smith's patients were in the slowest 10% to respond functionally. When the data are adjusted for severity of illness at baseline, however, Dr. Smith's profile is comparable with that of the other psychiatrists. Her choice of imipramine in treatment was more common than 80% of the other psychiatrists in the PPO. Although pharmaceutical costs were lower with imipramine, even after adjusting for severity, these savings were offset by more frequent visits.

## Applications of Outcome Assessment

The following goals of outcomes assessment are based on a composite agenda from areas of basic science, clinical practice, and policy: enhancing informed decision-making by government, providers, and patients; developing standards of care and protocols for treatment; making decisions about resource utilization; and assessing the effectiveness of different treatment interventions.

## Profiling Treatment Effectiveness

Three fundamental types of classification and analysis are necessary to assess treatment outcomes effectively. First, a *risk-adjustment scheme* is needed to identify systematically the differences in the severity of mental illness (e.g., the comorbidity of psychiatric substance abuse and medical problems and the social and biological variables in the targeted symptoms and functioning levels under treatment).

Second, a *treatment definition scheme* must be devised to describe the nature, duration, and intensity of the treatment interventions, including the context or setting in which treatment is delivered. Third, a set of *measurable outcome variables* must be designed to address a comprehensive range of outcomes that includes the degree of social functioning. Unless all three elements of analysis are considered, outcomes assessment efforts can be meaningless.

## Costs and Benefits

Cost consideration is perhaps most threatening to providers who fear that cost reduction rather than quality improvement will influence decision-making. Cost-benefit and cost-effectiveness analyses are two techniques that can answer questions by payers who want to maximize the return on their investment in mental health care.

In cost-benefit analysis, costs and benefits are expressed in the same units, generally monetary. The costs may be direct or indirect. In the case of Mr. Fine, direct costs included the actual dollars spent on imipramine and Dr. Smith's services. Indirect costs included the value of lost productivity due to Mr. Fine's illness. If the use of an SSRI allowed Mr. Fine to return to work more rapidly, the increased cost of this treatment would be balanced against the increased benefit of a reduction in lost work days. One problem in applying cost-benefit analysis to health care is the difficulty, if not impossibility, of placing a dollar value on imprecisely measurable benefits of health care, such as improved quality of life.

Cost-effectiveness analysis attempts to address this problem by expressing the benefits of treatments in nonmonetary measurements such as compliance, reduced symptoms, life satisfaction, or prolonged days of life. If Dr. Smith were to switch Mr. Fine to an SSRI, the increased cost might be offset by the enhanced treatment compliance and/or greater subjective improvements in Mr. Fine's mood. Cost-effectiveness analysis allows greater flexibility in making comparisons but does not capture outcomes in comparable units.

Conducting useful cost-benefit and cost-effectiveness analyses in outcomes research is extremely challenging for the following reasons: identifying and measuring all relevant costs is problematic, measuring multiple outcomes is required, and carrying out studies over sufficient time to assess results adequately is not always possible. Thus, a well-designed outcomes management system should balance costs and quality of care by monitoring effectiveness and not merely by reducing amounts of care or the costs of treatments.

## PERSPECTIVES INFLUENCING OUTCOMES ASSESSMENT

Outcomes assessment will play a major role in mental health care in the future, as indicated by the emphasis on quality measures and cost effectiveness in President Clinton's 1993 health care initiatives. Although sweeping reform has not taken place, incremental changes in the health care system will continue as insurers and employers demand accountability reports (6). In addition to demands for health care cost containment, competition among providers and the differences in medical and psychiatric procedures across geographic boundaries create incentives for better treatment evaluations. Assessing outcomes has been difficult for physicians in the past; however, the availability of computerized databases can provide the means to monitor outcomes that were not previously possible.

We can design standard quality measures to take into account the results of consumer satisfaction surveys. As discussed in Chapter 25, we can issue periodic guidelines to designate the most effective methods of disease prevention, diagnosis, treatment, and clinical management of disease, with cost information factored into the determination of effectiveness. A clearinghouse can be established to disseminate this information to providers. Measures of outcomes and costs of health care plans can

be made public to aid consumers in making choices (see Chapter 27).

Using a multidimensional perspective, Mirin and Namerow (7) have explored the application of general medical outcomes studies to the mental health field. Mental health providers will require outcomes data to ensure that health policy decisions are based on reasonable data. Important questions remain about the utilization of outcomes research that has been linked to sometimes conflicting objectives: limiting cost increases, setting reimbursement priorities, targeting appropriate treatments to different conditions, and monitoring hospitals and practitioners for quality of care. The American Psychiatric Association's new policy concerning managed care points out the need to provide interpretations of data used for political and cost containment purposes (8).

Outcomes assessment for mental health and substance abuse problems is considered multivariable: interventions result in multiple effects ("outcomes") and, most importantly, different observers may value each outcome differently. As a consequence, treatment outcomes must be evaluated from all of the following perspectives: patient, family, provider, employer, payer, community, local government, academia, and media.

### Patient Perspective

A patient seeking treatment is always in distress and is functionally impaired. A patient seeks help with a particular problem or problems in mind, and the resolution of these problems will determine the patient's evaluation of outcome. For example, in our case of Mr. Fine, his problems included depressed mood, insomnia, low energy level, and inability to concentrate.

During the course of treatment, the patient may articulate further problems, and the degree of resolution of these problems may influence the patient's measure of successful outcome.

From the patient's perspective, management for successful outcome will involve a treatment method that evokes the least amount of anxiety and causes the least amount of embarrassment or dehumanization. In our case, Dr. Smith was successful in creating a positive environment. Mr. Fine liked her pleasant manner and considered her office efficient and convenient.

The outcomes plan must give the patient an active voice in decision-making. Patients must be able to balance the side effects of the treatment with the potential for improvement. Mr. Fine was cautioned to expect certain side effects from imipramine, yet he indicated a willingness to tolerate any unpleasantness if the medication would lift his depression. Despite this decision, he reported unhappiness with the blurry vision and constipation associated with imipramine soon after beginning treatment.

Most important, realistic treatment expectations should be outlined; patients should not expect to return to 100% of their former functioning. Dr. Smith warned Mr. Fine that he might not be able to return to his usual work efficiency. Mr. Fine at first seemed to care little about whether he was able to work, but as time passed, his inability to attend to this responsibility became an increasing source of distress to him, despite Dr. Smith's warning.

## Family Perspective

Perspectives of patient and family may often, but not necessarily, coincide. Occasionally, the chief complaint comes from the family, with the patient experiencing little manifest discomfort (e.g., mania without insight). Mrs. Fine found her husband to be distant when depressed and she missed his companionship. His unemployment caused her considerable worry and she canceled plans for a vacation after tax season. Mr. Fine's daughter missed his help with her homework, was concerned about his health, and received lower grades as a result. The level of family burden is much higher for patients with more chronic mental illness. In all cases, the family's burden (loss of privacy, disruption of family homeostasis, limitations of family activi-

ties, and the pain of watching a family member's suffering and functional deterioration) can be separately articulated and considered in assessing outcomes.

The family often can provide the therapist with useful observations about behavioral changes that may not be obvious to the patient. In turn, the therapist can help the family achieve satisfactory outcomes separate from those observable in the patient. By asking the family to describe Mr. Fine's symptoms, Dr. Smith was furthering their understanding of the illness. Mrs. Fine's report on her husband's functional status at home and the extent to which he had recovered his usual personality gave her a role in the patient's care. Mrs. Fine was reassured and felt supported when Dr. Smith welcomed her observations. Attending to the family's perspective (and needs) helps to foster alliance, enhance compliance, and improve both family and patient satisfaction.

## Provider Perspective

The provider's perspective is based on an objective and theoretical understanding of the nature and probable causes of the patient's symptoms, as well as the expected prognosis of the disorder, and may result in goals limited to symptomatology. Disjunctions may occur between the perspectives of the provider, the patient, and the family, each of whom may desire different outcomes of treatment. For example, from Dr. Smith's perspective, a successful outcome was achieved as Mr. Fine was much better groomed and free of the substantial psychomotor agitation he had exhibited initially. Mr. Fine, on the other hand, seemed to be indifferent to those changes even when Dr. Smith attempted to point them out as favorable signs. Mrs. Fine and her daughter had not yet experienced the complete return of Mr. Fine to their family life. The provider must recognize the potential disparity between the patient's assessment of a successful outcome and the caregiver's goal. This awareness offers an opportunity to discuss treatment expectations from the different perspectives and may also widen the provider's perspective from improving symptoms to helping the patient recover, as much as possible, the most important goal—functioning.

## Employer Perspective

Perspectives beyond those of the consultation room include employers, whose concerns relate to the patient's productivity, dependability, safety, and ability to work collaboratively. For employers, short-term disability may be a burden, whereas long-term illness is a major personnel and economic problem. In the case of Mr. Fine, his employer wanted him to return to work quickly and to function at his previous level. His employer needed to know promptly if this was not possible so that a replacement worker could be found. An assessment of the patient's functional status, properly worded to protect confidentiality, should be provided to the employer early in the recovery process. If the patient is still at work, early assessment can alert supervisors to the need for modification of the workload. If the patient is unable to work, management may need to schedule replacements. Proper attention to the employer's needs is likely to improve the patient's situation at work and ultimately aid his recovery.

## Payer Perspective

The payer seeks "value" in treatment outcomes and has the difficult task of balancing competing demands with limited budgets. The value assigned to outcomes depends heavily on the identity of the payer who may be the patient, the family, the employer, an insurance carrier, the government, the provider (charity work), or an academic institution (research agency or company). The emphasis on particular outcomes and the interpretation of studies about them are powerfully influenced by the identity of the payer. In Mr. Fine's case, the payer was a PPO. Although the PPO supported the use of a low

cost, generic drug rather than an SSRI, they recognized that this differential cost would be reversed if extra visits with Dr. Smith were needed. The PPO also was concerned that both Mr. Fine and his employer were satisfied with the treatment, which could affect subscriber and contract retention. The outcomes assessment management program of the PPO must consider both the patient's health status and satisfaction with treatment outcome. Monitoring these aspects of their care affords the PPO an opportunity to identify and examine outliers who are dissatisfied and to target interventions to them. Monitoring outcomes of patients with similar conditions also provides the PPO with valuable information about treatment results and whether cost cutting—in this case, use of a less expensive drug—is likely to be an effective option.

## Community and Local Government Perspectives

The community's perspective generally involves concern about disruptive or dangerous behavior, homelessness, consumption of community resources, and employability. Disruptive behavior or homelessness may be seen as a public safety issue and as a reflection on the community's reputation. Citizens may react with dissatisfaction and turn that dissatisfaction upon political leaders. Mr. Fine's behavior was never considered dangerous or disruptive, but his failure to play his usual role in the annual library fund drive, for example, was a serious setback to that organization.

A variety of institutions, agencies, and organizations (e.g., schools, religious groups) also have unique perspectives relevant to the fulfillment of their respective missions. To some extent, any individual patient's outcome, or the outcome of patients in general, may affect the financial well being, internal operations, and external reputation of a health plan, hospital, or clinic. Thus, any regular effort to follow the health status of a person with a mental disability will be likely to prevent the patient's decline to the point where he or she becomes a problem to the community.

From the perspective of local government, public safety, public opinion, community esthetics, and administrative burdens carried by the police, court system, and emergency medical resources are common concerns.

## Academia Perspective

Because the mission of academia is to further knowledge, outcomes of satisfaction important to the patient may seem less important to researchers than scientifically reliable and valid data, selected in ways that help answer critical theoretical questions. To improve outcomes studies, researchers should frame their inquiries about symptoms and functional impairment in such a way that they are not perceived by the patient as an invasion of privacy. Many patients also find it difficult to give researchers insightful answers about their own emotional and behavioral states. Bearing these problems in mind, researchers can reduce the chance of bias in their results that stem from patients refusing to cooperate in carrying out studies.

## Media Perspective

The media is influenced by matters of public interest and by the fact that some issues sell more newspapers than others. Reporters may be insensitive to the way their interaction with the patient affects outcome. Media reporting of successful recovery of functioning and well being among the mentally ill would enhance public awareness that such outcomes are possible and would help reduce the stigma that remains a confounding problem for those with such illness.

## CLINICAL IMPACT OF OUTCOMES ASSESSMENT

Outcomes assessments provide psychiatry with both opportunities and dangers. We discuss the potential impact of outcomes assessment on the following areas: a clinician's understanding of psychopathol-

ogy and therapeutics, education and certification, professional freedom and quality of life, a clinician's interaction with payers and with consumers, and documentation and service delivery.

Outcomes studies may foster clearer definitions of psychiatric illness. Long-term outcome studies on the subtypes of schizophrenia or mood disorders, for example, should provide clinicians with better predictive information about the etiology, pathologies, and treatment of diseases. A recent example is the observation of the effects of selective serotonergic agents on obsessive compulsive disorder, which helped to clarify the concept of this entity and increase our ability to treat it. Outcome studies may facilitate the identification and promotion of more effective therapies and help to identify ineffective treatment through the rapid dissemination of information. Pressure from managed care companies who may base their reimbursement policies on such data also may affect professional treatment practice.

Outcomes research may affect educational curricula and professional certification. Although variation and innovation in teaching methods will continue, a more uniform standard of practice may be adopted based on a specific body of knowledge that, in turn, may result in better outcomes predictability. Furthermore, the standard of practice adopted for therapists who are forensic specialists may be determined more easily and reliably. Practitioners unfamiliar with outcome data may need to reeducate themselves before changing their practice style; some may find the new methods less consonant with personal philosophy, prior training, or preference at first, which may interfere with their sense of freedom and quality of life.

Outcomes research may lead to a better understanding between consumers and mental health practitioners. The credibility of psychiatric therapies may be improved, the range of effective approaches may be clarified, and unwanted differences among practitioners that reduce the effectiveness of care may be decreased. Standardized educational materials for patients may be developed whereby patients and families can receive clear and concise written, audio, and video materials on mental health disorders and their treatments.

Psychiatry's relationship to payers will be greatly affected by increased availability of outcome research data. For example, there has been concern that payers will support somatic treatments but will not cover psychotherapy because of the rapid symptom reduction achieved by the former and the relative lack of research support for the latter. Outcomes research, demonstrating that somatic therapies improve symptoms but not necessarily functioning or that symptom reduction and compliance with medication is sustained and/or enhanced by psychotherapy, would add to the medical credibility of psychotherapy and establish the value of that form of care in the minds of the payer community.

On the other hand, the constraints of research techniques on outcomes assessment may favor those therapies that are effective in the short term and produce changes that are measured easily and reliably. The field may be biased toward the promotion of somatic therapies at the expense of treating conditions that may respond better to long-term psychosocial approaches or supportive rather than acute care. Thus, outcomes research may ignore many patients who suffer chronic disability from a minor affective disorder or personality disorder. "Cure" may take precedence over "care." The degree of success in establishing a "therapeutic alliance," for example, has had limited application for research (especially outcomes research) even though it is widely believed to be an important ingredient in therapeutic efficacy. Although demonstrating the effectiveness of psychotherapy for certain conditions is a challenge, the inherent difficulties of such research make its accomplishment slow to achieve; meanwhile, lack of proof of efficacy

causes the profession to retreat further from providing long-term psychotherapy in favor of the more easily validated somatic therapies.

Purchasers of psychiatric services will most likely welcome the availability of outcome data that ease their decision-making and clarify the range of effective approaches. For the practicing clinician, this may lead to a new scenario: justification of treatment of routine acute cases with somatic therapies may actually become easier, whereas justification of ongoing, long-term subacute or chronic care, particularly involving psychotherapy, may become more difficult. Third-party payment for psychotherapy may be decreased accordingly, influencing psychiatrists to further allocate this work to nonmedical colleagues.

Documentation and service delivery are likely to become more fully standardized once reliable outcome data become widely available to payers and consumers. Although it may not be necessary to document cases in greater detail, the "standard of practice" for documentation will probably become clearer, and clinicians will be expected (for legal as well as clinical purposes) to include specific information (e.g., the presence or absence of melancholic symptoms when antidepressants are prescribed). Each institution may develop individual databases, or a national database may be constructed that would prompt clinicians to supply missing information or explore unmentioned areas. An online information system might suggest therapies based on clinician input, as well as provide up-to-date figures on response probability. Clinicians who are part of the billing profile of an institution may be under pressure to compete with current norms for faster or more effective results to gain the interest of payers.

## CONCLUSIONS

If professional involvement becomes standard at all levels of implementation, outcome studies can be conducted correctly and interpreted wisely. Specifically, we recommend that psychiatrists and other mental health professionals be involved in the design, implementation, and interpretation (especially significance and limitations) of such studies; the development of guidelines for payment rates based on outcome studies for managed care companies; and the design of a simple appeal procedure for a clinician who believes a patient's course of treatment is more complex than indicated by those guidelines.

An example of such a psychiatrist-assisted data collection is detailed in Chapter 26. A representative group of psychiatrists throughout the United States was asked to report periodically on their professional activities using a structured survey. By actively participating in the process of shaping the outcomes management movement as it affects psychiatrists and their patients, clinicians can play a significant role in improving the quality of services while protecting professional standards of care.

Our case study of Mr. Fine and Dr. Smith demonstrates the use of outcomes information to resolve a potentially developing impasse. Both agreed that the diagnosis of depression was correct. Concerned that the treatment had not progressed as well as she had expected after several weeks, Dr. Smith reviewed with her patient the course of treatment they had agreed to follow. At this point, Mr. Fine acknowledged that as he had begun to feel better, side effects from imipramine (dry mouth, blurry vision, and constipation) caused him to take his medication only sporadically in the past 2 weeks. Dr. Smith inquired about patient compliance after learning from the PPO manager that her treatment results were out of the normal range. Aware that the difficulties associated with imipramine were hampering his recovery, she proposed a change in medication to an SSRI. Within 3 weeks of this change, Mr. Fine's symptoms had im-

proved significantly. Dr. Smith continued the cognitive-behavioral therapy to help Mr. Fine develop some new strategies to cope with his tendency to be overly self-critical. Mr. Fine acknowledged that turning 50 years old and experiencing this crisis of depression had stimulated him to think about his life and what he wanted to accomplish in the future. He returned to work, though not yet at his previous level of functioning. Mr. Fine initiated a discussion with his employer for a change in his duties at work once tax season had passed. In addition, Mr. Fine realized that he and his wife had been ignoring their relationship at a time when they would soon find themselves alone. Their daughter was a junior in high school and preparing for college. Mr. and Mrs. Fine decided to pursue a time-limited (six-session) couples therapy with a clinical social worker, a colleague of Dr. Smith. Approval for these visits was sought and received from the PPO. The patient, his family, and his employer had all been affected by this process.

As a result of the "scrutiny" Dr. Smith had received, she initiated a discussion with the PPO's medical director concerning more effective utilization of the information she and her colleagues provided. Instead of bringing rapid closure to the questions or problems of Dr. Smith's clinical decision-making in this case, the payer sensed an opportunity for a dialogue. Dr. Smith and her colleagues used this case as an example in their attempts to assess the effectiveness of their different interventions, to develop guidelines supporting their clinical decisions, and to adapt to the changes in health care. In so doing, outcomes management served to enhance individual patient care, improve the general delivery of clinical care, and establish a method by which the inevitable future changes in the technology and financing of mental health care could be met with an open mind by clinicians, payers, and the public.

## REFERENCES

1. Docherty JP, Butler SF. A comprehensive system for value accounting in psychiatry. Unpublished data, 1993.
2. Krupnick JL, Pincus HA. The cost-effectiveness of psychotherapy: a plan for research. Am J Psychiatry 1992;149:1295–1305.
3. Stewart AL, Ware JE Jr. Measuring functioning and well-being. Durham: Duke University Press, 1992.
4. Ellwood P. Shattuck Lecture—Outcomes management: a technology of patient experience. N Engl J Med 1988;318:1549–1556.
5. Smith GR, Rost K, Fisher E, et al. Assessing the effectiveness of mental health care in routine clinical practice: characteristics, developments, and uses of patient outcomes modules. Unpublished data, 1994.
6. Steinwachs DM, Wu AW, Skinner EA. How will outcomes management work? Health Affairs 1994;13:153–162.
7. Mirin SM, Namerow MJ. Why study treatment outcome? Hosp Community Psychiatry 1991;42:1007–1013.
8. American Psychiatric Association. American Psychiatric Association policy concerning managed care. Psychiatric News, January, 1994.

# CHAPTER 7

# Evaluating Health Status

*Barbara Dickey, Hendrik Wagenaar*

## EVALUATING HEALTH STATUS

Better evaluation of mental health care is vitally important today in light of calls for reform: improve quality, contain costs, and increase access. The purpose of this chapter is twofold. The first purpose is to argue that research on the effectiveness of proposed changes in the organization and financing of mental health services should not be limited to econometric analyses but should incorporate the viewpoints of clinicians, patients, and patients' families. The second purpose is to propose a guide for the selection of outcome measures.

## MERGING TWO RESEARCH TRADITIONS

Analyses of treatment costs and treatment outcomes have traditionally taken place in two distinct arenas of research, health services research and clinical outcome trials, each with its own research goals, databases, and analytic styles (1). For example, health services research has relied on administrative databases to identify regional variations in treatment patterns (2–6) and to measure the effect of the introduction of diagnosis-related groups on the length of stay of psychiatric inpatients (7–11). These large databases have been extraordinarily useful in addressing policy issues confronting our health care system. Although the studies have been able to answer important questions, with few exceptions (12), they have failed to address quality of care and outcome issues.

In contrast, studies that have their roots in the research tradition of randomized clinical trials are far more likely to rely on primary data. Research is conducted to establish a causal connection between a program or treatment and the patient outcome of that program or treatment. Typically, the study design is experimental and homogeneity of subjects, rather than heterogeneity, is characteristic. Measurement is limited to the particular clinical effects under study. The collection of clinical outcome data is labor intensive, accounting in part for those studies' relatively small sample sizes.

Given the different research paradigms, the division of labor between clinical and health services researchers has produced work in which patterns of service use are studied without reference to clinical outcome, and the clinical outcome of discrete programs is studied in the absence of data about use. Interpretation of the findings in both cases is compromised, and neither approach alone is adequate to meet policy needs.

## ASSESSMENT OF PATIENT OUTCOME

The effects of structural changes in the delivery of health care on patients may go undetected unless the choice of "outcome" measures is grounded in theory about the relation between the policy that changes the system and the expected effect. Theory makes more precise our measurement of effect, helps us to interpret the data, and leads us to certain conclusions about system effectiveness.

The policy of deinstitutionalization led to hundreds of program evaluations that provided support for community care (13, 14). Two recent examples, the community support program and the Robert Wood Johnson program on chronic mental illness, introduced system change and then collected mental health status data about patients. However, in the absence of a rigorous design, the investigators described patient health status after the intervention but could not compare it with the health status of patients in other systems. Despite the positive findings of these evaluations, popular opinion indicates that the public mental health system, for all its successes in particular programs, still falls far short of providing adequate treatment and care to the many seriously mentally ill individuals who do not have access to our private mental health system.

Changing our thinking from program evaluation to assessment of the system effectiveness means that all aspects of design and methods are challenged. Measurement precision is a high priority in the selection of outcome instruments. The selection decision is complicated by the need for measures that can capture a broad range of health and illness states found in individuals who seek treatment across the system. Interest is growing in one category of self-report measurement, health status.

Fortunately, a good deal of theoretical and psychometric work has already been accomplished in the field of health status assessment (15–18). Large health services research studies, such as the health insurance experiment and the medical outcomes study, have used health status measures to identify links between key features of financing and organizational arrangements and favorable outcomes (18–20). In these studies, self-reports of health status were included.

Stewart and Ware (18) based their work on the original description by the World Health Organization (WHO) of health as "a state of complete physical, mental, and social well-being and not merely the absence of disease or infirmity" (21). The scales seek to measure not just illness states but also well-being states. This approach expands our understanding of system changes from the patient's point of view by including questions about mental health, that is, the capacity to experience personal growth and change, to care for self and others, and to engage in productive work. Contemporary studies have referred to the work of Jahoda (22), who stresses the need to understand the positive aspects of mental health in her review of the mental health literature for WHO. Jahoda concludes that mental health is not just the absence of disease or the presence of certain desirable behaviors but some subjective assessment of how we see ourselves in relation to how we believe we should be.

This definition of health status does not distinguish between the professional judgment of clinicians and the self-reported experience of patients or their families. However, the idea that these are distinctly different points of view is supported by other researchers in the fields of medical sociology and anthropology (23, 24). A careful distinction is drawn between the concept of disease, that which physicians diagnose and treat, and the concept of illness, that which patients experience, for example, pain and suffering. These investigators point out that the families of individuals with serious mental illness suffer more than just emotional anguish; they may also develop health problems or have difficulty in maintaining steady work performance themselves.

The matter of perspective has long been viewed as simply the difference between objective and subjective data, implying that a construct that can be quantified and measured precisely and reliably (e.g., disease) is objective; all of the remaining data is subjective. We do not argue that some data can be more precisely measured than others, but the implication of this assumption is that objective data play a superior role in research. If self-report data are labeled subjective, then legitimate feelings and perceptions tend to be discounted. Perhaps a better approach for services researchers is to set aside the subjective/objective data debate and shift to the informative perspective.

To underline the importance of this approach, we offer the following argument. A professional's description of a clinical syndrome is quite distinct from a patient's description of how he or she feels. Each perspective is important, and the data are not interchangeable. Some individuals have "everything" but still view life as overwhelmingly difficult and distressing. Others have significant health and social problems but still maintain a positive outlook and a realistic appraisal of their own capabilities and limits (25). By giving equal weight to the clinician's observation of disease, the patient's report of his or her illness, and the family's report of the burden, there is no implication that one perspective is more valued than another.

Current emphasis on biomedical research reflects the increasing sophistication of our understanding of the neurobiological aspect of mental disorders but minimizes the feelings and experiences of the person whose biomedical problem may also have devastating social and emotional consequences. Exclusive reliance on biomedical treatments are unlikely to alleviate the social and emotional problems associated with illness, creating an important reason to supplement clinical outcome assessments with patient and family reports.

Theoretically, and most importantly, views promulgating the theory that community treatment policies are more humane and normalizing should be empirically tested by examining a patient's own report of health status. These reports are at least as important as a professional's observation about patient success in adapting to community life.

Another important perspective that should be considered is that of the community. However, a discussion on this subject is beyond the scope of this chapter and will be saved for the future.

## DEVELOPING A MEASUREMENT OF HEALTH STATUS

A matrix can be developed based on the three key perspectives that determine the health status of an individual: clinical observations of disease, patient reports of the experience of illness, and family report of burden. Table 7.1 summarizes this measurement matrix and suggests specific topics for measurement within each cell of the matrix.

The usefulness of this matrix as a starting point in the measurement of health status is illustrated by the following example. Patient outcome measured by symptom reduction alone cannot fully reflect the effects of rehabilitation or social skills train-

**Table 7.1. Health Status**

| | Disease (Clinical Observation) | Illness (Patient Self-report) | Burden (Family Self-report) |
|---|---|---|---|
| SOCIAL | social network role functioning | social support role satisfaction | social support role satisfaction |
| MENTAL | neuro-psych status symptoms and signs | feelings moods | feelings concerns about future |
| PHYSICAL | morbidity mortality | perceived fitness pain | stress-related illness |
| GENERAL | overall health: severity of illness | overall health: felt need for services | overall health: felt need for services- |

ing. Even staff-rated functioning of patients in these programs may not change if disability is long standing. Further, patients who participate in community support programs may report no satisfaction with specific aspects of their own daily functioning, but change may be measured in their reports of their own feelings of psychological well being or distress. This is especially important for patients with chronic illnesses in whom subtle changes in feeling states may assume greater significance.

The matrix assumes that everyday life can be easily divided into measurement domains. Although these domains are arbitrary, their use has support. For example, in the separation of social health from mental health, if we accept the definition of mental health as the capacity to love and to work, then the boundaries between mental and social health are certainly blurred. Social health is widely accepted as an essential dimension of health status, but psychometrically sound measurement as an independent construct has been elusive (18, 20). Undoubtedly, the problems of individual values and varying definitions of normative role functioning contribute to the difficulties.

Separate measurement of mental and social health best serves our comprehensive approach by making possible certain analyses that address the complex links between social support systems, help-seeking behavior, and mental health. Sherbourne and Stewart (26) found that observations by professionals of the breadth and depth of social networks is likely to have a low correlation with the level of social support believed to exist by the patient. On the other hand, they found that patient-reported emotional and instrumental support from others appears to mediate the negative impact of severe mental illness. The widespread introduction of case managers may have considerable effect on the extent to which a patient believes that support is available, even if the size of the observed "social network" may not have changed.

Social health also encompasses the satisfaction individuals experience in their different roles when community integration, as part of the "normalization" policy, is incorporated into changes in the system of care. A professional's assessment of role functioning provides a perspective that is distinctly different from patient's reports of his or her own role satisfaction. Family members also may find that their parenting or spousal roles will change in response to changes in care, and thus their satisfaction with those roles will change.

Physical health, which is frequently ignored in mental health services studies, is critically important to the overall well being of patients with mental disorders. Measures of physical health must be included to account for the excess medical co-morbidity that is widely observed (27, 28). Other reasons for including physical health status are the interactions between physical illness, mental illness, and treatment that may result in compromised well being and functioning or in complications in treatment response. Family members (especially the primary caregiver) may report stress-related illness, a reduction in vigor, or an increase in pain if their caregiving activities increase substantially under different policy options.

In addition to including mental, social, and physical health in the WHO definition of health status, a fourth dimension is considered especially important in understanding help-seeking behavior: overall general health status (29). When reported by clinicians, it can be a substitute for the clinician's assessment of the patient's need for services. When patients are asked to report their general health status, it has been an important predictor of demand for treatment (29). Understanding demand is especially salient in the treatment of mental illness at the extreme ends of the treatment intensity spectrum: those most in need may deny any need at all and those with the fewest symptoms and life problems may demand considerable attention. The variation in compliance to treatment regimens and response rates might be explained by the fact that treated individuals use a broader base of information than do clinicians when reporting their overall health status, including more psychosocial aspects of their lives (30).

Our model is limited in several ways. First, our presentation of the issues might suggest that a single formula for outcome assessment will be adequate for all studies. To the contrary, every study can be improved by adding questions that link specific system changes to the factors most likely to be affected. Second, our measurement matrix assumes that theoretical links exist between specific macrolevel system changes and changes in patient health status scores. We have suggested some of those links, but tying changes in systems to specific effect on patients' health status is in its earliest stages. Scales were developed to measure multidimensional health status as part of the medical outcome study. A central purpose of the study was to link the scores to different system configurations (18, 19).

As mental health outcomes research expands, many questions can be addressed: How can we modify the matrix to accommodate the special needs of the elderly, children, and those who are developmentally delayed as well as mentally ill? How can we include the perspectives represented by those who may not be able to speak for themselves? What data collection methods are the most cost effective? What instruments are psychometrically sound and present minimal burden to the most seriously mentally ill?

## IMPLICATIONS FOR OUTCOMES ASSESSMENT

The word "reform" connotes looking forward to something better, a new and improved way of doing things. However, health care reform directed toward improving quality of care, containing costs, and increasing access creates a dilemma: attaining one goal may eliminate the chance to reach other goals. Many of the changes now being proposed are primarily motivated by financial objectives and may in fact deny access or inhibit the provision of care to the most vulnerable patients (31, 32). Reform must be accompanied by data to support claims of success or accusations of failure within the policy debate. Studies that include clinician, patient, and family reports about the effect of change must be integrated into that debate.

The preceding chapters have reviewed methods designed to encourage the integration of outcomes assessment into the clinical practice of mental health professionals. In the next section, we provide a systematic review of measurement instruments that assess the health status of adults and children from multiple perspectives and across the domains listed in Table 7.1. Several instruments are disease specific, but most are more generic in nature. Utilization of the instruments does not pose an unnecessary respondent burden; either the scales are relatively brief or they have been developed in stand-alone component parts that are easy to use. In almost all cases, the authors provided the material for the chapter or were given permission from others to write the chapter.

*Acknowledgments.* We thank Anita Stewart and Ann Hohmann for their careful reading and helpful comments on earlier drafts of this paper, Lydia Ratcliff for editorial support, and Elliot Mishler for his guidance. The work was supported by the Commonwealth Research Center at the Massachusetts Mental Health Center, Massachusetts Department of Mental Health.

## REFERENCES

1. Judd LL. Focus on mental health services research [untitled column]. Washington, DC: Foundation for Health Services Research, 1988;2:5.
2. Christiansen T, Pedersen KM, Harvald B, Rasmessen K, Jorgensen J, Svarer C. An investigation of the effect of regional variation in the treatment of hypertension. Soc Sci Med 1989;28:131–139.

3. Loft A, Andersen TF, Madsen M. A quasi-experimental design based on regional variations: discussion of a method for evaluating outcomes of medical practice. Soc Sci Med 1989;28:147–154.

4. McDermott W. Absence of indicators of the influence of its physicians on a society's health; impact of physician care on society. Am J Med 1981;70:833–843.

5. Wennberg JE, Freeman JL, Culp WJ. Are hospital services rationed in New Haven or overutilized in Boston. Lancet 1987;1:1185–1189.

6. Wennberg JE, Gittelsohn A. Variations in medical care among small areas. Sci Am 1982;246:120–134.

7. Frank RG, Lave JR. The impact of Medicaid benefit design on length of hospital stay and patient transfers. Hosp Community Psychiatry 1985;36:749–753.

8. Frank RG, Lave JR. A plan for prospective payment for inpatient psychiatric care. Hosp Community Psychiatry 1985;36:775–776.

9. Jencks SF, Goldman HH, McGuire TG. Challenges in bringing exempt psychiatric services under a prospective payment system. Hosp Community Psychiatry 1985;36:764–769.

10. McGuire TG, Dickey B, Shively GE, Strumwaaser I. Differences in resource use and cost among facilities treating alcohol, drug abuse, and mental disorders: implications for design of a prospective payment system. Am J Psychiatry 1987;144:616–620.

11. Mitchell JB, Dickey B, Liptzin B, Sederer L. Bringing psychiatric patients into medicare prospective payment system: alternatives to DRG's. Am J Psychiatry 1987;144:610–615.

12. Newhouse JP, Friedlander LJ. The relationship between medical resources and measures of health: some additional evidence. J Human Resources 1979;15:200–218.

13. Tessler RC, Goldman HH. The chronically mentally ill: assessing community support programs. Cambridge, MA: Ballinger Publishing Co., 1982.

14. Frank RG, Goldman HH, McGuire TG. A model mental health benefit in private health insurance. Health Aff (Millwood) 1992;11:98–117.

15. Bergner M. Quality of life, health status, and clinical research. Med Care 1989;27(3 Suppl):148–156.

16. Breslow L. Health status measurement in the evaluating of health promotion. Med Care 1989;27(3 Suppl):205–216.

17. Patrick DL, Deyo RA. Generic and disease specific measures in assessing health status and quality of life. Medical Med Care 1989;27(3 Suppl):217–232.

18. Stewart A, Ware JE Jr, eds. Measuring functioning and well-being. Durham and London: Duke University Press, 1992.

19. Tarlov AR, Ware JE Jr, Greenfield S, Nelson EC, Perrin E. The medical outcomes study. An application of methods for monitoring the results of medical care. JAMA 1989;262:925–930.

20. Ware JE Jr, Brook RH, Davies-Avery A, Williams KN, Stewart AL. Conceptualization and measurement of health for adults in the health insurance study. Model of health and methodology. Santa Monica: The Rand Corporation, 1980;1.

21. World Health Organization. Constitution. In: Basic documents. Geneva: World Health Organization, 1948.

22. Jahoda M. Current concepts of mental health. New York: Basic Books, Inc., 1958.

23. Eisenberg L, Kleinman A. Clinical social science. In: Eisenberg L, Kleinman A, eds. The relevance of social science to medicine. Boston: Reidel Publishing Co., 1981:1–26.

24. Twaddle AC. Sickness and the sickness career: some implications. In: Eisenberg L, Kleinman A, eds. The relevance of social science to medicine. Boston: Reidel Publishing Co., 1981:111–134.

25. Zola IK. Studying the decision to see a doctor: review, critique, corrective. Adv Psychosom Med 1972;8:216–236.

26. Sherbourne CD, Stewart AL. The MOS social support survey. Soc Sci Med 1991;32:705–714.

27. Farmer S. Medical problems of chronic patients in a community support program. Hosp Community Psychiatry 1987;38:745–749.

28. Koran LM, Sox HC Jr, Marton KI, et al. Medical evaluation of psychiatric patients. I. Results in a state mental health system. Arch Gen Psychiatry 1989;46:733–740.

29. Ware JE Jr, Davies-Avery A, Donald CA. Conceptualization and measurement of health for adults in the health insurance study. General health perceptions. Santa Monica: The Rand Corporation, 1978;5.

30. Connelly JE, Philbrich JT, Smith GR Jr, Kaiser DL, Wymer A. Health preceptions of primary care patients and the influence on health care utilization. Med Care 1989;27(3 Suppl):S9–S109.

31. Schlesinger M, Dorwart R. Ownership and mental-health services: a repraisal of the shift toward privately owned facilities. N Engl J Med 1984;311:959–965.

32. Ware JE Jr. Measures of a new era of health assessment. In: Stewart A, Ware JE Jr, eds. Measuring functioning and well-being. Durham and London: Duke University Press, 1992:3–24.

CHAPTER 8

# The MOS 36-Item Short-Form Health Survey (SF-36)

*John E. Ware*

---

*DESCRIPTION AND BACKGROUND*

*Formal Name*
The MOS 36-item Short-Form Health Survey (SF-36)

*Author*
John E. Ware, Ph.D.

*Key References*
Ware JE, Sherbourne CD. The MOS 36-Item Short-Form Health Status Survey (SF-36). I. Conceptual framework and item selection. Med Care 1992;30:MS253–MS265.

Ware JE, Snow KK, Kosinski M, Gandek B. SF-36 health survey manual and interpretation guide. Boston: New England Medical Center, The Health Institute, 1993.

---

## INTRODUCTION

The SF-36 is a multipurpose short-form measure of generic health status (1, 2). The development and validation of the SF-36 Health Survey was supported by a grant from the Henry J. Kaiser Family Foundation to the Health Institute, New England Medical Center. The SF-36 is a trademark of the not-for-profit Medical Outcomes Trust.

## DOMAINS AND NUMBER OF ITEMS

The SF-36 multi-item scales measure eight concepts commonly represented in widely used surveys: physical functioning, role limitations due to physical health problems, bodily pain, general health, vitality (energy/fatigue), social functioning, role limitations due to emotional problems, and mental health (psychological distress and psychological well being). It also includes a self-report of change in health during the past year. In addition to the eight-scale SF-36 profile, summary physical and mental health scales can be scored (3, 4). Both standard (4-week) and acute (1-week) recall versions have been published (2).

## APPLICATION

### Target Population

The SF-36 has been used successfully in general population surveys as well as cross-sectional and longitudinal studies of specific diseases and treatments.

### Data Collection Procedures

Survey forms for self-administration and scripts for personal interviews can be administered in 5–10 minutes and have been used with a high degree of acceptability and satisfactory data quality (2). Translations or adaptations are currently being evaluated in 29 countries (5).

### Psychometric Properties

Assumptions underlying the construction and scoring of SF-36 scales have been evaluated in more than three dozen studies in the United States and in other countries (5–8). The reliability of the eight scales and two summary measures has been estimated using internal consistency, test-retest, and alternate forms (Mental Health scale only) methods. With few exceptions, coefficients have exceeded the minimum standard of 0.70 recommended for measures used in group comparisons; most have exceeded 0.80 (2). Reliability estimates for physical and mental summary scores usually exceed 0.90 (3, 4).

These tests have been replicated across 24 different patient groups differing in sociodemographic characteristics and diagnosis. Although results indicate slight declines with more disadvantaged respondents, reliability coefficients consistently exceed recommended standards for group level analysis (2). Standard errors of measurement, 95% confidence intervals for individual scores, and distributions of change scores from test-retest and 1-year follow-up studies have been published (2, 3, 7). Estimates of sample sizes required to detect differences of various magnitudes have been documented for five different study designs (2, 3).

Because of the widespread use of the SF-36 across a variety of applications, evidence of all types of validity is relevant. The content validity of the SF-36 compares favorably with other widely used generic health surveys (2). Relative to the longer Medical Outcomes Study (MOS) measures they were constructed to reproduce, SF-36 scales typically have performed with about 80–90% empirical validity in cross-sectional and longitudinal studies. The validity of each of the eight scales and the two summary scales differ markedly as would be expected from factor analytic studies of construct validity (3, 4, 6). Specifically, the mental health, role-emotional, and social functioning scales and the mental health summary measure have been shown to be the best mental measures in numerous cross-cultural and longitudinal tests using the method of known groups validity (2, 3, 6).

Criteria used in the known groups validation of the SF-36, which include accepted clinical indicators of diagnosis and severity of depression, heart disease, and other conditions, are well documented in peer-reviewed publications and user's manuals (2–4, 6). The mental health scale has been shown to be useful in screening for psychiatric disorders (8), as has the mental health summary measure (3, 4). Relative to other published measures, they have performed equally or better in most tests published to date (2).

Predictive validity studies have linked SF-36 scales and summary measures to utilization of health care services, the clinical course of depression, and 5-year survival (2, 3). Validation studies using representative samples of the general U.S. population and patients with specific chronic conditions, including two foreign countries, are well documented in published articles and in the SF-36 user's manuals (2–8).

The SF-36 has been normed in the general U.S. population and for random samples from the United Kingdom, Sweden, and Germany using common translation and norming protocols developed by the International Quality of Life Association Project (5, 7, 8). Norming studies are underway in Australia, Denmark, France, Italy, and the Netherlands and will be completed in 1995 (8). In the United States, norms for age and sex groups have been published along with estimates of the effect of telephone interviews compared with self-administered versions (2).

## UTILITY

### Scoring Manual

Available information about the development and evaluation of the eight SF-36 scales, including content-based, norm-based, and criterion-based interpretation guidelines, have been published in a 320-page user's manual (1). A second manual focusing on the physical and mental summary measures includes a computer diskette for scoring and a test dataset (3).

## Automation

Computer-administered and telephone voice recognition interactive systems of administration are currently being evaluated. An optical scan card version of the SF-36 and accompanying software program are available to reduce the burden of data entry and analyses. An ASCII file can be generated automatically that can be downloaded for statistical analyses or for use with other datasets.

## Permission to Use

Permission to use and reproduce the SF-36 is routinely granted by the Medical Outcomes Trust (MOT) without charge. The trust is a nonprofit clearinghouse for widely used patient-based measures. Permission to reproduce SF-36 items and scoring algorithms has also been granted to computer software vendors and dozens of commercial survey and data processing firms offering a wide range of services based on standard SF-36 scoring algorithms and interpretation guidelines. The SF-36 Scoring Exercise available from the MOT includes a computer diskette with scoring algorithms and a test dataset (9).

Information can be obtained from The Medical Outcomes Trust, The Health Institute, New England Medical Center, Boston, MA, 02111. The telephone number is 617-426-4046.

## Description of Where and When Used

At last count, SF-36 user information packets had been sent to nearly 10,000 individuals and organizations. The SF-36 is currently being fielded in over 500 clinical trials; research topics are listed in the user's manual (2).

## SUMMARY OF STRENGTHS AND LIMITATIONS

Because of the widespread use of the SF-36 in a variety of applications, considerable information is accumulating about norms, benchmarks for comparing the burden of psychiatric and other conditions, and estimates of the benefits of various treatments. The SF-36 offers the option of scoring a profile and summary measures, which reduces the number of statistical comparisons and has advantages in the interpretation and presentation of results. Because general population surveys and clinical trials are currently underway worldwide, the SF-36 is likely to have an advantage in multinational studies for which comparative data are useful in interpretation.

Although a highly efficient and psychometrically sound measure, the SF-36 achieved its brevity by focusing on only eight health concepts and measuring each concept with a short-form scale. Some SF-36 scales have been shown to have 10–20% less precision than the long-form MOS measures they were constructed to reproduce. However, empirical studies of these tradeoffs suggest that the SF-36 provides a very practical alternative to many longer health outcomes measures and that the eight scales and two SF-36 summary scales rarely miss a noteworthy difference in physical or mental health status in group level comparisons.

REFERENCES

1. Ware JE, Sherbourne CD. The MOS 36-item short-form health status survey (SF-36). I. Conceptual framework and item selection. Med Care 1992;30:MS253–MS265.
2. Ware JE, Snow KK, Kosinski M, Gandek B. SF-36 health survey manual and interpretation guide. Boston: New England Medical Center, The Health Institute, 1993.
3. Ware JE, Kosinski M, Keller SD. SF-36 physical and mental component summary measures—a user's manual. Boston: New England Medical Center, The Health Institute, 1994.
4. Ware JE, Kosinski M, Bayliss MS, et al. Comparison of methods for scoring and statistical analysis of the SF-36 health profile and summary measures: results from the medical outcomes study. Med Care 1995;33:AS264–AS279.
5. Ware JE, Keller SD, Gandek B, Brazier J, Sullivan M, IQOLA Project Team. Evaluating translations of health status surveys: lessons from the IQOLA project. Int J Technol Assess Health Care (in press).
6. McHorney CA, Ware JE, Raczek AR. The MOS 36-item short-form health status survey (SF-36).

II. Psychometric and clinical tests of validity in measuring physical and mental health constructs. Med Care 1993;31:247–263.

7. Brazier JE, Harper R, Jones NMB, et al. Validating the SF-36 health survey questionnaire: new outcome measure for primary care. Br J Med 1992;305:160–164.

8. Berwick DM, Murphy JM, Goldman PA, et al. Performance of a five-item mental health screening test. Med Care 1991;29:169–176.

9. Medical Outcomes Trust. Scoring exercise for the SF-36 health survey with test dataset on diskette. 2nd ed. Boston: Medical Outcomes Trust, 1994.

CHAPTER 9

# Behavior and Symptom Identification Scale (BASIS-32)

*Susan V. Eisen*

---

*DESCRIPTION AND BACKGROUND*

*Formal Name*
  Behavior and Symptom Identification Scale (BASIS-32)

*Authors*
  Susan V. Eisen, Ph.D., and M. C. Grob

*Key References*
Eisen SV, Dill DL, Grob MC. Reliability and validity of a brief patient-report instrument for psychiatric outcome evaluation. Hosp Community Psychiatry 1994;45:242–247.

Eisen SV. Assessment of subjective distress by patients' self-report versus structured interview. Psychol Rep 1995;76:35–39.

Sederer LI, Eisen SV, Dill DL, Grob MC, Gougeon M, Mirin SM. Case-based reimbursement for psychiatric hospital care. Hosp Community Psychiatry 1992;42:1120–1126.

Eisen SV, Grob MC, Dill DL. Outcome measurement: tapping the patient's perspective. In: Mirin SM, Gossett J, Grob MC, eds. Psychiatric treatment: advances in outcome research. Washington, DC: American Psychiatric Press, 1991:213–235.

Eisen SV, Youngman D, Grob MC, Dill DL. Alcohol, drugs and psychiatric disorders: a current view of hospitalized adolescents. J Adolesc Res 1992; 7:250–265.

## INTRODUCTION

BASIS-32 was designed to assess outcome of mental health treatment from the patient's point of view. It is a brief but comprehensive measure of self-reported difficulty in the major symptom and functioning domains that lead to the need for inpatient psychiatric treatment. These include mood disturbances, anxiety, suicidality, psychotic symptoms, self-understanding, interpersonal relations, role functioning, daily living skills, impulsivity, and substance abuse.

BASIS-32 was empirically derived from psychiatric inpatients' reports of symptoms and problems that were cluster analyzed to arrive at the 32 items (1–3). It cuts across diagnoses, acknowledging the wide range of symptoms and problems that occur across the diagnostic spectrum.

Respondents are asked to indicate the degree of difficulty they have been experiencing on each item during the past week. Degree of difficulty is rated on a five-point scale as follows: 0, no difficulty; 1, a little; 2, moderate; 3, quite a bit; and 4, extreme. Assessments can be done at intake and at specified intervals during or after completion of treatment.

## DOMAINS AND NUMBER OF ITEMS

BASIS-32 consists of 32 items, and each is scored into one of five subscales: relation to self and others, daily living and role functioning, depression and anxiety, impulsive and addictive behavior, and psychosis. In addition, an overall average score is computed. Subscale and overall mean scores can range from 0 to 4.

## APPLICATION

### Target Population

Populations measured are midadolescents through adults receiving mental health treatment (ages 14 and up), excluding geriatric cases with severe dementia.

### Data Collection Procedures

Four different data collection procedures have been used successfully to obtain BASIS-32 assessments: structured interviews in which a staff member or volunteer reads the items to patients and elicits their ratings for each item, patient self-administration, telephone interviews, and mailed self-report questionnaires. Structured interviews and self-administration have been used at all time points (admission, discharge, and follow-up). Telephone interviews and mailed self-reports have been done for discharge and follow-up assessment.

Results of a recent study suggested that comparable participation rates are obtained for self-administered versus interviewer-administered methods (4). Comparison of mean subscale scores suggest that patients who self-administered the BASIS-32 reported more difficulty with respect to relation to self and others than patients who reported their ratings to an interviewer.

Published data regarding BASIS-32 were obtained through program evaluation projects implemented by evaluators who were separate from the clinical care providers. However, with increasing demands for outcome assessment, many facilities (including McLean Hospital, where BASIS-32 was developed) are now incorporating outcome assessment into the clinical care process and using clinical staff to collect data.

Time required for completion as a self-report ranges from 5 to 20 minutes. Self-administration takes less time than a structured interview, and most patients can complete it in 5–10 minutes. Administration as a structured interview generally takes 15–20 minutes. BASIS-32 is currently available in English and Spanish.

### Psychometric Properties

Psychometric properties of BASIS-32 were assessed on several samples of newly admitted psychiatric inpatients (1). Internal consistency (Cronbach's alpha) coefficients were computed for each subscale on a sample of 387 cases and were replicated on another sample of 144 cases, yielding the following results for each sample, respectively: relation to self and others, $r = 0.76$ and $0.77$; daily living and role functioning skills, $r = 0.80$ and $0.79$; depression and anxiety, $r = 0.74$ and $0.76$; impulsive and addictive behavior, $r = 0.71$ and $0.68$; and psychosis, $r = 0.63$ and $0.43$. Full-scale reliability was $r = 0.89$.

Test-retest reliability coefficients, computed on a separate sample of 40 cases, were as follows: $r = 0.80$ for relation to self and others, $r = 0.81$ for daily living and role functioning, $r = 0.78$ for depression and anxiety, $r = 0.65$ for impulsive and addictive behavior, and $r = 0.76$ for psychosis.

Concurrent validity was assessed by relating objective indicators of functioning at follow-up (6 months posthospital admission) with BASIS-32 follow-up scores. Two objective indicators—continued hospitalization or rehospitalization during the 6 months after admission and employment status at follow-up—were compared with patients' subjective reports of difficulty at the follow-up point. Consistent with their hospital status, patients who were discharged to the community and had remained so during the 6 months reported the least difficulty, whereas patients who were hospitalized at the 6-month follow-up point reported the greatest difficulty.

Regarding employment status among patients identified at admission as having a paid occupation, scores on the daily living and role functioning subscale at follow-up were expected to differentiate those who were working at follow-up from those who were not. Results supported this expectation; patients who were working reported significantly less difficulty with respect to daily living and role functioning than those who were not working.

Discriminant validity was assessed by analyzing whether specific BASIS-32 subscales predicted corresponding diagnoses.

As expected, results indicated that patients with a diagnosis of unipolar depression had significantly higher scores on the depression and anxiety subscale than patients with other diagnoses. Patients with a psychotic disorder had significantly higher scores on the psychosis subscale than patients who were not diagnosed with psychosis, and patients with a substance abuse disorder had significantly higher scores on the impulsive and addictive behavior subscale than patients without a substance abuse diagnosis.

BASIS-32 has also be shown to be sensitive to change. Comparison of admission scores with those obtained at a 6-month follow-up point were highly significant (1), as were changes during the course of a hospitalization (from admission to discharge) (5).

## UTILITY

### Scoring Manual

A BASIS-32 information packet is available from the authors. Contact Susan V. Eisen, Ph.D., Department of Mental Health Services Research, McLean Hospital, 115 Mill Street, Belmont, MA 02178, FAX: 617-855-2948. The packet includes sample copies of the measure, an instruction and scoring booklet, and a reference list.

Currently, three manual versions (BASIS-32A, B, and C), and one scan card version of BASIS-32 are available. BASIS-32A, designed to measure baseline symptomatology and functioning, includes ques-

tions regarding chronicity of each symptom or problem as well as demographic and employment information. BASIS-32B, designed for repeat assessment during or at completion of treatment, includes the 32 items with no additional information. BASIS-32C, developed for follow-up assessment, measures current employment status as well as current mental health treatment.

The scan card version of BASIS-32 was designed as a single "generic" measure that can be used at intake, during treatment, and/or at a follow-up point after termination of treatment. In addition to the 32 items, it includes demographic and employment information.

The manual versions of BASIS-32 can be scored by hand or by computer using the scoring algorithms provided in the instruction booklet. The scan card version of BASIS-32 is scored automatically using the Response Technologies (RT) scanner and accompanying software package described below under automation.

### Automation

Developed in collaboration with Response Technologies Inc., an optical scan card version of BASIS-32 and an accompanying software package are available. The scan card version works on the RT Survey Scan System, an easy to operate data collection program that uses an Optimal Mark Reader attached to any IBM-compatible PC. The scanner automatically reads the BASIS-32 ratings, eliminating the need for manual data entry. The accompanying software program computes scores for each of the five BASIS-32 subscales and an overall average score and prints out a graphic report of up to three sequential BASIS-32 assessments per person. The report also identifies extreme responses on six key items of potential clinical significance: adjusting to major life stresses; suicidal feelings or behavior; fear; anxiety or panic; drinking alcoholic beverages; taking illegal drugs or misusing drugs; and controlling temper, anger, or violence.

An ASCII file can be generated automatically and downloaded for combination with other datasets for statistical analysis.

## Permission to Use

BASIS-32 is copyrighted by The McLean Hospital Corporation, which has given mental health providers permission to reproduce and use the manual versions of BASIS-32 for the purpose of assessing outcomes of their own clients or patients. There is no charge for this use. Permission has not been granted for any such facility to sell BASIS-32 to others. However, nonexclusive licensing arrangements for commercial use of BASIS-32 by providers, insurance, managed care, pharmaceutical, software development, or consulting organizations can be made directly with McLean Hospital. Proposals should be submitted in writing to Susan V. Eisen, Ph.D., Department of Mental Health Services Research, McLean Hospital, 115 Mill Street, Belmont, MA 02178, FAX: 617-855-2948.

The automated BASIS-32 materials including scan card, accompanying software, hardware, and current pricing information can be obtained from Response Technologies Inc., 1485 South County Trail, East Greenwich, RI 02818, Telephone: 800-522-1440.

## Description of Where and When Used

BASIS-32 has been used most extensively with psychiatric hospital inpatients and less extensively with partial hospital and outpatient populations. It has been included in a list of recommended outcome measures distributed by the American Association for Partial Hospitalization.

The psychometric data reported in this chapter apply to psychiatric inpatients treated at McLean Hospital from 1985 through 1992. However, the measure has also been used in three multisite hospital outcome studies comprising a total of approximately 30 hospitals. Precise extent of use is not known, although the authors have filled requests for information from more than 600 different mental health facilities and providers within and outside the United States.

BASIS-32 has been used to assess patient's progress during the course of treatment and maintenance of improvement over a follow-up period. Change scores that adjust for degree of difficulty at baseline have been computed so that both patient and treatment predictors of good and poor outcome can be identified.

BASIS-32 has also been used to assess symptom patterns in different populations (e.g., adolescent and adult substance abuse) (6, 7), as well as to assess the impact of particular treatment cost reimbursement methods on patient outcome (5).

## SUMMARY OF STRENGTHS AND LIMITATIONS

There are several major strengths of BASIS-32. As a generic measure applicable to a wide range of people receiving mental health treatment, it is not limited to a particular diagnosis or symptom pattern. Second, all of the major symptom and problem domains that bring people to inpatient treatment are included. Third, staff and respondent burden are minimal because of the brevity and simplicity of the design.

There are limitations in BASIS-32. Generalizability of psychometric properties to more diverse populations is not yet known because of the lack of published studies from other settings. Three of the five subscales are relatively highly correlated with each other (0.58–0.66), suggesting limited discriminant validity of these subscales. Third, acutely psychotic, intoxicated, or demented patients may be unable to respond appropriately.

REFERENCES

1. Eisen SV, Dill DL, Grob MC. Reliability and validity of a brief patient-report instrument for psychiatric outcome evaluation. Hosp Community Psychiatry 1994;45:242–247.
2. Eisen SV, Grob MC, Dill DL. Outcome measurement: tapping the patient's perspective. In: Mirin SM, Gossett J, Grob MC, eds. Psychiatric treat-

ment: advances in outcome research. Washington, DC: American Psychiatric Press, 1991:213–235.

3. Eisen SV, Grob MC, Klein AA. BASIS: the development of a self-report measure for psychiatric inpatient evaluation. Psychiatr Hosp 1986;17:165–171.

4. Eisen SV. Assessment of subjective distress by patients' self-report versus structured interview. Psychol Rep 1995;76:35–39.

5. Sederer LI, Eisen SV, Dill DL, Grob MC, Gougeon M, Mirin SM. Case-based reimbursement for psychiatric hospital care. Hosp Community Psychiatry 1992;42:1120–1126.

6. Eisen SV, Youngman D, Grob MC, Dill DL. Alcohol, drugs and psychiatric disorders: a current view of hospitalized adolescents. J Adolesc Res 1992;7:250–265.

7. Eisen SV, Grob, MC, Dill DL. Substance abuse in an inpatient population. McLean Hosp J 1989; XIV:1–22.

# CHAPTER 10

# The Addiction Severity Index (ASI) and the Treatment Services Review (TSR)

*A. Thomas McLellan, John S. Cacciola, and Ian Fureman*

## INTRODUCTION

This chapter describes two instruments that have been used in the evaluation of substance abusing patients in both routine clinical care settings and, more often, in the course of performing outcome evaluation studies or quality assurance protocols. The instruments are designed as companion interviews, each with a related purpose. The Addiction Severity Index (ASI) is designed to evaluate the nature and severity of the problems presented by substance abusers at the start of their treatment and subsequently after discharge (1–5). The Treatment Services Review (TSR) was developed as a companion to the ASI to characterize the functions of a treatment program and is discussed in Part B of this chapter.

## Part A. The Addiction Severity Index (ASI)

### DESCRIPTION AND BACKGROUND

*Formal Name*
The Addiction Severity Index (ASI)

*Authors*
A. Thomas McLellan, Lester Luborsky, John Cacciola, and Ian Fureman.

*Key References*
McLellan AT, Cacciola J, Kushner H, Peters R, Smith I, Pettinati H. The fifth edition of the addiction severity index: cautions, additions and normative data. J Subst Abuse Treat 1992;9:461–480.

McLellan AT, Luborsky L, Cacciola J, Griffith J. New data from the addiction severity index: reliability and validity in three centers. J Nerv Ment Dis 1985;173:412–423.

McLellan AT, Luborsky L, O'Brien CP, Woody GE. An improved diagnostic instrument for substance abuse patients: the addiction severity index. J Nerv Ment Dis 1980;168:26–33.

## DOMAINS AND NUMBER OF ITEMS

The ASI provides information about aspects of a patient's life that may contribute to his or her substance abuse syndrome. The interview is based on the premise that addiction to drugs or alcohol is best considered in terms of the life events that preceded, co-occurred with, and/or resulted from the substance abuse problem. Thus, the ASI focuses on seven functional areas that have been widely shown to be affected among substance abusers: medical status, employment and support, drug use, alcohol use, legal status, family/social status, and psychiatric status.

Each of these areas is examined separately and individually by collecting parallel information regarding the frequency, duration, and severity of problem symptoms historically over the course of the patient's lifetime and more recently during the 30 days before the interview. Within each of the problem areas, the ASI provides both a 10-point, interviewer determined severity rating of lifetime problems and a multiitem composite score indicating the severity of the problems in the past 30 days.

The ASI contains 142 items that are divided into general demographics plus a common format for each of the seven problem areas.

## APPLICATION

### Target Population

The ASI is appropriate for all adult populations of alcohol, drug, multiple substance, and/or psychiatrically ill substance abusing individuals. Recent studies have shown that the ASI is not appropriate for use with very severe, chronic schizophrenics because the quality of their information is not found to be reliable or valid.

### Data Collection Procedures

The ASI is a semistructured interview and not a questionnaire. The development of rapport and trust is required to provide the most useful information. Therefore, the interview requires approximately 60–75 minutes to administer in a clinically sensitive manner. Follow-up interviews with the ASI are typically done at discharge and/or after treatment to measure change of status. These interviews require only a repeat of the past 30-day items, which takes only 15–20 minutes.

The ASI was designed for use by a research technician or a clinical caseworker or counselor. Although the ASI is available in a computerized format, it is designed as an interview and requires administration by a trained interviewer. Follow-up interviews with the ASI can be done over the telephone or in person; they cannot be mailed out for patient self-completion.

The ASI has been translated into 17 languages, including Japanese, French, Spanish, German, Dutch, and Russian. Administration manuals and most of the training aids are available in all of these languages.

### Psychometric Properties

The ASI has shown excellent test-retest and interrater reliability as tested by several investigators in this country and in three other languages. The instrument has also been shown to have predictive, concurrent, and discriminant validity across a range of patient types and treatment settings in this country. The key publications provide information on the reliability and validity testing. Normative data are available for a variety of subgroups, including males and females entering treatment for alcohol, opiate, and cocaine dependence; prison populations, homeless populations, pregnant substance abusers, and psychiatrically ill substance abusers (1).

## UTILITY

### Scoring Manual

Guidelines for each question on the ASI have been compiled in training materials, including two videos and three instructional manuals. Self-training can be accomplished using the video along with the administration manual, although a 1-day formal training seminar is recommended.

There are two types of "scores" on the ASI: the interviewer severity ratings and the problem composite scores. The severity ratings range from 0 (no problem) to 9 (extreme problem) and measure lifetime problems in each of the seven areas examined by the ASI. They are self-explanatory and easily derived. The composite scores are mathematically weighted combinations of items measuring the severity of each of these problems during the past 30 days. The composite scores range from 0 (no problem) to 1.0 (extreme problem) and can be compared from admission to follow-up to offer a sensitive indication of change in each of the seven areas. Scoring material is available from The Treatment Research Institute and provides directions on scoring.

### Automation

Two types of automation are available for the ASI. A free computer program is provided with the administration package that allows the user to set up a database for the ASI for subsequent use in developing clinical tracking and evaluation research protocols. This free software also scores the instrument.

The "Easy ASI" is a computer program developed by Christopher Henry and is not part of the standard information package provided by the ASI information service. The Easy ASI is designed for a laptop computer, enabling the interviewer to enter the ASI items (as well as comments) directly into computer storage (a relational database) as the interview is completed. The Easy ASI produces two reports from each interview. First, the clinical report is a narrative version of an admission note, describing the patient's condition in written text. Second, a director's report summarizes the demographic and background characteristics of a set of admissions.

**Permission to Use**

The ASI is in the public domain and there is no charge for its use. All materials for training and supporting the interview are available from ASI Information Service, c/o Treatment Research Institute, 2005 Market Street, Suite 1020, Philadelphia, PA 19103-7220. There is a small charge for reproducing, shipping, and handling the material. There is also an Information Support Service available to support users of the ASI. This toll-free telephone line offers general information on the use of the instrument and answers specific questions from 10:00 a.m. to 4:00 p.m. eastern time each weekday. The number is 1-800-238-2433. The Easy ASI software is not part of the ASI Information Service and is sold by Quickstart Computing, 11551 Forest Central Dr., Suite 134, Dallas, TX 72543, Telephone: 214-342-9020.

**Description of Where and When Used**

The ASI has been widely used in research and clinical practice.

**SUMMARY OF STRENGTHS AND LIMITATIONS**

The ASI is widely used clinically for assessing substance abuse patients at the time of treatment admission. Researchers have found the ASI useful because the composite scores and the individual variables can be compared within groups over time as a measure of improvement or between groups of patients at a posttreatment follow-up point as a measure of outcome from treatment.

There are two limitations to the ASI and both are linked to the nature of substance abuse: self-administration is not recommended for anyone and, for certain populations, especially those who are not seeking treatment. Even interview data are suspect.

In the search for faster and easier methods of collecting data, many clinicians and researchers have asked for a self-administered (either by computer or paper and pencil) version of the ASI. The use of a self-administered version has not been sanctioned for several reasons. First, we have tested the reliability and validity of the severity ratings by having raters use just the information that has been collected on the form—without the interview. This has resulted in very poor estimates of problem severity and essentially no concurrent reliability. Second, we have been sensitive to problems of illiteracy among segments of the substance abusing population. Even among the literate there are problems of attention, interest, and comprehension that are especially relevant to this population.

Disclosure about addictive behavior is likely to occur only in settings where help is sought and trust in the providers meets at least minimum standards. This means that the ASI is not appropriate for some subpopulations. The ASI is not suitable for adolescents because of its underlying assumptions regarding self- sufficiency and its failure to address issues (e.g., school, peer relations, family problems from the perspective of the adolescent) that are critical to an evaluation of adolescent problems. There is also reason to suspect denial, conclusion, or misrepresentation among those within criminal populations and those with chronic psychiatric disabilities.

# Part B. The Treatment Services Review (TSR)

---

*DESCRIPTION AND BACKGROUND*

*Formal Name*
The Treatment Services Review (TSR)

*Authors*
A. Thomas McLellan, Arthur I. Alterman, Lester Luborsky, and John Cacciola.

*Key References*
McLellan AT, Alterman AI, Woody GE, Metzger D. A quantitative measure of substance abuse treatments: the treatment services review. J Nerv Ment Dis 1992;180:100–109.

Alterman AI, McLellan AT, Shiffman RB. Do substance abuse patients with more psychopathology receive more treatment? J Nerv Ment Dis 1993;181: 576–582.

Alterman AI, McLellan AT. Inpatient and day hospital treatment services for cocaine and alcohol dependence. J Subst Abuse Treat 1993;10:269–275.

## DOMAINS AND NUMBER OF ITEMS

The TSR has 87 items that measure service provision to patients in the same seven problem areas that are measured in the ASI: medical status, employment and support, drug use, alcohol use, legal status, family and/or social status, and psychiatric status. The design premise of the TSR is that treatment programs can be effectively and usefully characterized in terms of the treatment services actually provided by the program in these problem areas. Each of these individual services and the problem composites are further categorized as coming either directly from the program (inprogram) or at another agency by referral (outprogram).

## APPLICATION
### Target Population

The TSR is appropriate for all populations of alcohol, drug, multiple substance, or psychiatrically ill substance abusing individuals who are receiving treatment or services from any program, agency, institution, or individual.

### Data Collection Procedures

The TSR is an interview that may be administered either in person or over the telephone and requires approximately 5–10 minutes to administer. The interview is typically repeated weekly or biweekly over the course of treatment to categorize the nature and number of services received.

The TSR was designed for use by a research technician or a clinical caseworker or counselor. Very little training is necessary for the interview, and guidelines for each question on the TSR have been compiled in training materials that include an instructional manual. Self-training can be accomplished with the administration manual and no formal training is recommended. Follow-up interviews with the TSR can be done over the telephone or in person; they cannot be mailed out for patient self-completion.

The TSR has been translated into nine languages, including French, Spanish, German, and Dutch.

### Psychometric Properties

The TSR has shown very good test-retest and interrater reliability and has also been shown to have predictive and concurrent validity across a range of patient types and treatment settings. Publications listed in the references provide information on the reliability and validity testing (6–11).

## UTILITY
### Scoring Manual

Scoring manuals are available in English and nine other languages. They are available through the Treatment Research Institute.

The TSR may be scored in two ways. Most users count the frequency of each of the individual treatment elements on a weekly basis, thus providing a face-valid measure of the pattern of services delivered. Summary measures of these individual elements have been constructed by simply adding the frequencies of each individual element within each problem area to obtain a composite score of the intensity of services provided. These scores can be further categorized as being delivered directly from the program (inprogram) or at another agency by referral (outprogram).

Scores for an individual patient are used clinically for tracking progress and for ensuring that the treatment plan is being followed. Average scores for randomly selected samples of patients within a treatment program are used to characterize the treatment program or the treatment intervention for research purposes.

### Automation

A free computer program is provided with the administration package that allows the user to set up a database for the TSR for subsequent use in developing clinical tracking and evaluation research protocols.

### Permission to Use

The TSR is in the public domain and there is no charge for its use. There are also no continuing charges or scoring fees. There is a minor charge for copies of the administration materials and the computer disk, although the instrument may be easily scored without a computer program. There is a small charge to cover the costs of reproducing and mailing these materials. There is also an Information Support Service available to support users of the TSR. This toll-free telephone line offers general information on the use of the instrument and answers to specific questions 10:00 a.m. through 4:00 p.m. eastern time each weekday. The number is 1-800-238-2433.

All materials for training and supporting the interview are available from ASI

Information Service, c/o Treatment Research Institute, 2005 Market Street (Suite 1020), Philadelphia, PA 19103-7220.

### Description of Where and When Used

The TSR is widely used for assessing "quality-assurance" protocols of substance abuse treatment. Samples of patients are interviewed weekly to determine whether the nature and amount of services and treatments provided corresponds to the original treatment plan. The TSR has also been used by treatment outcome researchers and those performing clinical trials with different treatment interventions to ensure that the interventions under study have been applied in the manner intended, that is, to ensure the "fidelity" of the interventions (6–10). Finally, the TSR has been used by researchers who are interested in the costs and cost effectiveness of treatments.

### SUMMARY OF STRENGTHS AND LIMITATIONS

One of the strengths of the TSR is the broad scope of information provided about services received. We have chosen to evaluate services related to such areas as employment, family relations, and legal status for two reasons. First, many programs do provide (or at least offer) several of these services, and this trend is likely to continue over the coming years. Second, problems in these areas are often a major reason for relapse to substance abuse after treatment.

In an attempt to measure the nature and amount of treatment services, it was necessary to choose between competing perspectives. Qualities such as program philosophy, organizational structure, level of funding or support, and administrative competence of those in charge are obviously important contributors to the overall efficacy of treatments but are not measured by the TSR.

Although the TSR measures the quantity and frequency of services provided, there is no attempt to measure the quality of these services. This is obviously a significant limitation and it will be important in the future to develop methods to assess the quality of services provided during treatment. It is also reasonable to question the patient-focused orientation of the interview. It would have been possible to interview program staff and to record the types of services available within the program. Although the results to date have been encouraging, expanded evaluation is needed under a wider range of patient samples and treatment programs.

## REFERENCES

1. McLellan AT, Cacciola J, Kushner H, Peters R, Smith I, Pettinati H. The fifth edition of the addiction severity index: cautions, additions and normative data. J Subst Abuse Treat 1992;9: 461–480.

2. McLellan AT, Luborsky L, Cacciola J, Griffith J. New data from the addiction severity index: reliability and validity in three centers. J Nerv Ment Dis 1985;173:412–423.

3. McLellan AT, Luborsky L, O'Brien CP, Woody GE. An improved diagnostic instrument for substance abuse patients: the addiction severity index. J Nerv Ment Dis 1980;168:26–33.

4. McLellan AT, Luborsky L, Woody GE, Druley KA, O'Brien CP. Predicting response to alcohol and drug abuse treatments: role of psychiatric severity. Arch Gen Psychiatry 1983;40:620–625.

5. McLellan AT, Luborsky L, Woody GE, O'Brien CP, Druley KA. Increased effectiveness of substance abuse treatment: a prospective study of patient-treatment "matching." J Nerv Ment Dis 1983;171:597–605.

6. McLellan AT, Alterman AI, Woody GE, Metzger D. A quantitative measure of substance abuse treatments: the treatment services review. J Nerv Ment Dis 1992;180:100–109.

7. Alterman AI, McLellan AT, Shiffman RB. Do substance abuse patients with more psychopathology receive more treatment? J Nerv Ment Dis 1993;181:576–582.

8. Alterman AI, McLellan AT. Inpatient and day hospital treatment services for cocaine and alcohol dependence. J Subst Abuse Treat 1993;10: 269–275.

9. McLellan AT, Grissom G, Durell J, Alterman AI, Brill P, O'Brien CP. Substance abuse treatment in the private setting: are some programs more effective than others? J Subst Abuse Treat 1993;10:243–254.

10. McLellan AT, Alterman AI, Metzger DS, et al. Similarity of outcome predictors across opiate, cocaine and alcohol treatments: role of treatment services. J Consult Clin Psychol 1994;62:1–18.

11. McLellan AT, Arndt IO, Woody GE, Metzger D. Psychosocial services in substance abuse treatment? A dose-ranging study of psychosocial services. JAMA 1993;269:1953–1959.

CHAPTER 11

# Global Assessment of Functioning (GAF) Scale

*Robert L. Spitzer, Miriam Gibbon,*
*Janet B. W. Williams, Jean Endicott*

*DESCRIPTION AND BACKGROUND*

*Formal Name*
Global Assessment of Functioning
(GAF) Scale

*Authors*
Robert L. Spitzer, M.D., Miriam Gibbon, M.S.W., Janet B. W. Williams, D.S.W., and Jean Endicott, Ph.D.

*Key References*
American Psychiatric Association. Diagnostic and statistical manual of mental disorders. 4th ed. Washington, DC: American Psychiatric Association, 1994.

Jones SH, Thornicroft G, Coffey M, et al. A brief mental health outcome scale: reliability and validity. Br J Psychol 1995;166:654–659.

## INTRODUCTION

The history of the GAF Scale begins with the 1962 publication by Luborsky (1) of the Health Sickness Rating Scale, the first attempt to evaluate psychological health/sickness on a single 100-point scale. Modifications were made in the descriptions of the 10 levels, including elimination of diagnostic concepts as anchor points (e.g., severe neuroses). This resulted in the development of a new instrument with behavioral descriptions for each decile called the Global Assessment Scale (GAS) (2). In 1987 the GAS was modified to include examples taken from an earlier version for

use with children, the C-GAS (3). In the new version, the highest level, 91–100, was eliminated and some minor changes in wording were made. A new scale, called the Global Assessment of Functioning (GAF) Scale, was created, which became Axis V for DSM-III-R (4). In DSM-IV (5), the 91–100 decile was reinstated.

### DOMAIN AND NUMBER OF ITEMS

The GAF Scale, Axis V of DSM-IV, is a 100-point single-item rating scale for evaluating overall psychosocial functioning (psychological symptoms and occupational and social functioning) during a specified time period on a continuum from psychological sickness to health. There is a specific instruction to exclude impairment due to physical or environmental limitations.

The GAF scale values range from 1 to 100, representing the hypothetically sickest person to the hypothetically healthiest. The scale is divided into 10 equal 10-point intervals; the defining characteristics of each interval comprise the scale. The two highest intervals, 81–90 and 91–100, measure those individuals who are not only without psychopathology but who also exhibit superior functioning, a wide range of interests, social effectiveness, warmth, and integrity. The next interval, 71–80, rates individuals with minimal or no psychopathology who do not demonstrate many of the positive mental health features noted above. Although some individuals who are rated above 70 may occasionally seek treatment, the vast majority of those patients in treatment for emotional disturbance will be rated between 1 and 70. Most outpatients will be rated in the range of 31–70, and most inpatients are rated between 1 and 40. At the lowest level, 1–10, treatment is urgently needed because of the immediate danger of possible suicide, harm to others, or an inability to maintain minimal personal hygiene.

Ordinarily, the time period for the GAF rating is "current," often operationalized as the lowest level of functioning during the week before the evaluation. Other intervals may be used, such as the time of best or worst functioning during the previous year.

## APPLICATION

### Target Population

The GAF is used to assess psychiatric patients at the time of admission to an inpatient or outpatient mental health facility, as a part of a DSM-IV multiaxial assessment.

### Data Collection Procedures

The information needed to make a rating may come from a single source or multiple sources: direct, structured, or unstructured interview of a patient; interview with an informant; or a case record. Completion of a GAF, after obtaining the necessary information, takes only a few minutes at most. The GAF can be used by clinical psychologists, psychiatrists, and other mental health professionals at the time of admission, discharge, or other time points of interest. The GAF is available in all of the languages into which the DSM-IV has been translated.

### Psychometric Information

In the original article describing the GAS, the reliability of the scale (intraclass correlation coefficient) ranged from 0.61 in a sample of nonpatients without a history of treated psychiatric disorder to 0.91 in a series of joint interviews of patients attending an aftercare clinic. Subsequent reliability studies by other investigators have yielded results in the same range. The reliability of the GAF evaluated during a test-retest study of the structured clinical interview for DSM-III-R in samples of patients and nonpatients ranged from 0.62 to 0.82

## UTILITY

### Scoring Manual

No scoring manual is available, but directions for using the scale and interpreting the scores are included in DSM-IV, Axis V.

### Automation

No automated version of the scale is available from the authors.

### Permission to Use

Permission for use is assumed as part of the multiaxial evaluation system in the DSM-IV classification.

## DESCRIPTION OF WHERE AND WHEN USED

The GAS and the GAF have been used in several hundred research studies to describe patient and nonpatient samples and to measure change in functioning over time, as in treatment outcome studies. It is recommended that clinicians using the GAF should compare their evaluations on a series of subjects with other clinicians in their facility to maximize consistent use of the scale.

## SUMMARY OF STRENGTHS AND LIMITATIONS

The GAF is widely used in clinical practice and in several hundred research studies. The scale's popularity is due to its use as a global measure of a key clinical concept (overall psychosocial health/sickness) and its adaptability to any standard evaluation in a mental health facility or study.

One limitation of the scale results from combining the level of role functioning and severity of psychopathologic symptoms that, in some cases, may result in low scores for high functioning patients who present with a single, severe symptom.

## REFERENCES

1. Luborsky L. Clinicians' judgements of mental health. Arch Gen Psychiatry 1962;7:407–417.
2. Endicott J, Spitzer RL, Fleiss JL, Cohen J. The global assesment scale: a procedure for measuring overall severity of psychiatric disturbance. Arch Gen Psychiatry 1976;33:766–771.
3. Shaffer D, Gould MS, Brasie J, et al. A children's global assessment scale (C-GAS). Arch Gen Psychiatry 1983;40:1228–1231.
4. American Psychiatric Association. Diagnostic and statistical manual of mental disorders. 3rd ed. Washington, DC: American Psychiatric Association, 1987.
5. American Psychiatric Association. Diagnostic and statistical manual of mental disorders. 4th ed. Washington, DC: American Psychiatric Association, 1994.

CHAPTER 12

# Life Skills Profile (LSP)

*Gordon Parker, Dusan Hadzi-Pavlovic, and Alan Rosen*

*DESCRIPTION AND BACKGROUND*

*Formal Name*
Life Skills Profile (LSP)

*Authors*
Gordon Parker, M.D., Ph.D., F.R.A.N.Z.C.P., Dusan Hadzi-Pavlovic, M. Psychol., and Alan Rosen, M.R.C. Psych., F.R.A.N.Z.C.P.

*Key References*

Rosen A, Hadzi-Pavlovic D, Parker G. The life skills profile: a measure assessing function and disability in schizophrenia. Schizophr Bull 1989; 15:325–337.

Parker G, Rosen A, Emdur N, Hadzi-Pavlovic D. The life skills profile: psychometric properties of a measure assessing function and disability in schizophrenia. Acta Psychiatr Scand 1991;83:145–152.

Parker G, Hadzi-Pavlovic D. The capacity of a measure of disability (the LSP) to predict hospital readmission in those with schizophrenia. Psychol Med 1995;25:157–163.

## INTRODUCTION

The Life Skills Profile (LSP) was developed to measure function and disability in adults with schizophrenia. Until recently, research has been relatively preoccupied with comparative evaluations of symptomatic treatments, but recent advances in vocational rehabilitation, family management, and social skills training suggest there is a need to chart accurately the general functioning of those with schizophrenia over time.

## DOMAINS AND NUMBER OF ITEMS

There are 39 items and five subscales that assess the general domain of disability in schizophrenia. The five subscales measure self-care, nonturbulence, social contact, communication, and responsibility.

## APPLICATION

### Target Population

The LSP is designed for those with schizophrenia of any type and at any phase of the disorder. The LSP can be used to assess social disability in a number of other chronic or relapsing mental illnesses.

### Data Collection Procedures

The scale takes about 5 minutes to complete by a respondent who knows the subject well or up to 20 minutes if the rater is required to interview the patient or a knowledgeable informant. The measure is not designed to be completed as a self-report. The item stems are jargon free and based on observed behaviors to allow the LSP to be completed by anyone who knows the subject well. Family members appear to rate subjects under the influence of a "burden of care" bias.

Although computerized versions have been developed to allow subscale and total scores to be calculated readily, rating and scoring of the paper-and-pencil version can be completed rapidly.

Permission has been given to German, French, Spanish, and Japanese researchers to translate the LSP. No formal examination of the LSP's properties has occurred in nonwestern cultures. The design of the LSP, with focus on constructs relevant to survival, function, and adaptation for those with schizophrenia, suggests that the items should not be culture specific. However, cultural factors presumably would influence community responses to manifest disability.

### Psychometric Properties

During the initial development of the scale, we (1) reported adequate variance in scores, with the means for each scale close to the respective medians; no sex differences in derived scores; the relative independence of the five scales; and good internal consistency (Cronbach's α) of 0.79. Test-retest reliability, with a retest interval of 4 weeks, with parents, residential care workers, and caseworkers as raters generated a mean intraclass correlation coefficient of 0.89. In a second study (2) of interrater reliability, pairs of parents, caseworkers, and residential care workers were compared. Parents had the lowest level of agreement. Inclusion of several impact measures in the study established that the parents reporting more burden completed the LSP with a subjective bias, scoring their relative as more disabled. This finding does not suggest that parents are "inaccurate" raters but that their scores may reflect more emotional involvement in making ratings.

An additional concurrent validity study examined scores on the LSP measure against those generated on the Katz Adjustment Scale (KAS). Total scores were. linked (r = 0.65) with total KAS and were most strongly associated with LSP nonturbulence (r = 0.61) and low self-care (r = 0.47) scores.

Sensitivity to change has been demonstrated (3) in a sample of 64 patients from the community with chronic mental illness who were assigned for management by an assertive community mental health service. Over the first 6 months, significant improvements were observed on all LSP subscales and in total LSP scores.

Predictive validity has been demonstrated in a study of 118 subjects followed-up after discharge (4). Those readmitted had baseline LSP scores indicating significantly greater disability, with discriminant function analyses indicating that the total LSP score predicted 60% of the readmissions and 75% of those not readmitted.

### UTILITY

### Scoring Manual

No scoring manual is provided, but scoring instructions are included in the article in *Schizophrenia Bulletin* (1). Items are scored on a scale of 1–4, and the total LSP (and the subscales) are summed item scores. Subscales are labeled in the direction of least disability to emphasize "functional" levels. Greater disability is indicated by lower LSP scores. None of the ratings involves clinical interpretation on the part of the rater, which increases score interpretability. Instead, the items are based on observed behaviors. For example, the following items are included: Does this person generally have problems (e.g., friction, avoidance) living with others in the household? Does this person generally neglect his or his health.

### Automation

Computer versions have been produced (e.g., New South Wales Department of Health) that have the advantage of storing and computing scores electronically. The authors do not, however, provide computerized software for the LSP.

### Permission to Use

The measure is copyrighted by the authors Parker and Rosen, so that permission to use should be sought from them. Forms are available from Professor Parker ($1 per form, $0.50 for photocopied forms; costs are waived in certain circumstances).

Correspondence should be addressed to Gordon Parker, M.D., F.R.A.N.Z.C.P., Professor and Head, School of Psychiatry, The University of South Wales, The Prince of Wales Hospital, High Street, Randwick, NSW 2031 Australia, Telephone: (02) 399-4372, FAX: (02) 398-7783.

### Description of Where and When Used

Published studies have mostly involved patients with schizophrenia. Studies underway include broader diagnostic groups of those with long-term severe mental illness. Although we anticipate the measure will have utility in such groups, that expectation will require testing to ensure that its psychometric properties are not compromised.

### SUMMARY OF STRENGTHS AND LIMITATIONS

The strategy of restricting LSP items to distinct behaviors rather than general domains has improved its psychometric properties and broadened the scope of respondents who could complete the scale. A related strength of the instrument is the clear wording of the items in behavioral language that avoids value judgments on the part of the rater.

The measure has strong psychometric properties, requires only a brief period for completion, and provides useful information on social impairment in those with schizophrenia.

One limitation of the scale is that the psychometric properties of the LSP when used with those with severe mental illness other than schizophrenia have not yet been established.

REFERENCES

1. Rosen A, Hadzi-Pavlovic D, Parker G. The life skills profile: a measure assessing function and disability in schizophrenia. Schizophr Bull 1989; 15:325–337.
2. Parker G, Rosen A, Emdur N, Hadzi-Pavlovic D. The life skills profile: psychometric properties of a measure assessing funding and disability in schizophrenia. Acta Psychiatr Scand 1991;83: 145–152.
3. Hambridge JA, Rosen A. Assertive community treatment for the seriously mentally ill in suburban Sydney: a programme description and evaluation. Aust N Z J Psychiatry 1994;28:438–445.
4. Parker G, Hadzi-Pavlovic D. The capacity of a measure of disability (the LSP) to predict hospital readmission in those with schizophrenia. Psychol Med 1995;25:157–163.

# CHAPTER 13

# Psychiatric Outcomes Module: Depression (DOM)

*G. Richard Smith, Jr., Robin L. Ross, and Kathryn M. Rost*

## DESCRIPTION AND BACKGROUND

*Formal Name*

The Depression Outcomes Module (DOM)

*Authors*

G. Richard Smith, Jr., M.D., M. Audrey Burnam, Ph.D., Barbara J. Burns, Ph.D., Paul Cleary, Ph.D., and Kathryn M. Rost, Ph.D.

*Key References*

Smith GR, Burnam MA, Burns BJ, et al. The depression outcomes module. University of Arkansas for Medical Sciences, Little Rock: Centers for Mental Healthcare Research, 1995.

Rost K, Smith GR, Burnam MA, Burns BJ. Measuring the outcomes of care for mental health problems: the case of depressive disorders. Med Care 1992;30:MS266–MS273.

## INTRODUCTION

This scale was developed using a multi-institutional, multidisciplinary panel to advise the scale developers on relevant clinical and methodological issues surrounding the treatment and outcomes of depression. The scale incorporates items or scales from previously developed measurement work or new items (1) when no appropriate items existed.

## DOMAINS AND NUMBER OF ITEMS

The DOM measures the types of care received for major depression, the outcomes of that care, and the patient characteristics that influence outcome and type of care. Four different forms comprise the module: the Patient Baseline Assessment, the Clinician Baseline Assessment, the Patient Follow-up Assessment, and the Medical Record Review Form.

The depression module measures outcome by monitoring changes in symptoms of depression and general functioning over time. Severity of depressive symptoms in the last 2 weeks are measured. Prognostic variables predicting outcome, also known as case-mix variables, are included as a separate component in the depression module to allow for more confident interpretation of the relationships between treatment and outcomes.

The fourth component of the depression module measures types of treatments (i.e., pharmacotherapy, individual therapy, group therapy, electroconvulsive therapy), the intensity (i.e., dose, frequency, duration, number of session), and setting (i.e., primary care, specialty care, emergency room, day treatment, hospital). This component also includes questions about treatment received outside the system as reported by patients.

The Patient Baseline Assessment consists of 80 items and includes verification of diagnostic criteria, measures of outcome, and measures of prognostic variables. The DOM is administered to those individuals who either have screened positive on the patient screener or have received an initial clinical diagnosis. It measures diagnosis at baseline using the DSM-IV criteria, general functioning status using the SF-36 items (2), initial levels of depression symptom severity, number of bed days, sociodemographic characteristics, and psychiatric history.

The Clinician Baseline Assessment consists of 20 items and assesses diagnosis at baseline using the DSM-IV criteria, including exclusion criteria, prognostic characteristics, and treatment information on psychotropic medication prescribed at the initial visit.

The Patient Follow-up Assessment consists of 83 items, is completed every 4 months after baseline until the depressive diagnosis is resolved, and provides information on treatment the patient has received since baseline.

The Medical Record Review consists of 11 items and is completed every 4 months after baseline by a trained clerical worker until the depressive diagnosis is resolved.

## APPLICATION

### Target Population

This measure is intended for adults treated for depression.

### Data Collection Procedures

The Patient Baseline Assessment and the Patient Follow-up Assessment each require 25 minutes to complete. The clinician is asked to provide information at baseline only with the Clinician Baseline Assessment, which requires 5 minutes to complete. When the Medical Record Review is included in the outcome management system, 10 minutes are required if the review is completed by hand or less time if the medical record is computerized.

All segments of the Depression Outcomes Module are self-administered, except for the Medical Records Review. If conditions necessitate, sections of the module can be mailed out or administered over the telephone.

The DOM has not been tested in culturally diverse populations and is available in English only.

### Psychometric Properties

The diagnostic component of the DOM has been designed to provide the highest possible sensitivity and specificity when compared to Depression Section of the Structured Clinical Interview for DSM-III-R (SCID) (3). Early versions of the module achieved a 100% sensitivity with a specificity of 77.8% at baseline assessment in a specialty care population.

In specialty care patients, test-retest reliability for severity of depression symptoms measured 1 week apart had a correlation coefficient of $r = 0.87$ ($P < 0.0001$). The two-item measure of suicidality was somewhat less reliable at retest ($r = 0.56$). Internal consistency for the depression severity scale was high (alpha coefficient of 0.87). Two research assistants achieved 100% concordance for interrater reliability on the Medical Record Review.

Depression severity correlated with clinician ratings of depression using the Hamilton-D ($r = 0.41$, $P < 0.01$), the number of depression symptoms on the SCID ($r = 0.60$, $P < 0.01$), and the number of depression symptoms on the Diagnostic Interview Schedule (DIS) interview ($r = 0.56$, $P < 0.01$). Changes in depression symptoms correlated strongly with three general measures of health: change in bed days ($r = 0.56$, $P < 0.005$), change in social functioning ($r = -0.52$, $P < 0.01$), and change in emotional functioning ($r = -0.47$, $P < 0.01$). One study comparing patients with and without pharmacotherapy treatment demonstrated a tendency for greater improvement in patients receiving pharmacotherapy (4).

### UTILITY

### Scoring Manual

The DOM user's manual includes scoring algorithms for the major diagnostic, case-mix, and outcome variables. Scoring information is not provided for the Medical Record Review because most sites will use these variables without extensive recoding. Score interpretation is straightforward.

## Automation

Velocity Healthcare Informatics has developed a computerized version to facilitate analysis (DM Wesley, personal communication with David M. Wesley, President/CEO, Velocity Healthcare Informatics, Minnetonka, MN, 1994).

## Permission to Use

The DOM is protected under copyright and is available for unlimited free use provided that no charge is made for its use. Contact G. Richard Smith, Jr., M.D., Centers for Mental Healthcare Research, Department of Psychiatry, University of Arkansas for Medical Sciences, 4301 W. Markham, Little Rock, AR 72205.

## Description of Where and When Used

The DOM can be used in the specialty mental health setting as well as in the primary care setting. Because studies have shown that general medical providers probably detect less than 50% of those patients thought to have clinically significant depression (5, 6), the authors of the module developed a simple case-finding strategy. In a primary care setting, all patients periodically complete a three-item screener. Patients who screen positive for a likely depressive disorder are then asked by their provider to complete the DOM. Research studies in the specialty care and the general medical settings have used the DOM to measure changes in severity of symptoms between patients who receive pharmacological intervention concordant with treatment guidelines (7, 8) and patients who do not (1, 4).

## SUMMARY OF STRENGTHS AND LIMITATIONS

The DOM can identify a homogeneous group of patients, particularly in specialty care settings. The module measures key constructs with sufficient reliability and validity to discern clinical improvement in groups of patients based on differences in treatment. These strengths will allow clinicians to use outcomes data to optimize treatment and will help patients to make informed decisions about how to alleviate their symptoms and improve their functioning. Administrators and payers will be able to better identify and provide the most effective forms of care for improving the health status of the consumer.

One limitation is that the DOM is in its early stage of development. Data are not yet available on special populations, on the relative burden the instrument might have when used in clinical (not research) populations, and on national (age and sex adjusted) norms. Further study is also needed to increase the reliability of the measure of suicidality.

REFERENCES

1. Rost K, Smith GR, Burnam MA, Burns BJ. Measuring the outcomes of care for mental health problems: the case of depressive disorders. Med Care 1992;30:MS266–MS273.
2. Ware JE Jr, Snow KK, Kosinski M, Gandek B. SF-36 health survey manual and interpretation guide. Boston: The Health Institute, New England Medical Center, 1993.
3. Spitzer RL, Williams JBW. User's guide for the structured clinical interview for DSM-III-R. Washington, DC: American Psychiatric Press, 1990.
4. Rost K, Wherry J, Williams C, Smith GR Jr. The process and outcomes of care for major depression in rural family practice settings. J Rural Health (in press).
5. Perez-Stable EJ, Miranda J, Munoz RF, Ying Y. Depression in medical outpatients: underrecognition and misdiagnosis. Arch Intern Med 1990;150:1083–1088.
6. Schulberg HC, Saul M, McClelland M, Ganguli M, Christy W, Frank R. Assessing depression in primary medical and psychiatric practices. Arch Gen Psychiatry 1985;42:1164–1170.
7. Depression Guideline Panel. Depression in primary care: vol 1. detection and diagnosis. Clinical Practice Guideline No. 5. Washington, DC: U.S. Department of Health and Human Services, Public Health Service, 1993. [AHCPR Publ. No. 93-0550.]
8. Depression Guideline Panel. Depression in primary care: vol 2. treatment of major depression. Clinical Practice Guideline No. 5. Rockville, MD: U.S. Department of Health and Human Services, 1993. [AHCPR Publ. No. 93-0551.]

# CHAPTER 14

# Psychiatric Outcomes Module: Substance Abuse Outcomes Module (SAOM)

*G. Richard Smith, Jr., Robin L. Ross, and Kathryn M. Rost*

## DESCRIPTION AND BACKGROUND

*Formal Name*

The Substance Abuse Outcomes Module (SAOM)

*Authors*

G. Richard Smith, Jr., M.D., Thomas Babor, Ph.D., Audrey Burnam, Ph.D., Kathryn M. Rost, Ph.D, Robert Drake, M.D., and Kim Heithoff, Sc.D.

*Key Reference*

Smith GR, Babor T, Burnam A, Rost KM, Drake R, Heithoff K. The substance abuse outcomes module. Little Rock: Centers for Mental Healthcare Research, University of Arkansas for Medical Sciences, 1995.

## INTRODUCTION

The SAOM was developed using a multi-institutional, multidisciplinary panel to advise the module developers on relevant clinical and methodological issues surrounding the treatment and outcomes of substance abuse. It is a hybrid of outcomes modules, one on alcohol abuse and one on drug abuse previously developed by the authors. The new scale combines the most psychometrically sound and clinically relevant measures and scales from both of these modules.

## DOMAINS AND NUMBER OF ITEMS

The SAOM measures the types and amount of care received for substance abuse, the outcomes of the care received, and the prognostic characteristics that influence outcome, including readiness to change. The module assesses diagnostic criteria to identify a diagnostically homogeneous group of patients and measures whether the subject meets diagnostic criteria for substance abuse or dependence by his or her own report.

Outcome is measured by monitoring the change in consumption, symptoms of dependence, and general functioning change over time. General functioning is measured by the SF-36 (1) (also known as the Health Status Questionnaire and as the RAND-36 [2]). Scales assess physical functioning, physical and emotional role functioning, bodily pain, general health, vitality, social functioning, mental health, and health transitions. The module supplements the SF-36 by measuring particular aspects of functioning relevant to substance abuse. Prognostic variables that predict treatment seeking, choice of treatment modality, and outcomes of care are included in the substance abuse module to allow for more confident interpretation of the relationships between treatment and outcomes. The fourth component of the SAOM measures the following treatment components: type (pharmacotherapy, individual therapy, group therapy, 12-step programing), extent (dose, frequency, duration, number of sessions), and setting (specialty care and primary care, inpatient, outpatient, residential, aftercare, emergency room). The module is designed to measure both treatment provided by the system as recorded in medical records and treatment received outside the system as reported by patients.

The module's structure is similar to the Depression Outcomes Module, with baseline and follow-up components available. The Patient Baseline Assessment consists of 97 items (including items in the SF-36) and is administered after the initial diagnosis or the start of a new episode of substance abuse treatment. It measures diagnosis at baseline using the DSM-IV criteria, general functioning using the SF-36, initial levels of symptom severity, bed days, days lost from work due to substance abuse, readiness to change, consequences of substance abuse, and prognostic factors. The prognostic characteristics measured by the baseline assessment are severity of dependence, including age of onset (3–6), previous treatment history (7–9), parental substance abuse (5, 10), social support (11, 12), support for sobriety (13, 14), and co-occurring psychiatric conditions (10, 15–17).

The Patient Follow-up Assessment, consisting of 75 items, is completed every 4–6 months after baseline for a minimum of 18 months. The Follow-up Assessment also provides information on the treatment that the patient has received since baseline, as well as the patient's general functioning, symptom severity, bed days, and days lost at work.

The Medical Record Review, consisting of six items, is completed at 4–6 months after the Patient Baseline Assessment by a trained clerical worker. This information characterizes the treatment the patient received in the preceding months from the major provider of care or treatment covered by a third-party payer. The only outcomes measure on this assessment is mortality, including cause of death.

## APPLICATION

### Target Population

The target population is adult substance abusers in public and private specialty care networks. Patients with cognitive deficits or literacy problems can be surveyed in face-to-face interviews.

### Data Collection Procedures

The Patient Baseline Assessment and the Patient Follow-up Assessment each require 30 minutes to complete. The respondent burden involves only the time it takes for the patient to complete the questionnaires. When the Medical Record Review is included in the outcome management system, 10 minutes are required if the review is completed by hand or less time if the medical record is computerized. The Baseline and Follow-up Assessment are designed to be completed by patients who have not been drinking or using drugs on the day of administration.

All segments of the SAOM are self-administered, except for the Medical Records Review. If conditions necessitate, sections of the module can be mailed out or administered over the telephone.

The module is available in English only and has not been tested in culturally diverse populations.

### Psychometric Properties

The diagnostic component of the SAOM is consistent with the DSM-IV criteria has good test-retest reliability (intraclass correlation coefficient [ICC] = 0.70) and good agreement with the Composite International Diagnostic Interview-Substance Abuse Module (18) ($\kappa$ = 0.95).

The 20-item Consequences of Drug and Alcohol Use scale is a modified version of the DrinC (WR Miller, JS Tonigan, R Longabaugh, unpublished data, 1994). It assesses physical, social, intrapersonal, impulse, and interpersonal consequences of both drug and alcohol use. Similar to the psychometric properties reported from Project MATCH data (19), the five subscales of the 20-item modified version continued to demonstrate adequate test-retest reliability (ICCs ranging from 0.75 to 0.87) and internal consistency (coefficient $\alpha$ range from 0.72 to 0.94).

The measure of alcohol consumption

(quantity $\times$ frequency of drinking in past month) incorporated into the module showed excellent test-retest reliability (ICC = 0.87) and concurrent validity using consumption estimates made using the Timeline Followback Assessment (20) (Pearson r = 0.74). The quantity of drug use other than alcohol is not assessed because previous efforts have demonstrated that patient self-report is neither reliable nor valid (21).

The four-item Severity of Illness Scale, which assesses physical and social problems that have resulted from drug and alcohol use in the past 3 months, has good test-retest reliability (ICC = 0.73) and internal consistency (Cronbach's $\alpha$ = 0.72) and correlates highly with number of dependent symptoms (Pearson r = 0.83). Similarly, the five-item Social Support Scale demonstrates adequate test-retest and internal consistency (ICC = 0.67 and coefficient $\alpha$ = 0.87, respectively). Finally, although the SAOM attempts to measure support for sobriety as a prognostic indicator, the internal consistency of the items was found to be poor ($\alpha$ = 0.43) with marginal test-retest reliability (ICC = 0.67).

## UTILITY

### Scoring Manual

The SAOM user's manual includes scoring algorithms for the major diagnostic, case-mix, and outcome variables. Scoring information is not provided for the Medical Record Review because most sites will use these variables without extensive recoding. Score interpretation is straightforward.

### Automation

The SAOM is not available on an interactive computer program.

### Permission to Use

The SAOM is protected under copyright and is available for unlimited free use provided that no charge is made for its use. Additional information about the scales is available from the authors by telephone (501-686-5600) or FAX (501-686-8154).

### Description of Where and When Used

The module is being pilot tested for use by a national corporation as part of a study of their employee assistance program referral patterns.

## SUMMARY OF STRENGTHS AND LIMITATIONS

A strength of the module is the use of subscales from Project MATCH for assessing motivation for treatment, readiness for change, and consequences of drug and alcohol abuse. A national database is provided for the comparison of results. The module also measures key constructs with good reliability and validity that allows users to discern clinical improvement in groups of patients based on differences in treatment.

One limitation of the module results from the authors not yet completed studies to allow for testing the validity of consumption and treatment self-reports in subjects with psychiatric comorbidities. However, as the items have been drawn from scales with robust psychometric properties, we anticipate similar results.

Although the current literature has identified case-mix variables that are important predictors of outcomes, further research will delineate whether these variables should be differentially weighted. This process could greatly influence the utility of outcomes monitoring. Another limitation of the module is that two subscales (support for sobriety and social support network) were derived according to the face validity of the items and therefore do not have a proven standard for comparison.

REFERENCES

1. Ware JE Jr, Snow KK, Kosinski M, Gandek B. SF-36 health survey manual and interpretation guide. Boston: The Health Institute, New England Medical Center, 1993.
2. Rand 36-item health survey 1.0, RAND Health Sciences Program. Santa Monica: The RAND Corporation, 1992.
3. Butynski W, Canova D. An analysis of state alcohol and drug abuse: profile data. Washington, DC: National Association of State Alcohol and Drug Abuse Directors, 1988.

4. Stein JA, Newcomb MD, Bentler PM. Structure of drug use behaviors and consequences among young adults: multi-trait–multi-method assessment of frequency, quantity, work site, and problem substance use. J Appl Psychol 1988;74: 595–605.

5. Correa EL, Sutker PB. Assessment of alcohol and drug behavior. In: Ciminero AR, Calhoun KS, Adams HE, eds. Handbook of behavior assessment. New York: John Wiley and Sons, 1986:446–495.

6. Pavkov TW, McGovern MP, Geffner ES. Problem severity and symptomatology among substance misusers: differences between African-Americans and caucasians. Int J Addict 1993; 28:909–922.

7. Condelli WS, Hubbard RL. Relationship between time spent in treatment and client outcomes from therapeutic communities. J Subst Abuse Treat 1994;11:25–33.

8. Hawkins JD, Catalano RF Jr. Aftercare in drug abuse treatment. Int J Addict 1985;20:917–945.

9. French MT, Zarkin GA, Hubbard RL, Rachal JV. The impact of time in treatment on the employment and earnings of drug abusers. Am J Public Health 1991;81:904–907.

10. McLellan AT, Kushner H, Metzger D, et al. The fifth edition of the addiction severity index. J Subst Abuse Treat 1992;9:199–213.

11. Booth BM, Russell DW, Yates WR, Laughlin PR, Brown K, Reed D. Social support and depression during alcoholism treatment. J Subst Abuse Treat 1992;4:57–57.

12. Gordon AJ, Zrull M. Social networks and recovery: one year after inpatient treatment. J Subst Abuse Treat 1991;8:143–152.

13. Olson DH, Tiesel JW. Assessment of family functioning. In: Rounsaville BJ, Tims FM, Horton AM Jr, Snowder BJ, eds. Diagnostic source book on drug abuse research and treatment. Rockville, MD: U.S. Department of Health and Human Services, 1993:59–78.

14. Orvaschel H. Social functioning and social supports: a review of measure suitable for use with substance abusers. In: Rounsaville BJ, Tims FM, Horton AM Jr, Sowder BJ. eds. Diagnostic source book on drug abuse research and treatment. Rockville, MD: U.S. Department of Health and Human Services, 1993: 79–92.

15. Kosten TR, Rounsaville BJ, Kleber HD. 2.5 year follow-up of depression, life crisis, and treatment effects of abstinence among opioid addicts. Arch Gen Psychiatry 1986;43:733–738.

16. Hesselbrock MN, Hesselbrock VM, Babor TF, Stabenau JR, Meyer RE, Weidenman M. Antisocial behavior, psychopathology and problem drinking in the natural history of alcoholism. In: Goodwin DW, Van Dusen KT, Mednick SA, eds. Longitudinal research in alcoholism. Boston: Kluwer-Nijhoff Publishing, 1983:197.

17. Rounsaville BJ, Dolinsky ZS, Babor TF, Meyer RE. Psychopathology as a predictor of treatment outcomes in alcoholics. Arch Gen Psychiatry 1987;44:505–513.

18. Cottler LB, Robins, LN, Helzer JE. The reliability of the CIDI-SAM: a comprehensive substance abuse interview. Br J Addict 1989;84: 801–814.

19. Project MATCH Research Group. Project MATCH: rationale and methods for a multisite clinical trial matching patients to alcoholism treatment. Alcohol Clin Exp Res 1993;17:1130–1145.

20. Sobell LC, Maisto SA, Sobell MB, Cooper AM. Reliability of alcohol abusers' self-reports of drinking behavior. Behav Res Ther 1979;17: 157–160.

21. Babor TF, Brown J, Del Boca FK. Validity of self-reports in applied research on addictive behaviors: factor or fiction? Behav Assess 1990: 12:5–31.

# CHAPTER 15

# Symptom Checklist-90-Revised (SCL-90-R®) and the Brief Symptom Inventory (BSI®)

*Virginia L. Smith*

## DESCRIPTION AND BACKGROUND

*Formal Name*
Symptom Checklist-90-Revised (SCL-90-R®) and the Brief Symptom Inventory (BSI®)

*Author*
Leonard R. Derogatis

*Key References*
Derogatis LR. Symptom Checklist-90-R (SCL-90-R) administration, scoring, and procedures manual. 3rd ed. Minneapolis: National Computer Systems, 1994.

Derogatis LR. Brief Symptom Inventory (BSI) administration, scoring, and procedures manual. 3rd ed. Minneapolis: National Computer Systems, 1993.

Derogatis LR, Lazarus L. SCL-90-R®, Brief Symptom Inventory and Matching Clinical Rating Scales. In: Maruish M, ed. Treatment planning and outcome assessment. New York: Lawrence Earlbaum Associates, 1994.

## INTRODUCTION

Symptom Checklist-90-Revised (SCL-90-R) is a self-report symptom inventory designed to measure psychological distress. The Brief Symptom Inventory (BSI) is a brief form of the SCL-90-R. These tests provide an overview of a patient's symptoms and their intensity. The SCL-90-R and BSI tests identify the level of distress that a patient is experiencing at a specific point in time ("the last 7 days" is the standard normative period for these tests).

Gender-keyed norms are available for each test for four groups: nonpatient adults, nonpatient adolescents, psychiatric outpatients, and psychiatric inpatients. There are different norms for the SCL-90-R and the BSI tests. In addition, a pair of matched clinician rating scales, the Derogatis Psychiatric Rating Scale (DPRS) and the SCL-90 Analogue Scale, are available to assess clinicians' judgements of patient status on the same nine symptom dimensions designed into the self-report scales (1–3).

## DOMAINS AND NUMBER OF ITEMS

The SCL-90-R and BSI tests measure nine primary symptom dimensions: somatization, obsessive-compulsive, interpersonal sensitivity, depression, anxiety, hostility, phobic anxiety, paranoid ideation, and psychoticism. Each test also provides three global indices of distress, including a Global Severity Index, which measures the current overall level of distress; a Positive Symptom Distress Index, which measures the intensity of distress; and a Positive Symptom Total, which indicates the number of patient-reported symptoms.

SCL-90-R has 90 items, and the BSI has a 53-item subset of the SCL-90-R's items. Each test measures nine primary symptom dimensions and three global indices.

## APPLICATION

### Target Population

The SCL-90-R and BSI are used by clinical psychologists, psychiatrists, physicians, and counseling professionals in mental health, medical, and educational settings as well as for research purposes. The tests can be used either as a screening tool during the initial evaluation of a patient at intake or as a measurement of patient progress during or after treatment.

### Data Collection Procedures

The SCL-90-R takes 12–15 minutes for patients to complete, whereas the BSI takes only 8–10 minutes. The tests can be taken in a paper-and-pencil format, audiocassette, or online computer administration.

National Computer Systems (NCS) publishes the SCL-90-R and BSI tests in Hispanic languages and French Canadian as standard products. In addition, there are numerous other foreign language translations that can be used only for research, not for clinical purposes. All requests for foreign translations other than Hispanic or French Canadian should be made in writing to the product manager at NCS.

The SCL-90-R and BSI tests are designed for use with adults and adolescents 13 years or older. The tests are written at a sixth-grade reading level.

### Psychometric Properties

Internal consistency for the SCL-90-R range from 0.77 to 0.90 and from 0.71 to 0.85 for the BSI for the nine primary symptom dimensions. Test-retest reliability ranged between 0.80 and 0.90 for the SCL-90-R with a 1-week interval between tests and between 0.68 and 0.91 for the BSI with a 2-week interval between tests. The BSI is slightly less reliable than the SCL-90-R because it has fewer items per construct.

There are also over 700 studies on the SCL-90-R and over 250 studies on the BSI attesting to the validity of these instruments. Bibliographies for the SCL-90-R and BSI tests are available from NCS upon request.

## UTILITY

### Scoring Manual

There are administration manuals for both the SCL-90-R and BSI tests to facilitate scoring and interpretation. Both the SCL-90-R and BSI tests can be scored via hand scoring or computer system software. The SCL-90-R report is also available via teleprocessing.

### Automation

NCS sells computer system software for the SCL-90-R and BSI, called MICROTEST or MICROTEST-Q. This software can be used to generate profile, interpretive, or progress reports.

The normative profile on the profile reports plots area T-scores for nonpatients and provides outpatient and inpatient T-scores for comparison. The interpretive report provides narrative text with the author's interpretation of the scores. The progress report tracks an individual's progress along the nine symptom dimensions and three global indices over time.

### Permission to Use

Both the SCL-90-R and BSI tests are exclusively published and distributed by NCS Assessments, 5605 Green Circle Drive, Minnetonka, MN 55343. They can be ordered by mail or by calling Customer Service at 800-627-7271, extension 5151. A fee is charged.

### Description of Where and When Used

When used for outcomes measurement, the SCL-90-R or BSI test is often administered at intake, during treatment, at discharge, and at follow-up. At intake, the tests can reflect the severity of illness and establish a baseline for progress evaluation. During treatment, the test quantifies the effect of care on changes in symptom severity and supports decisions about continuing, changing, or terminating treatment. At discharge, the test assesses readiness for discharge based on changes measured in symptom severity. It also establishes pretreatment and posttreatment comparisons for evaluation of outcomes and provider profiling. At follow-up, the test can measure the maintenance effect of care in evaluation of outcomes, medical cost offset, and provider profiling.

## SUMMARY OF STRENGTHS AND LIMITATIONS

These measurements are well researched and validated. The SCL-90-R and BSI tests effectively measure the constructs and have over 950 independently published research studies demonstrating their validity and utility.

Another strength is that the tests are brief and multidimensional. The SCL-90-R and BSI are among the only tests that cover a wide variety of psychological symptom dimensions with only a few questions.

The SCL-90-R and BSI are two of the most commonly used objective instruments for measuring the outcomes of mental health treatment. These tests can be repeated over time without the loss of validity. In particular, the BSI is often used as a single composite score to track patient progress over time.

The DPRS and SCL-90 Analogue are unique in that they allow the clinician to measure the same nine primary dimensions through an objective rating by a clinician and a rating by other nonclinical observers, as provided by the patient self-report SCL-90-R and BSI. The ability to measure common dimensions in different ways can increase the validity of the information collected and provide a more comprehensive assessment of these dimensions.

These tests are not used as a diagnostic tool. The SCL-90-R and BSI indicate current levels of symptomatic distress and need for further in-depth psychological evaluation. Another limitation is that they cannot be used with children under 13 years of age.

## REFERENCES

1. Derogatis LR. Symptom Checklist-90-R (SCL-90-R) administration, scoring and procedures manual. 3rd ed. Minneapolis: National Computer Systems, 1994.
2. Derogatis LR. Brief Symptom Inventory (BSI) administration, scoring, and procedures manual. 3rd ed. Minneapolis: National Computer Systems, 1994.
3. Derogatis LR, Lazarus L. SCL-90-R®, Brief Symptom Inventory and Matching Clinical Rating Scales. In Maruish M, ed. Treatment planning and outcome assessment. New York: Lawrence Earlbaum Associates, 1994.

# CHAPTER 16

# Eating Disorder Inventory-2 (EDI-2)

*David M. Garner*

---

## DESCRIPTION AND BACKGROUND

*Formal Name*
Eating Disorder Inventory-2 (EDI-2)

*Author*
David M. Garner, Ph.D.

*Key References*
Garner DM. Self-report measures for eating disorders. Curr Contents Soc Behav Sci 1993;25. (Also see Curr Contents Arts Human 1993;15:20.)

Garner DM, Olmsted MP, Polivy J, Garfinkel PE. Comparison between weight-preoccupied women and anorexia nervosa. Psychosom Med 1984; 4:255–266.

Garner DM, Olmsted MP, Davis R, Rockert W, Goldbloom D, Eagle M. The association between bulimic symptoms and reported psychopathology. Int J Eating Dis 1990;9:1–15.

Garner DM, Garner MV, Van Egeren LF. Body dissatisfaction adjusted for weight: the body illusion index. Int J Eating Dis 1992;12:263–271.

Shore RA, Porter JE. Normative and reliability data for 11 to 18 year olds on the eating disorder inventory. Int J Eating Dis 1990;9:201–207.

## INTRODUCTION

The EDI-2 is a widely used (1), standardized, self-report measure of psychological symptoms commonly associated with anorexia nervosa, bulimia nervosa. and other eating disorders (2). The EDI-2 does not yield a specific diagnosis of an eating disorder; rather, it is designed to measure psychological traits or symptom clusters presumed to have relevance to understanding and treating eating disorders. The psychological profile provided by the EDI-2 is consistent with the understanding of eating disorders as multidetermined and heterogeneous syndromes.

## DOMAINS AND NUMBER OF ITEMS

The original EDI, developed by Garner et al. in 1983, was comprised of 64 items organized into eight subscales (3). Three of the subscales were designed to assess attitudes and behaviors concerning eating, weight, and shape (drive for thinness, bulimia, body dissatisfaction); the remaining five subscales drew on more general organizing constructs or psychological traits clinically relevant to eating disorders (ineffectiveness, perfection, interpersonal distrust, interoceptive awareness, maturity fears). The current version retains the original 64 items and eight subscales, plus three additional subscales (27 new items) comprising the provisional subscales (i.e., asceticism, impulse regulation, and social insecurity). Thus, the EDI-2 consists of 11 subscales derived from 91 items presented in a six-point, forced choice format requiring respondents to answer whether each item applies "always," "usually," "often," "sometimes," "rarely," or "never."

Two descriptive examples of the EDI-2 subscales are provided: Drive for Thinness and Body Dissatisfaction. The Drive for Thinness subscale assesses the relentless pursuit of thinness, and the morbid fear of fatness have been described as cardinal features of eating disorders. The clinical manifestation of an intense drive to be thinner or fear of fatness are essential for a diagnosis of an eating disorder. Items on this subscale assess excessive concern with dieting, preoccupation with weight, and fear of weight gain.

Although body dissatisfaction is endemic to young women in western culture, in its extreme form it is considered to be a major factor responsible for initiating and then sustaining the extreme weight controlling behaviors seen in eating disorders. The Body Dissatisfaction subscale of the EDI-2 measures dissatisfaction with the overall shape and with the size of those regions of the body of extraordinary concern to those with eating disorders (i.e., stomach, hips, thighs, buttocks).

## APPLICATION

### Target Populations

In clinical settings, the EDI-2 provides individual patient profiles that may be compared against norms for eating disorder patients and nonpatient comparison samples. This information is particularly relevant in individual cases because of the emerging consensus that remarkable heterogeneity exists in the psychopathology associated with eating disorders. Administered at several points in time, the EDI-2 can provide valuable information about clinical status and response to treatment (1).

In nonclinical settings, the EDI-2 provides an economical means of identifying individuals who have subclinical eating problems or those who may be at risk for developing eating disorders. It can be administered easily in schools, athletic camps, or other institutional settings to screen for eating disorder symptomatology and other areas of distress.

The EDI-2 has been used with respondents as young as 11 years of age (2). The asceticism, impulse regulation, and social insecurity subscales of the EDI-2 are intended for adolescents 12 years of age or older.

### Data Collection Procedures

The EDI-2 is a self-report forced-choice measure that can be administered in individual and group settings. Most young adults are able to complete the test in 15 minutes or less.

In clinical settings and in other circumstances where detailed information about specific symptoms and symptom frequency is required for clinical or diagnostic purposes, respondents should be given the EDI-2 Symptom Checklist (EDI-2-SC). The EDI-2-SC provides data regarding frequency of symptoms such as binge eating, self-induced vomiting, use of laxatives, diet pills, diuretics, exercise patterns, weight, and menstrual history. Detailed information on the symptom areas assessed by the EDI-2-SC is necessary to determine whether patients meet formal diagnostic criteria for an eating disorder. The EDI-2-SC takes between 5 and 15 minutes to complete, depending on the number of symptom areas relevant to the respondent.

Administration should be conducted in a private setting and should be introduced as a measure of the respondent's attitudes, feelings, and behaviors related to eating and other areas in general. If respondents complete the EDI-2 at home, they should be reminded not to obtain assistance from others. In group administrations, respondents should be advised not to consult with others when answering the questions. Respondents should be informed that it is important to answer all items. They should be encouraged to explain any concerns or difficulties responding to items by writing their comments on the back of the test booklet. The EDI-2 is not intended to tap idiosyncratic item interpretations; respondents should be given the opportunity to ask questions and the examiner should provide any necessary clarification of items. The EDI-2 need not be administered by a professional trained in psychology. However, the examiner should have some understanding of the dimensions being used by the EDI-2 so that accurate clarification of any item can be provided.

Optimal use of the EDI-2 requires the completion of a number of demographic questions. Completion of these items is particularly important to gain information related to the respondent's weight history. Age, sex, and diagnostic status are critical to the choice of appropriate comparison samples.

The EDI-2 has been translated into Arabic, Chinese, Dutch, Estonian, Finnish, Flemish, French, German, Hebrew, Japanese, Portuguese, Spanish, and Swedish, among other languages. Validation of the instrument is in different stages in the various languages and cultures in which it has been applied. Further information on the official translations of the instrument can be obtained from Psychological Assessment Resources.

**Psychometric Properties**

Reliability coefficients (standardized $\alpha$) for the original EDI scales were between 0.83 and 0.92 for the eating disorder sample and between 0.83 and 0.93 for the female college comparison group (2). Eberenz and Gleaves (4) report similar reliability coefficients for the original EDI subscales (between 0.80 and 0.91) on a large eating-disorder patient sample. Both the original report (2) and the later study (4) revealed lower $\alpha$ for the provisional subscales for two eating-disorder samples (asceticism, 0.70 and 0.65; impulse regula-

tion, 0.77 and 0.75; and social insecurity, 0.80 and 0.73).

Test-retest reliability also has been established by several studies and is described in the EDI-2 manual. Welch et al. (5) reported retest reliability for EDIs administered 1 week apart to 70 student and staff nurses. The coefficients were 0.79–0.95 for all scales except for interoceptive awareness (0.67). The retest reliabilities after 3 weeks for 70 nonpatient university undergraduates reported by Wear and Pratz (6) were above 0.80, except the maturity fears subscale.

Validity of the instrument is supported by a significant body of literature indicating that the EDI-2 subscales measure clinically relevant dimensions of experience for eating-disorder patients (2). The original scales have demonstrated appropriate content and criterion validity. Considerable evidence exists for both convergent and discriminant validity for the original EDI scales (2, 7). More importantly, many of the findings from the original validation studies have been replicated and extended by subsequent research conducted in a wide range of different settings. The psychometric properties of the original instrument are sound and the constructs measure symptom domains that have clinical utility. Moreover, consistent evidence shows that the EDI is sensitive to clinical change. A recent factor analysis does not support the reliability or validity of three EDI-2 provisional scales (4). Recent research indicates that a significant proportion of eating-disorder patients suffer from characterological disturbance, and the items chosen for the impulse regulation and social insecurity subscales were specifically selected to tap content areas that typify this patient group. Further research will determine the clinical utility and predictive validity of these new subscales or their derivatives.

In addition to norms for eating disorder and female college students, the manual provides separate norms based on variables such as diagnostic status, gender, and age, which aid in the interpretation of individual EDI-2 profiles. As indicated earlier, patients with clinical eating disorders differ from comparison samples of nonpatient young women. Similarly, women and men differ substantially on some EDI-2 scales and different distributions of scores are found in younger, compared with older, adolescents.

## UTILITY

### Scoring Manual

The EDI-2 Item booklets, answer sheets, profile forms, symptom checklists, and professional manual can be obtained from Psychological Assessment Resources. Scoring of the EDI-2 is easily performed by tearing off the face sheet of the NCR answer sheets. The manual provides detailed information related to administration, scoring, and interpretation. It also provides descriptive statistics for different patients and nonpatient groups, data pertaining to norms on different samples, and data related to test reliability and validity.

Raw scores on EDI-2 subscales are plotted on profile forms that allow comparison with subscale norms derived from eating-disorder patients and a female college student comparison group. Shaded areas on the profile form are the 95% confidence intervals for these groups. Scores falling in the shaded ranges are not significantly different ($P = 0.05$ level) from the respective normative sample means. The EDI-2 subscale scores are most often evaluated using the norms for both eating-disorder and nonpatient comparison groups. EDI-2 profiles may also be evaluated in terms of relative subscale scores because the peaks and valleys provide the clinician with a picture of the respondent's areas of relative concern.

### Automation

A computer version of the EDI-2 is available from Psychological Assessment Resources. The EDI-2 computer version administers and scores the EDI-2 and produces a profile of the individual's test results compared with both eating-disorder

patient norms and nonclinical comparison group norms. In addition, the program provides interpretive statements for each EDI-2 scale. Responses can be directly entered by the client, or the clinician can enter a client's responses to the paper-and-pencil version of the test for scoring and interpretation. The computer version of the EDI-2 is usually completed in less than 15 minutes.

### Permission to Use

Psychological Assessment Resources, P.O. Box 998, Odessa, FL 33556 (Telephone: 1-800-331-8378) owns the copyright to the EDI-2 test materials and can provide information on current fees.

### Description of Where and When Used

In clinical settings, the EDI-2 can provide information helpful in understanding the patient, planning treatment, and assessing progress. The EDI-2 yields individual patient profiles that may be compared against norms for eating-disorder and comparison samples. It also may be used as a screening instrument to identify eating disorders in nonpatient populations and to distinguish individuals with serious emotional disturbances from normal dieters.

As a research tool, the EDI-2 provides descriptive information, allowing comparison of samples in one research setting to those from other research sites. It has been used both as an outcome measure and a prognostic indicator in treatment studies. The EDI-2 also has been used to track psychological functioning in prospective studies of individuals at risk for eating disorders. Subscales of the EDI-2 have been used to select or define criterion groups in studies of body satisfaction/dissatisfaction, weight preoccupation, and perfectionism.

## SUMMARY OF STRENGTHS AND LIMITATIONS

The EDI-2 is standardized and economical, and it does not require a trained interviewer. It can be completed in a relatively brief period of time and may be administered in groups. Research over the past decade has shown that the EDI is sensitive to clinical change and that it may play a valuable role in clinical evaluations of eating-disorder patients or those suspected of eating disorders. Less information is available on the EDI-2 provisional subscales (asceticism, impulse regulation, and social insecurity). Recently, concerns have been raised regarding the psychometric properties of these three subscales.

The EDI-2, like all self-report instruments, can be criticized as being vulnerable to potential distortion due to response-style bias, inaccurate reporting, defensiveness, and denial. The alternative, a structured interview, has the advantage of affording a more detailed appraisal of specific psychopathology and the opportunity for probing and clarifying the meaning behind certain responses. However, structured interviews are time consuming, require a trained interviewer, and may be impractical for many situations. Both types of data collection should be considered in a comprehensive assessment of eating-disorder symptomatology. Finally, the EDI-2 should not be considered an exhaustive sampling of psychopathological characteristics of eating disorders.

## REFERENCES

1. Garner DM, Rockert W, Garner MV, Davis R, Olmsted MP. Comparison between cognitive-behavioral and short-term psychodynamic therapy for bulimia nervosa. Am J Psychiatry 1993;150: 37–46.
2. Garner DM. Eating disorder inventory-2 professional manual. Odessa, FL: Psychological Assessment Resources, 1993.
3. Garner DM, Olmsted MP, Polivy J. Development and validation of a multidimensional eating disorder inventory for anorexia nervosa and bulimia. Int J Eating Dis 1983;2:15–34.
4. Eberenz KP, Gleaves DH. An examination of the internal consistency and factor structure of the eating disorder inventory-2 in a clinical sample. Int J Eating Dis 1994;16:371–379.
5. Welch GW, Hall A, Walkey FH. The factor structure of the eating disorders inventory. J Clin Psychol 1988;44:51–56.
6. Wear RW, Pratz O. Test-retest reliability for the eating disorder inventory. Int J Eating Dis 1987; 6:767–769.
7. Rathner G, Rumpold G. Convergent validity of the eating disorder inventory and the anorexia nervosa inventory for self-rating in an Austrian nonclinical population. Int J Eating Dis 1994;16: 381–393.

CHAPTER 17

# The Child Behavior Checklist (CBCL) and Related Instruments

*Thomas M. Achenbach*

---

## DESCRIPTION AND BACKGROUND

*Formal Name*
The Child Behavior Checklist (CBCL) and Related Instruments

*Author*
Thomas M. Achenbach, Ph.D.

*Key References*
Achenbach TM. Integrative guide for the 1991 CBCL/4-18, YSR, and TRF profiles. Burlington: University of Vermont, Department of Psychiatry, 1991.

Achenbach TM. Manual for the Child Behavior Checklist/4-18 and 1991 profile. Burlington: University of Vermont, Department of Psychiatry, 1991.

Achenbach TM. Manual for the Teacher's Report Form and 1991 pro-file. Burlington: University of Vermont, Department of Psychiatry, 1991.

Achenbach TM. Manual for the Youth Self-Report and 1991 profile. Burlington: University of Vermont, Department of Psychiatry, 1991.

Achenbach TM. Manual for the Child Behavior Checklist/2-3 and 1992 profile. Burlington: University of Vermont, Department of Psychiatry, 1992.

McConaughy SH, Achenbach TM. Manual for the Semistructured Clinical Interview for Children and Adolescents. Burlington: University of Vermont, Department of Psychiatry, 1994.

## INTRODUCTION

Separate versions of the CBCL are designed to obtain parents' ratings of children at ages 2–3 (CBCL/2-3) and 4–18 (CBCL/4-18). Related instruments are designed to obtain teachers' ratings of pupils at ages 5–18 (Teacher's Report Form, TRF), self-ratings by adolescents at ages 11–18 (Youth Self-Report, YSR), clinicians' ratings of 6–18 year olds during semistructured clinical interviews (Semistructured Clinical Interview for Children and Adolescents, SCICA), and observers' ratings of the behavior of 5–14 year olds in classrooms,

recess, and other group settings (Direct Observation Form, DOF). Forms are also available for assessing young adults via parent ratings (Young Adult Behavior Checklist, YABCL) and self-ratings (Young Adult Self-Report, YASR).

## DOMAINS AND NUMBER OF ITEMS

All measures are designed to assess behavioral and emotional problems in a standardized fashion, as reported by particular kinds of respondents. The wording of the items, definitions of points on the scales, and rating periods are geared to the types

97

of respondents and the conditions under which they see the subjects. In addition to problems, the CBCL/4-18, TRF, YSR, YABCL, and YASR also assess competencies, whereas the DOF records on-task behavior. All the instruments provide for obtaining open-ended descriptions of specific characteristics of the subjects, as well as scores for the structured items.

The standardized problem items range from 96 on the DOF to 118 on the CBCL/4-18 and TRF. The SCICA has 121 observational items and 114 self-report items for ages 6–18, plus an additional 11 items for ages 13–18. Competence items range from 10 on the YABCL to 20 on the CBCL. Subscales include empirically based syndrome scales ranging from 6 on the DOF to 9 on the CBCL and YSR. All instruments have empirically based internalizing, externalizing, and total problem scales. Competence scales range from 1 to 4.

## APPLICATIONS

### Target Populations

The target populations include both genders within the age range specified for a particular instrument and as seen by the type of respondent for which that instrument is designed. Normative data enable users to compare scores for individual subjects with those obtained by large samples of subjects who are not mentally retarded or physically disabled. Although the instruments can be used to assess mildly retarded and disabled subjects, the items and normative data are geared primarily to subjects who are not retarded nor physically disabled.

### Data Collection Procedures

The CBCL/2-3, CBCL/4-18, TRF, YSR, YABCL, and YASR take about 15–20 minutes to complete. The respondent scores items describing behavioral/emotional problems on three- or four-point scales. The scales require approximately fifth-grade reading skills for self-administration. They can be administered by an interviewer, but it is desirable for the respondent to view a copy of the form while the interviewer asks the questions. The DOF is designed for use by trained observers who make several 10-minute observations of the subjects, whereas the SCICA is designed for trained clinical interviewers who conduct interviews lasting about 60–90 minutes.

All the instruments are available in questionnaire format for completion by pen or pencil. Some are also available in machine readable and interactive computer entry formats.

For culturally diverse populations, translations of one or more forms are available in 43 languages.

### Psychometric Properties

The references listed above report reliability, validity, and derivation data for all the instruments. The test-retest reliabilities of most scale scores are in the 0.80's and 0.90's. For most of the instruments, the references provide extensive item-by-item and scale-by-scale statistical comparisons between clinically referred and demographically similar nonreferred subjects, analyses of demographic differences, correlations with other instruments, and research findings. The Bibliography of Published Studies (1) includes cross-cultural replications of the empirically based syndrome structure, plus reliability, validity, and research data from numerous cultures. To aid users, publications are listed under some 200 topics, such as outcome studies, specific medical conditions, ethnic groups, and psychiatric diagnoses. The Bibliography lists all authors of the published reports, as well as languages into which the forms have been translated.

## UTILITY

### Scoring Manual

Manuals are available for the CBCL/2-3, CBCL/4-18, TRF, YSR, and SCICA (see Key References). Basic data for the DOF, plus references to articles on the DOF, are provided in the manual for the CBCL/4-18. Pending publication of manuals for the YABCL and YASR, basic data can be obtained from Brown and Achenbach (1). Detailed scoring information is available for all instruments, including both hand scoring and microcomputer scoring. The manuals and other publications illustrate diverse applications for many purposes, including outcome assessments. A training videotape is available for the SCICA.

For users with at least a Master's degree level of training in standardized assessment, interpretation is made easy by the display of items and scale scores on hand-scored and computer-scored profiles. The manuals and other documentation provide guidelines and illustrations of use in multiple contexts.

Respondent burden is minimal because respondents merely need to complete structured items that have been refined through extensive use and feedback from diverse users.

### Automation

Automation options include key entry on microcomputers from forms completed by respondents, scoring of machine readable forms by optical scanners, and interactive key entry by the respondents themselves. Computer software is available for scoring all forms and for integrating data obtained from different respondents about the same subject.

### Permission to Use

All rating forms, profiles, books, and programs are copyrighted and must not be altered or reproduced without written permission. All materials are available for a fee from Child Behavior Checklist, 1 South Prospect Street, Burlington, VT, 05401-3456, Telephone: 802-656-8313 or 802-656-4563.

### SUMMARY OF STRENGTHS AND LIMITATIONS

The instruments described here were developed to meet the need for standardized, quantifiable, psychometrically sound, economical procedures that could be used to assess behavioral and emotional problems under diverse conditions. They were also designed to provide data from which syndrome scales could be empirically derived to capture the actual patterns of problems that co-occur in the populations to be assessed. The empirically derived scales have been shown to have numerous important correlates, to predict differences in long-term outcomes, and to be cross-culturally robust.

Because these instruments are based on a multiaxial assessment model, they are not viewed as the sole means of assessment. Instead, comprehensive assessment should also include procedures such as medical examinations, standardized tests of ability, achievement, perceptual-motor functioning, developmental histories, and data on family context. Finally, because of the instruments' longer time horizon, they may not be sensitive to short-term change.

REFERENCE

1. Brown JS, Achenbach TM. Bibliography of published studies using the child behavior checklist and related materials. Burlington: University of Vermont, Department of Psychiatry, 1995.

# CHAPTER 18

# Beck Depression Inventory (BDI™)

*Robert A. Steer, Aaron T. Beck*

---

*DESCRIPTION AND BACKGROUND*

*Formal Name*
Beck Depression Inventory (BDI™)

*Author*
Aaron T. Beck, M.D.

*Key Reference*
Beck AT, Steer RA. Manual for the Beck Depression Inventory. San Antonio: Psychological Corporation, 1993.

## INTRODUCTION

The BDI (1) is a revision of the original 1961 instrument that was developed by Beck et al. (2). Aaron T. Beck, M.D., copyrighted the revision in 1978 and assigned its distribution rights to The Psychological Corporation in 1987.

## DOMAINS AND NUMBER OF ITEMS

According to several surveys that have been conducted during the past 5 years (3–5), the BDI is one of the most widely used psychological tests for measuring the severity of depression. The BDI is a 21-item scale that includes the following depressive symptoms: mood, pessimism, sense of failure, self-dissatisfaction, guilt, punishment, self-dislike, self-accusations, suicidal ideas, crying, irritability, social withdrawal, indecisiveness, body image change, work difficulty, insomnia, fatigability, loss of appetite, weight loss, somatic preoccupation, and loss of libido.

Respondents are asked to rate themselves with a four-point scale that ranges from 0 to 3 for the past week, including today. A total score is calculated by summing the 21-item ratings. The total score can thus range from 0 to 63. Cognitive-affective and somatic-performance subscales may also be scored, respectively, by summing the ratings for the first 13 and last 8 symptoms (1). The former subscale is particularly useful for detecting and assessing depression in geriatric (6), medical (7), and substance abusing (8) patients whose somatic depressive symptoms might actually be attributable to their medical illnesses rather than to depression per se.

## APPLICATION

### Target Populations

The utility of the BDI for detecting, assessing, and monitoring changes in depression has been studied extensively with respect to a broad spectrum of normal and clinical populations throughout the world for both sexes (9). Caution should be used when using the BDI to screen for depression in normal adolescents and adults. High BDI total scores in normal populations, such as college students, may be indicative of adjustment problems instead of depression (10). In contrast, low BDI total scores in normal and psychiatric populations do not exclude the possibility of a depressive syndrome but may indicate atypical clinical depressions or other psychiatric problems (11). The BDI is most appropriately used for measuring severity in patients who have been clinically diagnosed with depression.

With respect to the demographic correlates of the BDI, the evidence is equivocal. Some studies have reported that age and education are significantly correlated with BDI total scores, whereas other studies have found that these characteristics are not significantly related to BDI total scores (9). However, one analysis (12) found that most of the 21 symptoms display little sex bias for either college students or psychiatric outpatients. Studies also vacillate about the effect of race on the BDI (9, 13). In other studies, adolescents tend to have higher total scores than adults (14).

## Data Collection Procedures

The BDI is usually self-administered and requires between 5 and 10 minutes to complete, whereas oral administration may take 15 minutes. According to a recent survey of 151 clinical psychologists (5), the paper-and-pencil BDI requires an average of 11 (SD = 6) minutes to administer, an average of 6 (SD = 5) minutes to score, and an average of 8 (SD = 6) minutes to interpret. The BDI imposes very little respondent burden with respect to the length of its administration or its symptom content. However, psychiatric patients may be concerned about the reasons they are asked about suicidal ideation, especially if they are undecided about committing suicide. Similarly, geriatric patients, if retired, and young adolescents, if not currently engaged in sexual activity, may raise questions about how to rate symptoms addressing work performance and loss of libido. For the symptom relating to work performance, such respondents should be encouraged to base their ratings on present daily activities or school work, whereas the ratings for the latter symptom should be based on sexual desire or interest.

Much information has been collected about administering the BDI in different formats, such as reading it out loud, using paper-and-pencil forms, or using online computer questions (13). The method of administration determines the amount of time that is required to complete the instrument, but the method of administration has little effect on the levels of the resultant total scores.

The Psychological Corporation is currently offering the BDI in hand scorable and optically scannable paper-and-pencil answer sheets along with an interactive personal computer version in either English or Spanish. However, the BDI has been translated into most major languages, such as French, German, Japanese, and Chinese. There are also numerous translations that have addressed the specific idioms and dialectics that are spoken in different Latin American and European countries (9).

The BDI has been effectively used to measure self-reported depression with a variety of culturally diverse populations such as inner-city pregnant adolescents (15) and inner-city intravenous drug abusers who are not currently in treatment (8).

## Psychometric Properties

Comprehensive reviews have not only addressed the psychometric properties of the BDI (9, 13) but also discussed its usage in psychotherapy outcome studies (16, 17). For example, in their metaanalyses of psychometric data drawn from published research studies that were conducted between 1961 and July 1986, Beck et al. (13) reported that the average internal-consistency estimates (coefficient $\alpha$) of the total scores were 0.86 for psychiatric patients and 0.81 for normals, respectively. The average correlation of the BDI total scores with clinical ratings of depression was >0.60 for both psychiatric patients and normal adults. The BDI also discriminates among subtypes of mood disorders, such as dysthymia and major depression (18), and symptoms, such as sadness and loss of libido, have differentiated psychiatric outpatients who were diagnosed with major depression and generalized anxiety disorders (19).

Finally, the BDI reflects a general syndrome of depression composed of highly intercorrelated first-order symptom dimensions whose number and compositions are dependent on the types of samples that are being investigated (13). In summary, psychometric analyses of the BDI for both normal and psychiatric populations (9, 13) have consistently indicated that this instrument is a reliable and valid measure of self-reported depression.

## UTILITY

### Scoring Manual

The BDI Manual presents detailed psychometric and comparative information about the use of the BDI with patients who were diagnosed with a variety of different psychiatric disorders (1). Suggested methods of administration, scoring, and interpretation are also provided along with a description of its development. According to the interpretative guidelines that are suggested in the 1993 edition of the BDI manual (1) for patients who have been clinically diagnosed with depression, total scores of 0–9 indicate minimal depression, total scores of 10–16 represent mild depression, total scores of 17–29 reveal moderate depression, and total scores of 30–63 reflect severe depression. With respect to screening for depression in normal populations, BDI total scores of 17–20 may suggest dysphoria, whereas total scores of 21 and above may be indicative of depression (10). The presence of dysphoria or depression, however, must be ultimately confirmed by a clinical interview.

In interpreting the BDI, the ratings for specific symptoms, especially those for hopelessness and suicide ideation, should be routinely evaluated. If a respondent has a rating of 2 or 3 for either of these two symptoms, he or she should assessed for suicide potential.

The BDI may be used in any situation in which the severity of a respondent's self-reported depression is required and the respondent's reading ability is at least at a fifth-grade level. It is a sensitive outcome measure when used to evaluate changes in depression (16, 17). When the BDI is used to evaluate change, then it should be administered at least 1 week apart to comply with the timeframe that is requested in the instructions. Importantly, the changes in the BDI total scores over time have been found to agree highly with those based on independent clinical observations (20). The BDI is also an excellent instrument for gathering symptom information to be discussed later during therapy sessions. For example, in cognitive therapy, patients frequently are asked to complete a BDI on a weekly basis so that the therapist and patient can both evaluate changes in specific depressive symptoms.

### Automation

The Psychological Corporation offers several methods for automating the administration, scoring, and interpretation of the BDI. Optically scannable paper-and-pencil answer sheets and personal computer software for interactive administration and subsequent interpretation are available. The software not only lists profile scores and comparisons with normative psychiatric populations but also generates a detailed narrative report that can be immediately printed or filed for editing. Importantly, the software retains historical data and reports about the respondent that may be incorporated into future outcome evaluations and progress reports.

### Permission to Use

The Psychological Corporation (555 Academic Court, San Antonio, TX 78204-2498, Telephone: 1-800-288-0752) sells the BDI to individuals whose credentials and training ensure that they are capable of professionally using psychological test data. A variety of pricing and scoring options are available, and the overall costs are based on the number of tests and types of options that are purchased. For example, the 1994 charge for a minimum order of a package of 25 paper-and-pencil, hand-scorable record forms was $25.50

## SUMMARY OF STRENGTHS AND LIMITATIONS

The BDI is one of the most widely used psychological tests in the world for measuring the severity of self-reported depression in adolescents and adults. It is rapidly administered and possesses an extensive database detailing its usage with a broad variety of normal and psychiatric populations. The instrument is highly consistent internally and correlates with other self-report measures and clinical ratings of depression. A plethora of outcome studies have been conducted with this instrument across diverse cultures.

With respect to its limitations, the BDI responses can be easily faked (1). No items are included to detect feigning or denying depression. Furthermore, the original 1961 instrument upon which the BDI is based was written before the 1994 release of the Diagnostic and Statistical Manual of Mental Disorders, 4th edition (DSM-IV) (21). Thus, the BDI does not contain several symptoms that are now purported by the DSM-IV to be criteria in the diagnosis of clinical depression, that is, increased sleep, appetite, and weight (22). However, the effectiveness of these three symptoms for differentiating clinical depression from other psychiatric syndromes is limited because they are frequently found in syndromes other than depression (23).

## REFERENCES

1. Beck AT, Steer RA. Manual for the Beck Depression Inventory. San Antonio, TX: The Psychological Corporation, 1993.
2. Beck AT, Ward CH, Mendelson M, Mock J, Erbaugh J. An inventory for measuring depression. Arch Gen Psychiatry 1961;4:561–571.
3. Archer RP, Maruish M, Imhof EA, Piotrowski C. Psychological test usage with adolescent clients: 1990 survey findings. Profess Psychol Res Pract 1991;22:247–252.
4. Piotrowski C, Keller JW. Psychological testing in applied settings: a literature review from 1982–1992. J Train Pract Profess Psychol 1992; 6:74–82.
5. Ball JD, Archer RP, Imhof EA. Time requirements of psychological testing: a survey of practitioners. J Pers Assess 1994;63:239–249.
6. Gallagher D, Nies G, Thompson LW. Reliability of the Beck depression inventory with older adults. J Consult Clin Psychol 1982;50:152–153.
7. Clark DA, Steer RA. Use of nonsomatic symptoms to differentiate clinically depressed and nondepressed hospitalized patients with chronic medical illnesses. Psychol Rep 1994;75: 1089–1090.
8. Steer RA, Iguchi MY, Platt JJ. Use of the revised Beck Depression Inventory with intravenous drug users not in treatment. Psychol Addict Behav 1992;6:225–232.
9. Steer RA, Beck AT, Garrison B. Applications of the Beck Depression Inventory. In: Sartorius N, Ban TA, eds. Assessment of depression. Geneva: World Health Organization, 1986: 121–142.
10. Kendall PC, Hollon SD, Beck AT, Hammen CL, Ingram RE. Issues and recommendations regarding use of the Beck Depression Inventory. Cognitive Ther Res 1987;11:289-298.
11. Joiner TE, Schmidt KL, Metalsky GI. Low-end specificity of the Beck Depression Inventory. Cognitive Ther Res 1994;18:55–58.
12. Santor DA, Ramsay JO, Zuroff DC. Nonparametric item analyses of the Beck Depression Inventory: evaluating gender item bias and response option weights. Psychol Assess 1994;6:255–270.
13. Beck AT, Steer RA, Garbin MG. Psychometric properties of the Beck Depression Inventory: twenty-five years of evaluation. Clin Psychol Rev 1988;8:77–100.
14. Teri L. The use of the Beck Depression Inventory with adolescents. J Abnorm Psychol 1982; 10:277–284.
15. Steer RA, Scholl TO, Beck AT. Revised Beck Depression Inventory scores of inner-city adolescents: pre- and postpartum. Psychol Rep 1990;66:315–320.
16. Edwards BC, Lambert MJ, Moran PW, McCully T, Smith KC, Ellington AG. A meta-analytic comparison of the Beck Depression Inventory and the Hamilton rating scale for depression as measures of treatment outcome. Br J Clin Psychol 1984;23:93–99.
17. Lambert MJ, Hatch DR, Kingston MD, Edwards BC. Zung, Beck, and Hamilton rating scales as measures of treatment outcome: a meta-analytic comparison. J Consult Clin Psychol 1986;54:54–59.
18. Steer RA, Beck AT, Brown G, Berchick RJ. Self-reported depressive symptoms that differentiate recurrent-episode major depression from dysthymic disorders. J Clin Psychol 1987;43: 246–250.
19. Steer RA, Beck AT, Riskind JH, Brown G. Differentiation of depressive disorders from generalized anxiety by the Beck Depression Inventory. J Clin Psychol 1986;42:475–478.

20. Taylor EB, Klein DN. Assessing recovery in depression: validity of symptom inventories. Cognitive Ther Res 1989;13:1–8.
21. American Psychiatric Association. Diagnostic and statistical manual for mental disorders. 4th ed. Washington, DC: American Psychiatric Association, 1994.
22. Vredenburg K, Krames L, Flett GL. Reexamining the Beck Depression Inventory: the long and short of it. Psychol Rep 1985;56:767–778.
23. Steer RA, Beck AT. Modifying the Beck Depression Inventory: a reply to Vredenburg, Krames, and Flett. Psychol Rep 1985;57: 625–626.

# CHAPTER 19

# Brief Psychiatric Rating Scale (BPRS)

*L. Stephen Miller, William O. Faustman*

---

## DESCRIPTION AND BACKGROUND

*Formal Name*
Brief Psychiatric Rating Scale (BPRS)

*Authors*
John Overall and D. R. Gorham.

*Key References*
Overall JE, Gorham DR. The brief psychiatric rating scale. Psychol Rep 1962;10:799–812.

Rhoades HM, Overall JE. The semistructured BPRS interview and rating guide. Psychopharmacol Bull 1988; 24:101–104.

Hedlund JL, Vieweg BW. The brief psychiatric rating scale: a comprehensive review. J Operational Psychiatry 1980;11:49–65.

Faustman WO. Brief psychiatric rating scale. In: Maruish ME, ed. The use of psychological testing for treatment planning and outcome assessment. Hillsdale, NJ: Lawrence Erlebaum Associates, 1994:371–401.

Overall JE, Gorham DR. The brief psychiatric rating scale (BPRS): recent developments in ascertainment and scaling. Psychopharmacol Bull 1988; 24:97–99.

## INTRODUCTION

The BPRS is an extensively used instrument that is well suited for outcomes research. Developed by Overall and Gorham (1), it is a clinician-based rating scale that provides an efficient means to evaluate a large number of psychiatric symptom constructs. Originally derived from inpatient subjects, it may be applicable in other settings as well. It emphasizes significant clinical syndromes (e.g., psychosis, depression, anxiety) often seen in psychiatric inpatients and sometimes seen in outpatients.

## DOMAINS AND NUMBER OF ITEMS

The original BPRS consisted of 16 items. It was later altered to its most modern and most widely used version by the addition of 2 items (2) for a total of 18. Each item is measured along a seven-point continuum from "not present" to "extremely severe." Users should be careful to note that some versions use a 0–6 scoring method, whereas others use a 1–method. For more extensive reviews of the BPRS and its development, psychometric properties, and research and clinical uses, there are general reviews (3, 4) and the BPRS authors' relatively recent review of its psychometric properties (5).

Each item on the scale is described to represent a psychiatric symptom with reasonably specific operational definitions. Psychiatric symptoms exhibited by a patient do not need to correspond to items on the BPRS in a one-to-one manner. For example, a given symptom, such as a bizarre grandiose delusion, may be rated under several BPRS items (e.g., grandiosity, unusual thought content).

A number of factor analytic studies (6–8) have identified and confirmed several related symptom constructs formed from combining items, the most consistent being thinking disturbance, withdrawal/retardations, hostile/suspiciousness, and anxious depression (9).

Various combinations of BPRS items also have been identified for use in a typological fashion (9–11), as well as for quantifying negative, positive, and depressive symptoms with some success (12–15). Additionally, several recently developed scales of psychopathology, such as The Positive and Negative Syndrome Scale (16), have included the BPRS with additional items thought to measure positive and negative symptoms.

## APPLICATION

### Target Population

The BPRS was originally developed because of the need to measure symptom change in early clinical drug studies (10). At that time, few, relatively short, efficient instruments were available to measure change in pervasive symptoms such as psychosis. Currently, the BPRS is used most commonly with persons expressing fairly significant symptoms such as those often noted in an inpatient psychiatric setting.

### Data Collection Procedures

Completion of the BPRS is based on an interview that follows the general format of a clinical interview conducted during routine assessment and treatment of a patient. Thus, it relies on a combination of the self-report of the patient and the observations of the clinician. Time of completion varies but typically takes 20–30 minutes; thus, only moderate demands are made on both the clinician and patient. The authors of the scale (1) have suggested spending approximately 3 minutes to develop rapport with the patient. This is followed by approximately 10 minutes of nondirective

interaction, in which clinical information can be obtained in an informal manner. The final 5–10 minutes of the interview are used then to ask specific questions to address topic areas not addressed adequately during the nondirective phase of the interview. Rhoades and Overall (2) presented a number of helpful sample questions for use with the BPRS, and others (17, 18) developed structured interview procedures as potential guides for its use.

Additional training requirements for experienced clinicians are minimal, though careful attention needs to be paid to the proper definitions of the item constructs. The BPRS also may be used by trained research assistants and clinical support staff, provided they are given adequate exposure and training with the operational definitions of each item.

Because the BPRS is a clinician-based scale, there are fewer standardization problems in its use internationally compared with purely self-report scales of psychopathology. The BPRS has been used in research in numerous countries and has shown suitable utility. Additionally, the BPRS has shown adequate cross-cultural reliability (7).

### Psychometric Properties

The BPRS has been well scrutinized. Both interrater and intrarater reliability have been shown for the BPRS (19). The BPRS has proven to have good discriminant validity in numerous controlled studies of medication response (2). Both the scale and its factor subscales have been shown to be sensitive to treatment effects of a range of antipsychotic medications in samples of schizophrenic patients (20, 21). It also has been shown to measure change in anticholinergic medication (22) and electroconvulsive therapy (23). Although the BPRS has been used in studies examining the clinical efficacy of medications in the treatment of depression (24), it may show less sensitivity in its documentation of antidepressant medication effects than other measures frequently included in those studies (25).

Concurrent validity has been shown in schizophrenic populations between the BPRS and other measures, such as the Minnesota Multiphasic Personality Inventory (26), the Scale for the Assessment of Positive Symptoms and the Scale for the Assessment of Negative Symptoms (13, 27), the Nurses' Observation Scale for Inpatient Evaluation (14), and the Hamilton Depression Scale (15).

## UTILITY

### Scoring Manual

Although there is no specific scoring manual, scoring guidelines, as well as exact item descriptions in the literature, have proven sufficient. The general face validity of the well-recognized symptom constructs that make up the BPRS, the easily presented severity scale for each item, the factor clusters, and the summative scoring format together create an easily scoreable and interpretable scale. It is important to keep in mind that the BPRS items are written in such a way as to necessitate being based on a specific time period. Patients typically are evaluated in the context of the week before the interview. Thus, the rating should not be applied as a "lifetime" measure of symptoms.

### Automation

The summative nature of the items in producing a total score and separate factor scores allows easy transformation to automatic scoring. However, the brevity of the scale generally does not necessitate such a need and it is easily hand scored.

### PERMISSION TO USE

The BPRS has been in the public domain since the 1960s (5) and can be used by virtually all qualified clinicians at no charge. A copy of the items and operational definitions are provided in Appendix B.

### Description of Where and When Used

The BPRS is widely used for monitoring symptom change during pharmacological or psychosocial treatment in a variety of settings, such as day hospitals, inpatient wards, and research units. Unlike some rating scales targeted for specific clinical diagnoses (e.g., schizophrenia, major depression), the BPRS can yield useful information in patients with a variety of significant psychiatric diagnoses (e.g., bipolar disorder, major depression, schizophrenia). Additionally, some research suggests that it also may be effective with outpatient populations, provided they show significant clinical symptoms (28).

### SUMMARY OF STRENGTHS AND LIMITATIONS

Overall, the BPRS has many advantages that support its use in outcome data collection in clinical settings. These include ease of use, adaptability for integration into varied clinical routines, and the moderate time and effort demands placed on both respondents and clinicians. Additionally, the minimum number of items makes the scale very efficient. It has a straightforward scoring design that results in a relatively high level of scoring reliability. The BPRS also has the advantage of extensive supportive psychometric and sensitivity literature in significantly ill patients. Finally, the items used by the BPRS are familiar to most mental health professionals.

The BPRS is not without its limitations. It takes some practice to become proficient in its use. Clinicians need to have a clear understanding of the operational definitions of the items being used. This includes the need for a method of calibration if used for research purposes. The BPRS also may have some limitations in its appropriateness for outpatients who have minimal rateable symptoms.

Finally, although summative, the BPRS is primarily descriptive in nature and does not readily translate into specific diagnostic categories. Most of these limitations can be addressed by the use of prudence and preparedness. Practice using the instrument and incorporating it into already established assessment routines within the clinical setting will increase its efficiency and cut down on time demands. Familiarization with the operational definitions of each item will minimize multiple or differing judgments as to both the presence and severity of any given symptom. Regularly scheduled, routine calibration meetings where clinical raters meet to restandardize their scoring can increase interrater reliability, as well as minimize individual clinical rater drift from established scoring guidelines.

An understanding of the range of symptoms represented and their minimal measurable level of severity (presence or absence) should guide appropriate decision-making about the instruments applicability to particular patient populations, such as in an outpatient setting. The descriptive nature of the items are best used as a global measure of change across symptoms rather than in detailed classification or specific diagnoses. When these limitations are accounted for, the BPRS remains one of the principal tools for the measurement of symptom change in the area of psychopathology.

*Acknowledgments.* We thank Dr. John E. Overall for graciously allowing the reprinting of the BPRS scale and its descriptors. Parts of this work were supported by the Department of Veterans Affairs and a grant (MH-30854) from the National Institute of Mental Health to the Stanford/VA Mental Health Clinical Research Center.

REFERENCES

1. Overall JE, Gorham DR. The brief psychiatric rating scale. Psychol Rep 1962;10:799–812.
2. Rhoades HM, Overall JE. The semi-structured BPRS interview and rating guide. Psychopharmacol Bull 1988;24:101–104.
3. Hedlund JL, Vieweg BW. The brief psychiatric rating scale: a comprehensive review. J Operational Psychiatry 1980;11:49–65.
4. Faustman WO. Brief psychiatric rating scale. In: Maruish ME, ed. The use of psychological testing for treatment planning and outcome assessment. Hillsdale, NJ: Lawrence Erlebaum Associates, 1994:371–401.
5. Overall JE, Gorham DR. The brief psychiatric rating scale (BPRS): recent developments in ascertainment and scaling. Psychopharmacol Bull 1988;24:97–99.
6. Overall JE, Hollister LE, Pichot P. Major psychiatric disorders. A four-dimensional model. Arch Gen Psychiatry 1967;16:146–151.
7. Dingemans PM, Winter MLF, Bleeker JAC, Rathod P. A cross-cultural study of the reliability and factorial dimensions of the brief psychiatric rating scale (BPRS). Psychopharmacology 1983;80:190–191.
8. Goldman RS, Tandon R, Woodard J, et al. Consistency of psychopathological dimensions in schizophrenia as determined by the BPRS: a multicenter factor analytic study. Biol Psychiatry 1991;29:45A (Abstr).
9. Overall JE, Klett CJ. Applied multivariate analysis. New York: McGraw-Hill, 1972.
10. Overall JE. The brief psychiatric rating scale in psychopharmacology research. In: Pichot P, ed. Psychological measurements in psychopharmacology: modern problems in pharmacopsychiatry. Basel: Karger, 1974:67–78.
11. Overall JE, Rhoades HM. Refinement of phenomenological classification in clinical psychopharmacology research. Psychopharmacology 1982;77:24–30.
12. Kulhara P, Chadda R. A study of negative symptoms in schizophrenia and depression. Comp Psychiatry 1987;28:229–235.
13. Thiemann S, Csernansky JG, Berger, PA. Rating scales in research: the case of negative symptoms. Psychiatry Res 1987;20:47–55.
14. Dingemans PM. The brief psychiatric rating scale (BPRS) and the nurses' observation scale for inpatient evaluation (NOSIE) in the evaluation of positive and negative symptoms. J Clin Psychol 1990;46:168–174.
15. Newcomer JW, Faustman WO, Yeh W, Csernansky JG. Distinguishing depression and negative symptoms in unmedicated patients with schizophrenia. Psychiatry Res 1990;31:243–250.
16. Kay SR, Fiszbein A, Opler LA. The positive and negative syndrome scale (PANSS) for schizophrenia. Schizophr Bull 1987;13:261–276.
17. Gabbard GO, Coyne L, Kennedy LL, et al. Interrater reliability in the use of the brief psychiatric rating scale. Bull Menninger Clin 1987;51:519–531.
18. Tarell JD, Schulz SC. Nursing assessment using the BPRS: a structured interview. Psychopharmacol Bull 1988;24:105–111.
19. Flemenbaum A, Zimmermann RL. Inter- and intra-rater reliability of the brief psychiatric rating scale. Psychol Rep 1973;36:783–792.
20. Borison RL, Sinha D, Haverstock S, McLarnon MC, Diamond BI. Efficacy and safety of tiospirone vs. haloperidol and thioridazine in a

double-blind, placebo-controlled trial. Psychopharmacol Bull 1989;25:190–193.

21. den Boer JA, Ravelli DP, Huisman J, Ohrvik J, Verhoeven WMA, Westenberg HGM. A double-blind comparative study of remoxipride and haloperidol in acute schizophrenia. Acta Psychiatr Scand 1990;82(Suppl 358):108–110.

22. Tandon R, Mann NA, Eisner WH, Coppard N. Effect of anticholinergic medication on positive and negative symptoms in medication-free schizophrenic patients. Psychiatry Res 1990;31: 235–241.

23. Abraham KR, Kulhara P. The efficacy of electroconvulsive therapy in the treatment of schizophrenia: a comparative study. Br J Psychiatry 1987;151:152–155.

24. Feighner JP, Merideth CH, Claghorn JL. Multicenter placebo-controlled evaluation of nomi-fensine treatment in depressed outpatients. J Clin Psychiatry 1984;45:47–51.

25. Raskin A, Crook TH. Sensitivity of rating scales completed by psychiatrists, nurses, and patients to antidepressant drug effects. J Psychiatr Res 1976;13:31–41.

26. Faustman WO, Moses JA Jr, Csernansky JG, White PA. Correlations between the MMPI and the brief psychiatric rating scale in schizophrenic and schizoaffective patients. Psychiatry Res 1989;28:135–143.

27. Gur RE, Mozley D, Resnick SM, et al. Relations among clinical scales in schizophrenia. Am J Psychiatry 1991;148:472–478.

28. Pull CB, Overall JE. Adequacy of the brief psychiatric rating scale for distinguishing lesser forms of psychopathology. Psychol Rep 1977;40: 167–173.

# CHAPTER 20

# The Family Burden Interview Schedule–Short Form (FBIS/SF)

*Richard C. Tessler, Gail M. Gamache*

### DESCRIPTION AND BACKGROUND

*Formal Name*
    The Family Burden Interview Schedule-Short Form (FBIS/SF).

*Authors*
    Richard C. Tessler, Ph.D., and Gail M. Gamache, Ph.D.

*Key References*
Tessler RC, Gamache GM. Toolkit for evaluating family experiences with severe mental illness. Cambridge, MA: Human Services Research Institute, 1995.

Tessler RC, Gamache GM. Continuity of care, residence and family burden in Ohio. Milbank Q 1994;72:149–169.

## INTRODUCTION

The FBIS/SF was developed in the tradition of a line of research on the family experience going back to the early days of deinstitutionalization in which family caregiving was conceptualized as a burden (1). The FBIS/SF is a specially modified version of the longer Family Experiences Interview Schedule (2).

## DOMAINS AND NUMBER OF ITEMS

The measurement of the burdensome aspects of caregiving hinges largely on the definition of burden. Burden is a very general concept, referring to a broad range of difficulties (3). The consequences of being related to someone suffering from severe mental illness can be roughly divided into the obligation to offer long-term care and the emotional distress and worries associated with a family member with mental illness. Some family members may provide a great deal of assistance and yet feel quite content, whereas others may do less objective caregiving and yet feel very unhappy about the load they are carrying.

The FBIS/SF takes a multidimensional approach and distinguishes different aspects of burden from one another. The following objective and subjective dimensions of burden associated with caring for or caring about a relative with mental illness are measured: care given with the activities of daily life, supervision of bothersome or troublesome behaviors (3), impact on daily routines (4), financial expenditures (5), and worry. There are 65 items.

## APPLICATION

### Target Population

The target population consists of primary family caregivers of adults aged 18–64 with severe mental illness and residing in the same home or elsewhere in the community. It is also appropriate for other family members. This protocol is not intended for studies of caregiving to minor children with serious emotional disorders or to the elderly with dementia.

### Data Collection Procedures

The interview can be conducted face to face or over the telephone. The time frame for most questions is the past 30 days. Interviewers do not need to have a clinical background but do require training in structured interviewing. Each question is to be read exactly as it is worded and in the order in which it appears in the questionnaire. Underlined words are to be emphasized. Interviewer instructions appear in capital letters, enclosed by parentheses and are not to be read to the respondent. When the interviewer instructions are underlined, that means to substitute a word, usually a person's name for the word or phrase in capital letters. Thus, "(NAME)" in this interview would be substituted by the name of the patient. We estimate the interview would take about 15 minutes to administer. When a question ends with a question mark (such as questions about financial expenditures), the interviewer stops at that point without reading any responses and records the answer as given by the respondent. When the stem or lead-in question ends with a colon, the fixed responses are read to the respondent so they can choose the one that best fits their experience.

The FBIS/SF is available in English only. It was used with ethnically diverse families in the evaluation of the Robert Wood Johnson Foundation (RWJF) Program on Chronic Mental Illness (6).

### Psychometric Properties

Although researchers may choose to modify the scales and indices somewhat based on their own psychometric analyses (e.g., to delete a given item if it does not meet a chosen criterion), the recommendation is to use the measures as described to ensure comparability across studies. Prior analyses (including factor analyses) have indicated acceptable psychometric properties. Reliability coefficients were computed for two independent samples: 305 family members as part of the evaluation of the RWJF Program on Chronic Mental Illness and 176 family members as part of the assessment of the Assertive Community Treatment Program in Connecticut. Cronbach's $\alpha$ for the two samples are objective assistance in daily living, 0.777 and

791 0.791; for subjective assistance in daily living, 0.742 and 0.761; objective supervision, 0.650 and 0.612; subjective supervision, 0.638 and 0.676; impact, 0.568 and 0.564; and worry, 0.891 and 0.798. The low internal consistency coefficients reported for supervision were not unexpected because issues of control occur much more sporadically than problems in daily living, especially within a 30-day period. The supervision measures are more properly viewed as indices rather than scales. Impact is considered an index measure of the quantitative impact on family respondents' daily routines. The low $\alpha$ indicate that disruption in one area does not necessarily imply disruption in another area. Financial expenditures is a summary total of dollar amounts given, and thus computing a reliability coefficient is not appropriate.

## UTILITY

### Scoring Manual

The design of the FBIS/SF includes five modules related to the negative aspects of caregiving. The items in each module are numbered separately so that modules may be used independently of each other. For example, assistance with the activities of daily living has a theoretical range of 0–4, where 0 is not at all, 1 is less than once a week, 2 is once or twice a week, 3 is three to six times a week, and 4 is everyday. The scores for the items in this module are averaged. Thus, a mean score of 1.5 on the ADL Care Scale (items A1a, A2a, A3a, A4a, A5a, A6a, A7a, and A8a) indicates that the average frequency of ADL caregiving was about once a week.

### Automation

There is no automated version.

### Permission to Use

No fee is charged for its use, and permission to use is granted by contacting Richard Tessler, Ph.D., Sociology Department, Thompson Hall, University of Massachusetts, Amherst, MA 01003-7525, Telephone: 413-545-5980.

## Description of Where and When Used

An expanded version of the FBIS, the Family Experiences Interview Schedule, was used in an evaluation of the RWJF Program on Chronic Mental Illness in three cities in Ohio (6). A number of other investigators have also used, or are presently using, the longer version (2).

## SUMMARY OF STRENGTHS AND LIMITATIONS

The FBIS/SF addresses an important topic of increasing interest as cost-containment efforts in both the private and public sector limit professional intervention. These cost-containment efforts are likely to shift some of the caretaking currently provided by professionals to family members. Other strengths of the FBIS/SF are that it is brief and easy to use by nonprofessionals, it does not require interviewer judgment in the scoring, it is multidimensional in scope, and there is a low respondent burden.

The limitation of the short-form version is that some domains available in the longer version are not included: the modules for measuring respondent and patient background, contact, family enumeration, stigma, the benefits and gratification of caregiving, and attitudes toward professionals.

## REFERENCES

1. Fisher GA, Benson PR, Tessler RC. Family response to mental illness: developments since deinstitutionalization. In: Greenley JR, ed. Mental disorder in social context. Greenwich, CT: JAI Press Inc., 1990:203–236.
2. Tessler RC, Gamache GM. Toolkit for evaluating family experiences with severe mental illness. Cambridge, MA: Human Services Research Institute, 1995.
3. Creer CE, Sturt E, Wykes T. The role of relatives. In: Wing JK, ed. Long-term community care: experience in a London borough. London: Cambridge University Press, 1982:29.
4. Platt SA, Weyman A, Hirsch S, Hewitt S. The social behavior assessment schedule: rationale, contents, scoring and reliability of a new interview schedule. Soc Psychiatry 1980;15:43–55.
5. Franks DD. Economic contribution of families caring for persons with severe and persistent mental illness. Admin Policy Mental Health 1990;18:9–18.
6. Tessler RC, Gamache GM. Continuity of care, residence and family burden in Ohio. Milbank Q 1994;72:149–169.

CHAPTER 21

# Clinician Rating Scales: Alcohol Use Scale (AUS), Drug Use Scale (DUS), and Substance Abuse Treatment Scale (SATS)

*Robert E. Drake, Kim T. Mueser, Gregory J. McHugo*

## DESCRIPTION AND BACKGROUND

*Formal Name*

Alcohol Use Scale (AUS), Drug Use Scale (DUS), and Substance Abuse Treatment Scale (SATS).

*Authors*

Robert E. Drake, M.D., Ph.D., Kim T. Mueser, Ph.D., and Gregory J. McHugo, Ph.D.

*Key References*

Drake RE, Osher FC, Noordsy DL, Hurlbut SC, Teague GB, Beaudett MS. Diagnosis of alcohol use disorders in schizophrenia. Schizophr Bull 1990;16:57–67.

McHugo GJ, Drake RE, Burton HL, Ackerson TH. A scale for assessing the stage of substance abuse treatment in persons with severe mental illness. J Nerv Ment Dis (in press).

## INTRODUCTION

Over the past decade, families clinicians, and mental health administrators have become increasingly aware of the problem of co-occurring substance use disorders in persons with severe mental illness, also termed dual diagnosis (1, 2). Research has established several key findings regarding co-occurring disorders. First, substance disorder in persons with severe mental illness is extremely common (3). Second, substance abuse among persons with severe mental illness often has extremely negative clinical effects, such as precipitating relapses and increasing suicidality or violence; adverse medical consequences, such as vulnerability to human immunodeficiency virus infection; precipitating psychosocial instability, such as financial problems and homelessness; and higher treatment costs (4–8). Third, evidence continues to emerge that substance abuse in this population responds to treatment when mental health and substance abuse interventions are integrated at the clinical level (9). Fourth, because of numerous problems in assessing substance abuse in this population, reliable and valid assessment depends on close clinical observation (10).

## DOMAINS AND NUMBER OF ITEMS

The AUS and the DUS were developed to help clinicians assess and monitor substance use in persons with severe mental illness. Each scale incorporates Diagnostic and Statistical Manual for Mental Disorders, 3rd edition, revised (DSM-III-R) criteria, which can be modified in accordance with further revisions of the DSM. The AUS and DUS use a clinicians' rating to classify patients in categories that correspond to DSM-III-R criteria and to clinical distinctions that are considered meaningful for this population: abstinent, use without impairment, abuse, dependence, and dependence with institutionalization. Consistent with DSM-III-R criteria, abuse is defined as a pattern of substance use that leads to significant impairment or distress in vocational, social, emotional, or medical functioning or results in recurrent use in situations that are physically hazardous. These criteria can be tailored to persons with severe mental illness because they typically experience negative effects such as an inability to manage mental illness, money, housing, or rehabilitation when they are abusing a substance. Dependence involves greater severity of the addiction process; when patients have difficulty maintaining themselves outside of institutional or homeless settings because of their involvement with substances, they are rated as severely dependent.

The ratings document an individual's pattern of use for all psychoactive substances, not just the usual categories of abused drugs. Because dually diagnosed patients improve over months and brief changes are often not predictive, we recommend a time frame of 6 months for the ratings.

A companion scale, the SATS, was developed to aid in matching dually diagnosed persons with appropriate interventions and to assess and monitor their progress toward recovery from substance disorders (11). Empirical observations by clinicians and patients' self-reports indicated that persons with severe mental illness typically recover from substance use disorders in a sequential fashion. The SATS differentiates eight stages, defined with behavioral criteria, that corresponded to treatment needs and behavioral progress.

## APPLICATION

### Target Population

The clinician rating scales are intended for use with individuals with severe mental illness—those who are typically treated in state mental health systems because of severe disability, heavy service utilization, and lack of private insurance. Their diagnoses typically include schizophrenia and related disorders, severe bipolar and other mood disorders, and severe personality disorders.

### Data Collection Procedures

To use the clinician rating scales effectively, clinicians must be trained to understand the effects of alcohol and other drugs, the specific anchors used on these scales, and the DSM criteria for substance abuse and dependence. Furthermore, clinicians should supplement their direct observations of the patient with interviews using standardized instruments, information from collaterals (e.g., other providers, family members, law enforcement officers), regular urine drug testing, history as recorded in clinical records, and familiarity with available psychiatric assessments.

This procedure relies on the clinician to be active in pursuing and synthesizing information from multiple sources. It assumes that case managers or other clinicians know their patients well, understand the various clinical presentations of substance use disorders, are trained to use the instruments, and are unbiased in their assessments. Once trained, clinicians can classify their patients on the clinician rating scales in a few minutes.

Clinician ratings should always be validated by other data in a research study and, when the study involves a comparison of programs, clinician ratings should be examined separately from more objective measures of substance abuse.

Currently, the rating scales are available in English only.

### Psychometric Properties

The AUS is reliable, sensitive, and specific when used by case managers who follow their mentally ill patients over time in the community (12, 13). Test-retest reliabilities over a period of 1–2 weeks on small samples have been close to 100%. Interrater reliabilities, established by comparing ratings of clinical case managers and team psychiatrists, have yielded κ coefficients between 80 0.80 and 95 0.95 for current use on the AUS and DUS (7). When AUS ratings were compared with consensus diagnoses generated by a team of experienced psychiatrists using all clinical, research, and treatment data available for each patient to establish a current diagnosis of substance abuse or dependence, the AUS achieved a high sensitivity (94.7%) and specificity (100%) (14). An independent study used the AUS and the DUS to rate recent and past alcohol and drug use disorders, each separately, and found intraclass coefficient correlations ranging between 58 0.58 and 82. 0.82 (15).

Initial studies of the SATS also indicate high interrater and test-retest reliability, typically with intraclass correlations around 90. 0.90 (11). Clinician ratings of the SATS also correspond strongly to ratings made by researchers (average correlation = 70) 0.70). Correlations are in the 3 to .6 0.3–0.6 range on measures of similar constructs, such as patient self-reports about alcohol and drug use obtained via the Time-Line Follow-Back (16), used to assess convergent validity. As a measure of discriminant validity, SATS ratings are correlated with assessments of progress in other functional domains in the 0–0.3 range. In our field trials, trained case managers who have caseloads of 35 or less and work with their patients in the community are able to make ratings with a high degree of validity.

## UTILITY

### Scoring Manual and Ease of Interpretation

No scoring manual is necessary as both the instructions and the rating categories appear on the scales themselves. The ratings should be treated as ordinal and not interval or ratio scores. Training in the use of clinician substance abuse assessment scales can be divided into five steps: introduction to the concepts, description of the specific scale, practice and discussion using the scale (including vignettes and actual patients), reliability checks, and validity checks. Mental health clinicians who are familiar with the effects of alcohol and other drugs can learn to use these scales reliably within 1 hour of additional train-

ing. Validity depends on the time and energy a clinician has to acquire multimodal data. Norms for culturally diverse groups are not available.

### Automation

No automated version has been developed.

### Permission to Use

The scales are in the public domain, and no permission is required for their use. The AUS, DUS, SATS, and related publications are available from the New Hampshire-Dartmouth Psychiatric Research Center, Main Building, 105 Pleasant Street, Concord, NH 03301. They can also be obtained as part of a detailed assessment toolkit from the Health Services Research Institute, 2336 Massachusetts Avenue, Cambridge, MA 02140.

### Description of When and Where Used

The clinician rating scales described in this chapter were originally developed at the New Hampshire-Dartmouth Psychiatric Research Center for case managers to use in assessing their patients' substance use status. Subsequently, the scales have been used for clinical and research purposes across the United States, and many are now incorporated as part of standardized data collection in the New Hampshire mental health system. The scales can also be used in research evaluations if formal instruments and explicit decision rules are established for combining data into these ratings.

## SUMMARY OF STRENGTHS AND LIMITATIONS

Clinicians have access to a great deal of relevant information about the patients they wish to rate, and these scales provide a structured format for using multiple types and sources of data to assess substance disorder and its treatment. Although individual substance abuse assessment instruments have poor reliability and validity in this population, these clinician rating scales offer a brief, simple format for evaluating patients, offering them appropriate treatments, and monitoring their progress over time.

A limitation of the clinician rating scales is that they are not intended to serve the function of a comprehensive evaluation for the purpose of treatment planning. A more complex approach, suitable for a thorough clinical assessment of the dually diagnosed patient, includes the four tasks of detection, classification, detailed assessment, and treatment planning in a process of reciprocal feedback (10).

Another limitation of the clinician rating scales is that they are currently tied to DSM-III-R criteria rather than DSM-IV criteria. This occurs because we are in the middle of studies using the current scales and because the criteria of destabilizing emotional adjustment or a medical disorder (including psychiatric disorder) have been dropped between versions of the DSM. For users in clinical programs, DSM-IV criteria can easily be substituted into the scales.

## REFERENCES

1. Lehman AT, Dixon L, eds. Substance abuse among persons with chronic mental illness. New York: Harwood Academic Publishers, 1995.
2. Minkoff K, Drake RE, eds. Major mental illness and substance disorder. San Francisco: Jossey-Bass, 1991.
3. Mueser KT, Bennett M, Kushner MG. Epidemiology of substance abuse among persons with chronic mental disorders. In: Lehman AF, Dixon L, eds. Substance abuse among persons with chronic mental illness. New York: Harwood Academic Publishers, 1995.
4. Bartels SJ, Teague GB, Drake RE, Clark RE, Bush P, Noordsy DL. Substance abuse in schizophrenia: service utilization and costs. J Nerv Ment Dis 1993;181:227–232.
5. Clark RE. Family costs associated with severe mental illness and substance use: a comparison of families with and without dual disorders. Hosp Community Psychiatry 1994;45:808–813.
6. Cournos F, Empfield M, Horwath E, et al. HIV seroprevalence among patients admitted to two psychiatric hospitals. Am J Psychiatry 1991; 149:1225–1229.
7. Drake RE, Wallach MA. Substance abuse among the chronic mentally ill. Hosp Community Psychiatry 1989;40:1041–1046.
8. Yesavage JA, Zarcone V. History of drug abuse and dangerous behavior in inpatient schizophrenics. J Clin Psychiatry 1983;44:259–261.
9. Drake RE, Mueser KT, Clark RE. The course and treatment outcome of substance disorder in patients with severe mental illness. Am J Orthopsychiatry (in press).
10. Drake RE, Mercer-McFadden C. Assessment of substance abuse among persons with severe mental disorder. In: Lehman AT, Dixon L, eds. Substance abuse among persons with chronic mental illness. New York: Harwood Academic Publishers, 1995.
11. McHugo GJ, Drake RE, Burton HL, Ackerson TH. A scale for assessing the stage of substance abuse treatment in persons with severe mental illness. J Nerv Ment Dis 1995;183:560–565.
12. Drake RE, Osher FC, Noordsy DL, Hurlbut SC, Teague GB, Beaudett MS. Diagnosis of alcohol use disorders in schizophrenia. Schizophr Bull 1990;16:57–67.
13. Drake RE, Osher FC, Wallach MA. Alcohol use and abuse in schizophrenia: a prospective community study. J Nerv Ment Dis 1989;177: 408–414.
14. Drake RE, Osher FC, Noordsy DL, Hurlbut SC, Teague GB, Beaudett MS. Diagnosis of alcohol use disorders in schizophrenia. Schizophr Bull 1990;16:57–67.
15. Mueser KT, Nishith P, Tracey JI, Degiralamo J, Mulinaro M. Expectations and motives for substance use in schizophrenia. Schizophr Bull (in press).
16. Sobell LC, Sobell MB, Leo GI, Cancilla A. Reliability of a timeline method: assessing normal drinkers' reports of recent drinking and a comparative evaluation across several populations. Br J Addict 1988;83:393–402.

# CHAPTER 22

# Quality of Life Interview (QOLI)

*Anthony F. Lehman*

## INTRODUCTION

The purpose of the QOLI is to assess the recent and current life circumstances of persons with severe mental illnesses. Interest in assessing the quality of life among patients is increasing as treatment shifts to community-based services, even for the most seriously mentally ill.

## DOMAINS AND NUMBER OF ITEMS

The QOLI contains 153 items that measure global life satisfaction as well as objective and subjective QOL in eight life domains: living situation, daily activities and functioning, family relations, social relations, finances, work and school, legal and safety issues, and health. The sections on each life domain are organized so that information first is obtained about objective QOL and then about level of life satisfaction in that life area. This pairing of objective and subjective quality of life indicators by domain is essential to the quality of life assessment model (1).

Examples of objective QOL indicators are length of time at current residence, quality of living circumstances, frequency of social contacts, current employment status, victim of violent or nonviolent crime during the past year, and general health status. Examples of subjective QOL indicators are satisfaction with living situation, family relations, social relations, work, and health.

## APPLICATION

### Target Population

The QOLI was developed for use with persons with severe and persistent mental illnesses, primarily in community-based settings, but it has been adapted for use with patients in long-term institutions.

### Data Collection Procedures

The QOLI is a structured interview administered by trained lay interviewers and requires approximately 45 minutes to administer. A brief 15-minute version is currently under field testing. It is not formally available in languages other than English, although investigators elsewhere have adapted it to Spanish and French. It has been used with patient groups in the United States, Canada, Britain, and various other European countries. In the United States, patient populations have consisted primarily of caucasians and African-Americans.

## Psychometric Properties

Internal consistency reliabilities range from 0.79 to 0.88 for the life satisfaction scales and from 0.44 to 0.82 for the objective QOL scales. These reliabilities have been replicated in two separate studies of persons with severe mental illnesses (1). Test-retest reliabilities (1 week) are 0.41–0.95; objective QOL scales are 0.20–0.98.

Construct and predictive validity have been assessed as good by confirmatory factor analyses and multivariate predictive models (2). The QOLI differentiates between patients living in hospitals and supervised community residential programs in the United States and Britain (3, 4). Individual life satisfaction items clearly discriminate between persons with severe mental illness and the general population (5). Further construct validation has been assessed in studies of predictors of QOL among day treatment patients in Britain (6) and the relationship between QOL and feelings of empowerment among persons with severe mental illness in the United States (7). Convergent validity of the Lehman QOLI with the Heinrichs-Carpenter Quality of Life Scale is significant (8).

A variety of methodological papers has explored other issues, such as the relationship between QOL and clinical symptoms (9), gender and age (10), and housing type (11, 12). Factor analyses of the pooled objective QOL items have not been done because they have quite different formats and their contents address quite different issues (e.g., income level, number of arrests, frequency of family contacts). The intercorrelations among these objective domains tend to be minimal in this population. Exploratory and confirmatory factor analyses of the subjective QOLI items, in general, have strongly supported the hypothesized structure of the life satisfaction domains.

## UTILITY
### Scoring Manual

The QOLI can be used for cross-sectional group comparisons, longitudinal monitoring of within group QOL, and longitudinal comparisons of between group outcomes. A scoring manual is available. A users toolkit will also become available from the Health Services Research Institute in 1995.

All of the life satisfaction scores are based on a seven-point Likert scale, ranging from delighted to terrible. The objective indicators include Likert scales that rate, for example, frequency of social contacts; common quantitative units of amount of income in dollars or number of types of common daily activities undertaken in the past week; or categorical responses such as the respondent's type of residence, whether the respondent has been a crime victim, or whether the respondent has been arrested. Norms have been published for various subgroups of patients with severe and persistent mental illnesses (10) and comparisons with national norms of life satisfaction for the general population have been made (13).

### Automation

No automated version exists.

### Permission to Use

The QOLI is available in the public domain at nominal cost for a single copy. There are no users' fees.

### Description of Where and When Used

The QOLI was first developed in 1980 for use in a survey of severely mentally ill persons living in large board and care homes in Los Angeles (2, 5). Subsequently, the QOLI was used to compare the QOL experiences of severely mentally ill persons living in state hospital and community residential settings in Rochester, New York

(3). More recently, the QOLI has been adapted by the author for use in the national evaluation of the Robert Wood Johnson Program on Chronic Mental Illness (13), for a study of dually diagnosed patients in Baltimore (Lehman, Postrado, Kernan, Scott, unpublished data), and for an evaluation of Assertive Community Treatment Programs in Baltimore (14). In addition, the QOLI has been used by a number of researchers throughout the United States and in various other countries, particularly in Canada and Europe.

## SUMMARY OF STRENGTHS AND LIMITATIONS

The major strengths of the QOLI are its broad-based assessment of QOL, specifically for persons with severe and persistent mental illnesses; its potential value in research settings; and it use in service planning for individuals. Its psychometric properties have been well studied and are rated good to excellent. Normative data are available for various subgroups of patients, and the life satisfaction items can be compared with national norms in the general population.

The limitations include its length, a large number of variables generated without an overall summary score, and the fact that it has not been used with the general population or with other nonmentally ill patient groups.

## REFERENCES

1. Lehman AF. A Quality of Life Interview for the chronically mentally ill. Eval Prog Planning 1988;11:51–62.
2. Lehman AF. The well-being of chronic mental patients: assessing their quality of life. Arch Gen Psychiatry 1983a;40:369–373.
3. Lehman AF, Possidente S, Hawker F. The quality of life of chronic mental patients in a state hospital and community residences. Hosp Community Psychiatry 1986;37:901–907.
4. Simpson CJ, Hyde CE, Faragher EB. The chronically mentally ill in community facilities: a study of quality of life. Br J Psychiatry 1989; 154:77–82.
5. Lehman AF, Ward NC, Linn LS. Chronic mental patients: the quality of life issue. Am J Psychiatry 1982;139:1271–1276.
6. Levitt AJ, Hogan TP, Bucosky CM. Quality of life in chronically mentally ill patients in day treatment. Psychol Med 1990;20:703–710.
7. Rosenfield S, Neese-Todd S. Elements of a psychosocial clubhouse program associated with a satisfying quality of life. Hosp Community Psychiatry 1993;44;76–78.
8. Lehman AF, Postrado LT, Rachuba LT. Convergent validation of quality of life assessments for persons with severe mental illnesses. Qual Life Res 1993;2:327–333.
9. Lehman AF. The effects of psychiatric symptoms on quality of life assessments among the chronic mentally ill. Eval Prog Planning 1983b; 6:143–151.
10. Lehman AF, Slaughter JC, Myers CP. Quality of life of the chronically mentally ill: gender and decade of life effects. Eval Prog Planning 1992; 15:7–12.
11. Slaughter JC, Lehman AF. Quality of life of severely mentally ill adults in residential care facilities. Adult Residential Care J 1991;5:97–111.
12. Lehman AF, Slaughter JC, Myers CP. The quality of life of chronically mentally ill persons in alternative residential settings. Psychiatric Q 1991;62:35–49.
13. Lehman AF, Postrado LT, Roth D, McNary, SW, Goldman HH. Continuity of care and client outcomes in the Robert Wood Foundation Program on Chronic Mental Illness. Milbank Q 1994;72:105–122.
14. Dixon LB, Krauss N, Kernan E, et al. Modifying the PACT model to serve homeless persons with severe mental illness. Psychiatr Serv 1995;46: 684–688.

CHAPTER 23

# The Client Satisfaction Questionnaire (CSQ) Scales and the Service Satisfaction Scale-30 (SSS-30)

*C. Clifford Attkisson, Thomas K. Greenfield*

---

## DESCRIPTION AND BACKGROUND

*Formal Names*
Client Satisfaction Questionnaire (CSQ-8, CSQ-18 Forms A and B, and CSQ-31) and the Service Satisfaction Scale-30 (SSS-30)

*Authors*
C. Clifford Attkisson and Daniel L. Larsen in collaboration with William A. Hargreaves, Maurice LeVois, Tuan D. Nguyen, Robert E. Roberts, and Bruce Stegner (CSQ); and Thomas K. Greenfield, C. Clifford Attkisson, and Gregory C. Pascoe (SSS-30).

*Key References*
Attkisson CC, Greenfield TK. The Client Satisfaction Questionnaire-8

and the Service Satisfaction Questionnaire-30. In: Maruish ME, ed. The use of psychological testing for treatment planning and outcome assessment. Hillsdale, NJ: Lawrence Erlbaum Associates, 1994.

Attkisson CC, Pascoe GC, eds. Patient satisfaction in health and mental health services. Eval Prog Planning 1983;6(Suppl 3 and 4):185–418.

Greenfield TK, Attkisson CC. Progress toward a multifactorial Service Satisfaction Scale for evaluating primary care and mental health services. Eval Prog Planning 1989; 12:271–278.

## INTRODUCTION

Consumer satisfaction has achieved the status of an important measurement domain in health and human service outcome assessment. Recent reviews and compendiums of outcome measures for health, mental health, and human services emphasize the value of information about consumers' satisfaction with services (1-3). Since 1975, a team of investigators at the University of California, San Francisco (UCSF) has used standard scale development methods to construct measures for assessing consumer satisfaction with health and human services. The products of this research program, the CSQ and the SSS scales, are

direct measures of service satisfaction designed to be used with a wide range of client groups and service types.

The CSQ instruments are self-report questionnaires constructed to measure satisfaction with services received by individuals and families. The scales have been broadly adopted, nationally and internationally, by investigators and service program personnel who use the instruments for scientific work, evaluation research, and program planning. The most important of the early scales included the CSQ-8 and the CSQ-18 (the latter having parallel Forms A and B).

The Service Satisfaction Scale-30 (SSS-

30) was designed to assess multiple factors of service provision with a special focus on those conceptual factors identified as most salient by consumers of health and human services. Items were written "generically" so as to make their content apply meaningfully across a broad range of health, mental health, and chemical dependency services.

## DOMAINS AND NUMBER OF ITEMS

### The CSQ

Using a logic model, items were drawn from a large pool of items written by Larsen et al. (4) covering nine conceptual domains of client satisfaction: physical surroundings; procedures; support staff; kind or type of service; treatment staff; quality of service; amount, length, or quantity of service; outcome of service; and general satisfaction. Factor and item analyses, conducted across a series of studies, resulted in several unidimensional measures, each having somewhat different applied utility. In addition to an eight-item version, called the CSQ-8 (5), alternate forms of the CSQ-31 were constructed, each containing 18 items (6). The parallel 18-item forms (the CSQ-18A and CSQ-18B) are suitable for test-retest applications. Form B of the CSQ-18 includes the CSQ-8 items. Finally, shorter versions have been used for applications in which a very brief indicator is required (e.g., the CSQ-4 [7] or the CSQ-3 [8]).

### The SSS-30

The SSS-30 uses items that are less global and more specific than the CSQ item sets. In combination with the changed scaling, the introduction of more differentiated item content has yielded a strong foundation for a multifactorial instrument. With the SSS-30, we achieved the capacity to discriminate among service-related components with a scale that can measure differential levels of satisfaction with several components of the service delivery process. Factor analyses of consumer ratings within primary care and mental health outpatient services yielded two stable, replicated SSS-30 subscales: Practitioner Manner and Skill (nine items) and Perceived Outcome (eight items). Two additional though less stable dimensions were also found. However, these latter factors were not consistently identified across settings: Office Procedures (five items) and Accessibility (four items).

## APPLICATION

### Target Populations

The measures have been adopted in quality assurance, evaluation research, and services research studies across a wide range of health and human services (7, 9–11). Service settings studied include mental health and public health center clinics, primary care health clinics and health maintenance organizations, employee assistance programs, mandatory short-term alcohol abuse treatment programs for drunk drivers, residential alcoholism treatment programs, community-based residential care, case management for the individuals with severe mental disorder, and with AIDS self-support and psychoeducational groups (9, 12–21).

### Data Collection Procedures

Data gained from the CSQ scales are typically self-reported, but aural responses have been collected from individuals with serious mental disorder in hospital acute care, day treatment, and case management studies (21). Before presentation of the CSQ scale items, standard instructions are presented to respondents: "Please help us improve our program by answering some questions about the services you have received. We are interested in your honest opinions, whether they are positive or negative. Please answer all the questions. We also welcome your comments and suggestions. Thank you very much, we really appreciate your help."

Following presentation of the CSQ items, service recipients are thanked and invited to give additional open-ended comments: "The thing I have liked best about my experience here is... What I liked least was... If I could change one thing about the service it would be...."

Administration of the CSQ and SSS scales is relatively straightforward. Mail survey methods have sometimes been used for collecting the data (10). The main disadvantage of mail surveys is low response rates, 40–50% being the highest typically achieved in instances with one follow-up postcard reminder (7). The recommended approach is to use point of service surveys with a designated scale administrator or a receptionist trained in procedures for systematically soliciting voluntary participation from sampled clients. Various sampling approaches have been used: systematic or random samples of client rosters, samples stratified by duration or quantity of services received, and census samples of all clients seen during a specific time frame (17, 18). The latter approach has the advantage of assuring that most eligible clients are included. Completion rates tend to be above 90% when this approach is used. This method, however, tends to bias the sample toward clients who are in the initial phase of care, and it is important to stratify sampling to include sufficient numbers of service recipients across the spectrum of service provision.

Follow-up surveys after cessation or completion of services is also very important. The practical problem of surveying satisfaction at increasing time intervals after termination or cessation of services is the expected attenuation in response rate—a problem likely to confound interpretation of results. Most studies have used anonymous methods, though some have not and instead have included code numbers allowing linkage to service data. One methodological study with the CSQ found optionally identified (name written in at the option of the recipient) forms did not result in lower response rate or higher reported satisfaction (10). Despite the range of alternative approaches, the standard waiting room method meets well the simplicity and uniformity of implementation criterion.

## Psychometric Properties

The scales have highly desirable psychometric properties, including high levels of internal consistency and excellent consumer acceptability. The scales also function well in comparison with other methods of assessing service satisfaction (9, 12–15, 22). Twelve published studies report findings from surveys of 8,000 subjects in the scale development and refinement phase (3):

1. Internal consistency. The CSQ-8 and the CSQ-18A and 18B have demonstrated very high levels of internal consistency, as measured by Cronbach's $\alpha$ coefficients, which range from 0.83–0.93.
2. Item-total correlations. Moderately high item-total correlations were also reported and are consistent with the underlying single factor structure of the CSQ scales derived from factor analyses of the underlying data. These findings support the conclusion that the CSQ scales measure a global satisfaction construct.
3. Correlations among scale items. Interitem correlations were only moderately high, suggesting that beyond the global satisfaction factor there is additional variance due to error of measurement and/or differential responses to item content detected by respondents.
4. Comparison with other measures and methods. Various alternative methods were compared, including ranking methodologies (12, 14) and indirect and direct approaches to assessing satisfaction (15).
5. Negatively skewed score distributions. The CSQ scales almost always produce negatively skewed rating distributions when total raw scores or mean of item means are analyzed. Approximately 10% of respondents are generally found to be dissatisfied; however, it is difficult to distinguish degrees of satisfaction among the majority of respondents whose ratings accumulate at the most satisfied levels and cannot easily be distinguished from one another. These

findings stimulated our interest in continuing to develop multifactorial satisfaction measures that yield bell-shaped score distributions within factorial components.

During the second scale development phase, we wrote more refined and specific item pools and combined item pool enhancement with adoption of the Andrews and Withey (8) scaling approach used in the successful development of quality of life measures (13, 23, 24). This work culminated in the SSS-30 (13). The SSS-30 contains a broad array of specific items pertaining to the consumer experience of service access, acceptability, provision, and outcome. Second phase studies addressed several major problems:

1. Normalization of score distributions. To "normalize" the distribution of scores, alternative rating procedures have been introduced. Instead of the four-level rating scale used in the CSQ, the SSS instrument uses five- (and in one study, seven-) level anchored scales similar to those originally used in quality of life studies (10, 25). Work with the SSS series demonstrated that use of the more extreme "Delighted" and "Terrible" anchors reduced the ceiling effect and negative skew typical of CSQ results. Improved item scales and anchors used within the SSS scales result in less skewed item and subscale distributions that are suitable for multivariate and parametric analyses.

2. General versus specific factors. For subscales to have validity and interpretability (i.e., similar meaning) across settings, a basic requirement is that the factors on which they are based should have a high degree of replicability. Greenfield and Attkisson (18) and Greenfield (19, 20) provided evidence of factorial invariance across a range health and mental health service settings. Across several distinctly different types of service, the major factors of practitioner manner and skill satisfaction and perceived outcome satisfaction are well confirmed. Factors involving constructs such as satisfaction with office procedures and access to needed services appear much less stable across research study sites.

3. Psychometric properties. Available data on psychometric performance of the SSS-30 include norms from a general population primary-care medical outpatient service, a student mental health service (17, 18, 23), an employee assistance program (17), and repeat DUI offenders in a mandatory 15-session treatment program (19, 20). The SSS-30 total score can serve as a composite satisfaction measure with high internal consistency: Cronbach's $\alpha$ values have ranged from 0.93 to 0.96. In addition, several factor-based subscales have been identified in a series of studies. The two main subscales also have good internal reliability. Cronbach's $\alpha$ ranged from 0.83 to 0.93 (average 0.88) for the 9-item practitioner manner and skill subscale and from 0.80 to 0.90 (average 0.83) for the eight-item perceived outcome subscale. Internal reliability coefficients for the two smaller subscales are lower, ranging from 0.69 to 0.83 (average 0.74) for the five-item office procedures satisfaction subscale and from 0.60 to 0.75 (average 0.67) for the four-item access satisfaction subscale.

4. Correlation with the CSQ-8. The validity of the CSQ-8 as a general satisfaction measure is more well established than for the SSS-30 scale. The correlation between the SSS-30 total score (as a composite satisfaction indicator) and the CSQ-8 was examined in a drinking driving treatment program. The SSS-30 total raw score correlated 0.70 with the CSQ-8 total raw score, lending empirical support for the construct validity of the composite SSS-30 measure. In the drinking driving treatment study, the mean CSQ-8 score for treatment recipients was 27.21 (SD = 4.03) compared with the CSQ norm-group mean of 27.09 (SD = 4.01) (5).

## UTILITY
### Scoring

Scoring the closed-ended part of the CSQ and the SSS-30 scales involves unweighted summation of the direction-corrected response values (1–4 for all the CSQ scales and 1–5 for the SSS-30) for the total scales) and calculation of measures of central tendency (such as mean, standard deviation, median, and mode) of the individual item ratings and for the total scale scores and or for the SSS-30 factor scores. Scoring is not complicated and involves calculation of total score across all items for each subject and analyzing item and total score distributions across groups of subjects. Because of the scale's single factor structure, interpretation of CSQ-8 data involves a straightforward comparison of results obtained for a given service or client group with external data that constitute an appropriate norm, for example, the multiservice setting means and standard deviation results presented in Nguyen et al. (5).

### Automation

There are no published computer programs or automated methods available for use with the CSQ scales. The scales are easily scored and scanning may often be more time consuming than key-to-disk data entry for large-scale applications. All scanning applications must have prior permission from the authors because such automation requires use and modification of the authors' intellectual property.

### Permission to Use

Written permission is required for use of the CSQ and SSS-30 scales, and use is strictly limited to individuals and institutions who formally request permission directly from the authors. Prior written permission and payment of "per use" fees are required of all users. Because of the volume of requests received, it is not possible to respond to phone or voice mail requests. In addition, volume purchases are required, and the prepaid per use cost is currently 50¢ (U.S.) per use for the minimal order of 500 uses ($250 U.S.) with subsequent orders of 250 uses or more at 30¢ (U.S.) per use. Prices are subject to change to accommodate price increases for related supplies and materials. There are no exceptions to these policies. Specific inquiries and requests to use the scales must be addressed to the authors and sent via mail services or by FAX (415-476-9690 for Dr. Attkisson or 510-642-7175 for Dr. Greenfield). Response to initial inquiry is rapid and includes a current price schedule and reprints of basic published materials on the scales. Inquiries regarding the CSQ family of scales should be addressed to Dr. Attkisson and inquiries about the SSS-30 should be addressed to Dr. Greenfield.

The authors frequently receive requests for permission to modify the wording of scale items. Permission is never granted because such changes infringe on intellectual property of the authors; void or limit the normative comparisons available in the published literature; and may have significant effects on the psychometric performance of the items, scale factors, and the overall integrity of the scales. Users are asked to create their own site-specific items, if they deem it necessary to do so, and administer them after the satisfaction scale or separately as a part of a battery of measures.

### Description of Where and When Used

The CSQ-8 has received frequent citation in the scientific and professional literatures and has been adopted extensively for applied use within service settings and in research. The primary use of the CSQ scales, within practice settings, is to assess the aggregate satisfaction of groups of respondents and only rarely is the focus on the individual service recipient or surrogate. Although satisfaction scores have sometimes been treated as individual-level outcome measures, the usual application is to measure aggregate satisfaction levels of a group of consumers. The satisfaction scores have typically been used as outcome performance indicators for a service organization, clinic, or system of care. In these instances, it is critical to compare obtained scale scores (usually raw scale totals summed across all items and/or the mean of item means) against comparative norms from other service settings or from other time frames within the same setting. Using sampling and time-series methods, satisfaction levels can be compared across different service modalities, duration of service, types of clients, providers, or specific facilities.

The CSQ scales have been used with various subpopulations and language groups in the United States and abroad. Several of the CSQ scales have been translated into French, Spanish, and Dutch (26–29). The CSQ, translated using culturally sensitive translation methods, performed equivalently across several national and cultural groups. The most extensive cross-cultural work has been done in Spanish with Mexican-American and Latino populations (27, 30, 31).

The SSS-30 is intended for primary care medical settings and outpatient mental health services. Improved item scaling and content of the SSS-30 have resulted in factor-based subscales with improved psychometric properties that have enhanced suitability for multivariate and parametric analyses. Italian language versions of the SSS scales have been developed in Italy and empirical reports have been published (32, 33).

## SUMMARY OF STRENGTHS AND LIMITATIONS

The various phases of the UCSF research program have yielded important findings regarding use and interpretation of the CSQ and SSS measures. Scale development work has been primarily organized by empirical and practical considerations. The research has a strong conceptual framework and has produced measures that are face valid, thereby aiding specificity of assessment by consumers (24). Although our efforts have focused on improving the psychometric

properties of the measures and to control for threats to reliability and validity, investigation of the satisfaction construct has been a principal research agenda. Though our studies have emphasized examination of antecedent factors affecting service satisfaction, we have also turned to methods of studying behavioral consequences of patient satisfaction, for example, enrollment and disenrollment in health plans, compliance with medical regimens, prospective service use, and the relationship of early satisfaction to subsequent service use and outcome. The next generation of research studies will report on the use of the service satisfaction construct as an independent variable in relation to service use, cost, and outcome. The organizational structure of the system of care may also be strongly related to initial and long-term service satisfaction and service satisfaction may well be an important determinant of consumer behavior within the care system (28). These important relationships will be an inviting focus in future research.

In future research, investigators must also introduce improved control for variables that function as covariates of satisfaction: demographic and personal characteristics, socioeconomic status, and attitudes about health care. Age and gender effects are perhaps the most important candidates as covariates that may contribute variance to service satisfaction ratings (5, 22, 24), whereas life satisfaction and general attitudes toward the health care system have not been found in our research to be significantly related to direct measures of service satisfaction (16). Nevertheless, concurrent measurement of health care attitudes, life satisfaction ratings, and self-assessment of general health status can add significantly to overall precision and utility of a consumer satisfaction study. Within this framework, service satisfaction measures take an important place within the core array of outcome measures, health and functional indicators, and demographic classifications used in services research (3).

## REFERENCES

1. Ciarlo JA, Brown TR, Edwards DW, et al. Assessing mental health treatment outcome measurement techniques. Washington, DC: U.S. Government Printing Office, 1986. [DHHS Pub. No (ADM)6-1301.]
2. Hargreaves WA, Shumway M. Effectiveness of mental health services for the severely mentally ill. In: Taube CA, Mechanic D, Hohmann A, eds. The future of mental health services research. Washington, DC: U.S. Government Printing Office, l989. [DHHS Pub. No (ADM) 89-1600.]
3. Rosenblatt A, Attkisson CC. Assessing outcomes for sufferers of severe mental disorder: a conceptual framework and review. Eval Prog Planning 1993;16:347–363.
4. Larsen DL, Attkisson CC, Hargreaves WA, et al. Assessment of client/patient satisfaction: development of a general scale. Eval Prog Planning 1979;2:197–207.
5. Nguyen TD, Attkisson CC, Stegner BL. Assessment of patient satisfaction: development and refinement of a Service Evaluation Questionnaire. Eval Prog Planning 1983;6:299–313.
6. LeVois M, Nguyen TD, Attkisson CC. Artifact in client satisfaction assessment: experience in community mental health settings. Eval Prog Planning 1981;4:139–150.
7. Greenfield TK. The role of client satisfaction in evaluating university counseling services. Eval Prog Planning 1983;6:315–327.
8. Andrews FM, Withey SB. Social indicators of well-being: American perceptions of life quality. New York: Plenum, 1976.
9. Attkisson CC, Zwick R. The Client Satisfaction Questionnaire: psychometric properties and correlations with service utilization and psychotherapy outcome. Eval Prog Planning 1982; 5:233–237.
10. Kurtz LF. Measuring member satisfaction with a self-help association. Eval Prog Planning 1990;13:119–124.
11. Lebow JL. Research assessing consumer satisfaction with mental health treatment: a review of findings. Eval Prog Planning 1983;6:211–236.
12. Attkisson CC, Roberts RE, Pascoe GC. The Evaluation Ranking Scale: clarification of methodological problems and procedural issues. Eval Prog Planning 1983;6:349–358.
13. Pascoe GC. Consumer satisfaction with primary health care services: field test of a causal model (Doctoral Dissertation. University of California, San Francisco). Dissertat Abstr Int 1984;46: 1672–B.
14. Pascoe GC, Attkisson CC. The Evaluation Ranking Scale: a new methodology for assessing satisfaction. Eval Prog Planning 1983;6:335–347.
15. Pascoe GC, Attkisson CC, Roberts RE. Comparison of indirect and direct approaches to measuring patient satisfaction. Eval Prog Planning 1983;6:359–371.
16. Roberts RE, Pascoe GC, Attkisson CC. Relationship of service satisfaction to life satisfaction and perceived well-being. Eval Prog Planning 1983b;6:373–383.
17. Attkisson CC, Greenfield TK. The Client Satisfaction Questionnaire-8 and the Service Satisfaction Questionnaire-30. In Maruish ME, ed. The use of psychological testing for treatment planning and outcome assessment. Hillsdale, NJ: Lawrence Erlbaum Associates, 1994.
18. Greenfield TK, Attkisson CC Progress toward a multifactorial Service Satisfaction Scale for evaluating primary care and mental health services. Eval Prog Planning 1989;12:271–278.
19. Greenfield TK. Consumer satisfaction with the Delaware Drinking Driver Program in 1987–1988 (Report to the Delaware Drinker Driver Program). University of California, San Francisco, Department of Psychiatry, 1989.
20. Greenfield TK. Consumer satisfaction with the Delaware Drinking Driver Program in 1993. Berkeley, CA: Western Consortium for Public Health, 1994.
21. Schaefer SM. An evaluation of a multi-center hospital-based HIV case management pilot program at St. Paul Ramsey Medical Center/HIV Clinic and the University of Minnesota Hospital/HIV Clinic. Master's thesis. St. Mary's College Graduate Center, Minneapolis, Minnesota, 1992.
22. Attkisson CC, Pascoe GC, eds. Patient satisfaction in health and mental health services. Eval Prog Planning 1983;6(Suppl 3 and 4):185–418.
23. Attkisson CC, Greenfield TK, Spradling K. Consumer satisfaction study results: UCSF Student Health Service. San Francisco, CA: University of California, Graduate Division, 1986.
24. Pascoe GC. Patient satisfaction in primary care: a literature review and analysis. Eval Prog Planning 1983;6:185–210.
25. Lehman AF. A quality of life interview for the chronically mentally ill. Eval Prog Planning 1988;11:1–12.
26. de Brey H. A cross-national validation of the Client Satisfaction Questionnaire: the Dutch experience. Eval Prog Planning 1983;6:395–400.
27. Roberts RE, Attkisson CC. Assessing client satisfaction among Hispanics. Eval Prog Planning 1983;6:401–413.
28. Hirschman AO. Exit, voice, and loyalty: responses to decline in firms, organizations, and states. Cambridge, MA: Harvard University Press, 1970.
29. Sabourin S, Gendreau P, Frenette L. Le neveau de satisfaction des cas d'abandon dans un service universitaire de psychologie. Can J Behav Sci 1987;19:314–323.

30. Roberts RE, Attkisson CC, Stegner BL. A Client Satisfaction Scale: suitable for use with Hispanics? Hispanic J Behav Sci 1983a;5:461–476.

31. Roberts RE, Attkisson CC, Mendias RM. Assessing the Client Satisfaction Questionnaire in English and Spanish. Hispanic J Behav Sci 1984;6:385–396.

32. Ruggeri M, Dall'Agnola, Greenfield TK, et al. Factor analysis of the Verona Service Satisfaction Scale-82 and development of reduced versions. Int J Methods Psychiatric Res 1995;5: 147.1–147.16.

33. Ruggeri M, Greenfield TK. The Italian version of the Service Satisfaction Scale (SSS-30) adapted for community-based psychiatric patients: development, factor analysis and application. Eval Prog Planning 1995;18:191–202.

CHAPTER 24

# The Use of Outcomes Assessment in Managed Care: Past, Present, and Future

*Ronald D. Geraty*

## INTRODUCTION

The reform of the U.S. health care system now occupies a significant position on national, regional, and local political and business agendas. During the past few years, financing the cost of medical care has concerned consumers, payers, and providers. Efforts by employers to save money through "managing" care and by politicians to provide insurance for the uninsured have created a heightened public awareness about methods of health care delivery and strategies that can successfully provide care for everyone in need.

In particular, recent health care reform initiatives have focused on three primary goals: cost (including controlling the increase of costs), quality (including measuring and ensuring the quality of care), and access to care (including access for the uninsured). The private and public sectors have begun to focus attention on the use of managed care techniques; consequently, the reform movement has been accompanied by a closer scrutiny of managed care's ability to provide broad access to affordable, high-quality health care.

Within the field of mental health and substance abuse care, efforts to address the dilemmas of the health care system not only have reflected the existing concerns of all participants in the system but also have positively affected levels of sophistication as to the nature of the challenges presented and possible long-term solutions.

This chapter presents a historical perspective on the use of outcomes assessment in the management of mental health and substance abuse care by reviewing early methods for managing care delivery, discussing current managed care techniques and the study of outcomes, and providing a context for future investigation and implementation of outcomes assessment in a managed care environment.

## THE EVOLUTION OF MANAGED CARE

### Managed Access

During the early to mid-1980s, private sector mental health care consumers primarily accessed care through indemnity insurance policies that featured strong financial incentives toward the utilization of inpatient treatment. This reimbursement bias favoring expensive inpatient hospitalization over less restrictive care delivery settings—an imbalance that unfortunately bore only a limited relationship to fundamental concerns of clinical appropriateness and effectiveness—helped fuel an unintended growth in costs. In an attempt to control expenses, insurers contracted with utilization review (UR) firms to contain costs. Largely through administrative barriers, such as precertification requirements, the UR firms placed emphasis on restricting patient access to care. Limitations on access were designed to limit costs. Providers were essentially outsiders to the early UR process, which often employed nonclinical or nonpsychiatric reviewers. As a result, quality of care became the central point of contention by providers in an ongoing debate with proponents of UR.

Providers quickly became disenchanted with a disconnected process of nonpeer, third-party review that influenced professional practice via reimbursement decisions based on "confidential, proprietary" criteria. Many providers viewed UR cost containment measures as an unwarranted imposition on their ability to affect positive treatment results based on professional judgment and training. The atmosphere of the care delivery environment, therefore, was clouded by a conflict framed in terms of cost and access controls on the one hand and by reimbursement and quality concerns on the other. Worse yet, this system of *managed access* failed to contain costs appreciably.

**Managed Benefits**

Subsequently, the effort to gain control over runaway mental health care costs further evolved into a system of *managed benefits*. Within this framework, management companies used UR in conjunction with large discounted fee-for-service provider networks. The main emphasis was on management of patients' benefits through restrictions such as arbitrary annual coverage limitations, significant copays and deductibles, and benefit exclusions. Cost containment remained the overriding concern. Decreases in inpatient treatment costs were realized during the managed benefits era, but quality of care was not yet a prominent objective of the management mechanism. Precertification of treatment continued to be used, and treatment planning was a secondary consideration. Although providers, as members of networks, were "included" within the system, their care delivery was still "inspected."

Clinicians continued to harbor misgivings about the criteria and standards for reviewing the delivery of care, a situation exacerbated by a limited collegiality with those making UR decisions. From the clinician's point of view, the practice environment was further complicated by a multiplicity of external review agencies, each applying its own standards of necessary and appropriate care. Difficulties in attempting to deliver quality care to individual patients became amplified when each patient's treatment prospects were subject to one of a number of largely unknown review criteria sets. Given the absence of studies addressing the effect of UR activities on the outcome of mental health care, uncertainties about the clinical quality of the whole process intensified.

In 1994, a study examined data from the late 1980s on programs for the management of mental health and substance abuse care for 30 firms that employed approximately two million people (1). Findings revealed that very few of these firms used specialty behavioral managed care vendors and that for most of the firms the UR program for mental health and substance abuse was the same as UR for medical-surgical care in terms of vendor review, standards, and staff qualifications. Nonproprietary review criteria were used in only three of the programs. It was also found that as late as 1990, only 12 programs included outpatient review. After this time period, more advanced approaches began to take a stronger position in the care management industry.

**Managed Care**

The best efforts in managing the delivery of care next evolved into systems that could truly be characterized as *managed care*. As a core element of managed care systems, utilization management techniques are applied to quality-based provider networks. Greater emphasis is placed on treatment planning and quality management in cooperative relationships between providers and managers. To reach the goal of cost effectiveness, a focus on providing the most appropriate care in the most appropriate setting is needed. As opposed to previous stages in the evolutionary process of managed care, the approach has shifted toward identifying a more select cadre of high-quality, efficient providers and, at the same time, improving medically necessary access and benefits as the primary means of managing care while reducing costs.

In managed behavioral health care (as opposed to general medical-surgical managed care companies), individualized case management techniques applied by specialty trained clinicians lend an enhanced clinical focus to quality management of the care delivery process. Cases are individually managed by these clinicians through the use of medical necessity and appropriateness criteria developed specifically for mental health and substance abuse treatment. The application of quality-directed standards and criteria to treatment delivery has perhaps been the most ambitious undertaking of the managed behavioral health care industry.

Specialty managed behavioral health care companies have made great strides in reducing costs while improving access to care and maintaining quality, and today these firms manage care delivery under health coverages for over 100 million people in the United States. The managed behavioral health care approach (2) is distinguished by early intervention and specialty networks that cover a complete range of disciplines and offer access to a full continuum of care settings. It has been the experience of managed behavioral health care that quality treatment, delivered effectively, yields the cost efficiencies of optimized treatment results. In 1989, a comparison study of specialized behavioral health care approaches and nonspecialized UR methods revealed that specialty management significantly reduced costs without negatively affecting quality (3). Although demonstrations conducted at that time showed that specialty managed care techniques produced no adverse effects on quality, this was hardly an indication of the ability of practice standards and guidelines to raise the level of clinical efficiency and effectiveness.

**The Need for Better Quality Standards.** The manner in which care was provided under the earliest managed care systems varied in quality and organization. Traditional clinical processes that relied on local practice customs and individualized judgments and professional precepts remained. Under these conditions, ensuring predictable quality for broad patient populations was an overwhelming task. The absence of adequate definitions and standards of quality made effective quality management an elusive goal.

The lack of practical care quality standards was not endemic to managed care environments alone. Wide variations in preferred treatment methods and philosophy within the psychiatric community preceded attempts to manage care and, in fact, were major reasons for the growing sense that care delivery needed to be managed. In response to this state of affairs, many managed behavioral care companies individually decided to create management criteria and care delivery guidelines for use in their provider networks. Typically, standards reflecting the best knowledge and experience of advisory boards, expert panels, and staff and network practitioners were translated into guidelines to be applied in structuring clinical activity. In this way, managed behavioral care companies successfully improved the delivery process that, in turn, helped to achieve the goals created by an increase in affordable, quality care.

The introduction by managed behavioral health care of quality management methods and guidelines was an important step in promoting an awareness of increased accountability. Although rationalizing the delivery process created the potential for further advances in clinical care, much work remained in the effort to elevate the quality of delivered treatment. The salient shortcomings of quality approaches in early managed care systems and in the broader psychiatric community arose from the same void—the lack of reliable data on the clinical outcomes of treatment. As managed behavioral health care became more sophisticated, processes for tracking clinical outcomes were instituted. Specifically, adverse occurrence monitoring has provided a useful means of improving on negative or unanticipated patient treatment results. By identifying clinical sites at which clinicians repeatedly achieve substandard outcomes and by tracing patterns of negative events, assessment and proactive management of provider network quality and performance is possible. In 1994, a Foster Higgins survey revealed that 93% of the members of the American Managed Behavioral Health care Association (AMBHA), the trade association of the nation's leading specialty managed behavioral health care companies, regularly measured adverse occurrences (4). The key adverse events recognized in the industry (5) are as follows:

- Unexpected death of a hospitalized patient or severe suicide attempts;
- Readmission of a chemical dependency or depressive illness patient within 30 days of discharge;
- Inpatient hospitalization of a patient within 30 days of initial authorization of outpatient services;
- Lack of outpatient follow-up within 30 days of discharge.

Beyond these key indicators, a number of other clinical, medical, and psychopharmacological occurrences are monitored by AMBHA members.

The Foster Higgins survey also demonstrated that AMBHA members appear to be well ahead of the managed care industry as a whole in the collection of outcome data, with 93% of surveyed firms conducting outcome programs. Data collected at intake, during treatment, posttreatment, and later follow-up intervals are used to measure functionality and changes in behavior. The most frequently used collection methodologies are therapist observations and patient self-reports, and studies are performed in both a retrospective and prospective manner (4). Although most of the outcome studies conducted by AMBHA

members are relatively rudimentary, as are other studies within the broader psychiatric field, the pace and sophistication of such activity are accelerating.

As positive as these developed quality and outcome methods have proven to be, progress has been restricted mainly to demonstrations of the relative efficacy of treatment as applied within managed care systems and the identification of clinicians who fall below levels of performance generally expected of the provider network. The limited scope of this work to date merely reflects the fact that managed behavioral health care initially was established as an antidote to runaway costs, a fundamental malady in the health care system. The objective of consumers and payers was access to available care at a reasonable price. Managed behavioral health care has achieved unprecedented success in meeting this market demand (2), and that success is leading to higher quality in behavioral health care. Successful cost reductions have given the market and care managers the leeway to concentrate greater energies on the ultimate goal of the behavioral health care system—optimal treatment outcomes. Moreover, the enhanced efficiencies of better outcomes will be the source of cost improvements.

**Assessing Quality and Outcome.** To improve the process of assessing the delivery of mental health care, refinement of quality definitions and outcome measurements is required. Although serving a valuable purpose, previously used quality parameters, such as avoidance of adverse occurrences and adherence to practice standards of the psychiatric community, do not address the outcome and effects of particular treatments. Specific outcome data of applied treatment for specific patients with specific disorders are needed to advance the practice patterns of the profession.

Two elements in the accomplishment of successful outcomes have been suggested (6): efficacy of treatment and effectiveness of treatment. Efficacy of treatment is demonstrated by controlled research studies that yield the results of treatment approaches used with patients under conditions of carefully followed protocols. In contrast, effectiveness of treatment is gauged by studies designed to reveal how treatments work when applied in "real world" situations. To purchasers of care who seek value for their dollar, the effectiveness of treatment is the more immediate concern. As managed behavioral health care continues to expand, the impact of these systems of care on treatment effectiveness raises increasingly important issues. Managed behavioral care has served patient populations as well as, or better than, any other known system; however, more data on the specific effects of its inherent characteristics are needed. As previously mentioned, at the very least, specialized behavioral care has not adversely affected care. However, a closer examination of managed care system techniques can allow greater insights into the merits of such systems and the possibilities of elevating levels of quality and positive outcomes.

A typical feature of managed care programs, including managed behavioral health care, is the delivery of care on a capitated, prepaid basis as opposed to the fee-for-service arrangements of indemnity reimbursement. A 1990 analysis compared mental health outcomes under a managed care plan with a fee-for-service plan, covering identical ranges of services (7). The study examined outcomes of psychological distress and psychological well being. No clinically significant differences were seen in the mental health outcomes of the two groups. Clearly, one study cannot answer whether outcomes differ in prepaid and fee-for-service financing systems. However, ongoing studies of this kind can help to determine whether and when allocation of treatment resources based on prepayment will have a neutral impact on the effectiveness of treatment.

As used with mental health coverage for the persistently mentally ill, capitation payment may hold particular promise for effective treatment delivery. Preset funding for the care of these patient populations creates incentives to efficiently manage allocation of treatment resources toward effective outcomes. Flexible allocation of funds permits the utilization of less restrictive, less expensive, and more community-oriented treatment settings. This flexibility also allows for more specific customization of treatment plans to meet the needs of individual patients.

Recently, the results of a mental health demonstration project's capitation payment system were evaluated (8). The study compared the outcomes of an experimental group of chronically mentally ill patients under a capitation payment system with the outcomes of control patients under a fee-for-service system. Three outcome variables were analyzed: number of hospital days, level of symptoms, and level of functioning. Overall, patients in the experimental capitated group spent less time as hospitalized inpatients than the control group, but no significant differences in levels of symptoms and functioning were found. Although outcomes for the capitated group were not demonstrated to be superior, the knowledge that outcomes were not adversely impacted does promote further exploration of more flexible treatment approaches, and valuable insights into the need for future research were gained. Furthermore, an accompanying cost-benefit analysis showed that patients under a capitated system can be returned to the community and be maintained with a significant reduction in costs (9). The demonstrated cost-effectiveness of more flexibly allocated resources does encourage additional investigation of a wider range of potential paths to enhanced effectiveness of treatment. Again, individualized case management of treatment delivery at all necessary and appropriate points on a full continuum of care has been a distinguishing facet of the managed behavioral health care approach. With the deployment of a full continuum, elimination of medically unnecessary inpatient utilization has been attained. Although the favorable cost implications are evident, decreases in inpatient lengths of stay (LOS) have raised some questions about the potential impact of reduced LOS on patients' well being. Despite this finding, studies have found no variation in outcomes as a result of shorter hospitalizations (10, 11). The appropriate use of alternative settings, such as partial hospitalization or intensive outpatient treatment, does not increase recidivism or adverse occurrences.

Is there evidence that the case management process affects treatment outcome? One study identifies five essential functions of case management programs (12):

- Assessment of patients' needs;
- Development of treatment plans;
- Linkage of patients to services;
- Monitoring of the provision of services;
- Evaluation of patients' progress.

Based on practical experience and individually observed applications, case management has become widely used in clinical practice as a reliable means of monitoring and facilitating continuity of care. The advantages of this technique are particularly applicable in the treatment of long-term, severely mentally ill patients, as demonstrated in one controlled study of patients participating in a rehabilitation-oriented case management program (12). Outcomes for the experimental patient group after discharge from an inpatient setting (as gauged by occupational functioning, living situation isolation, and hospital recidivism) were compared with a matched group of control patients. At the 2-year postdischarge follow-up interval, participants in the case management program were much more likely to have better occupational functioning and to be less socially isolated than the control group. Although other studies have yielded less favorable results (13, 14), these analyses recognize either the presence of potentially confounding factors or the strong possibility that components missing from the continuum of care (i.e., 24-hour crisis intervention, crisis beds, respite beds, and so on) may have affected the results. The studies referenced here further recognize that examination of additional functional variables or program characteristics is needed to gain a clearer picture of case management's influence.

## Managed Outcome

Clearly, proof of improved outcome and quality, and not simply cost savings, is mandated by new demands for more treatment value in the emerging mental health care environment. For managed behavioral health care, systems such as managed outcome, which can integrate improved efficacy with effectiveness of treatment, will be the most successful. Competition among the various systems will be based on improved quality of care and patient outcomes.

A variety of competitive market forces is shaping the current behavioral health care environment at this time. As managed care organizations affiliate with each other and manage a diverse array of services and providers expand their services to include a comprehensive continuum of care, an increasing overlap of the roles of providers and managed care organizations will be created (15). With a concurrent growth in the trend toward more capitation and risk assumption in the delivery of care, both providers and managers are in positions of greater financial accountability for the outcomes of treatment. Well-developed management skills will be needed as management of risk increases and managed behavioral health care companies and providers develop a stronger relationship to achieve needed efficiencies. For example, sophisticated, integrated systems for gathering data on diverse patient populations; patient and payer satisfaction; delivery costs; and treatment settings, modalities, and efficacy will be a primary necessity. A movement toward such integrated behavioral health care systems has already begun.

The shift of public sector payers to manage care is another major market force. Rapidly increasing costs and fiscal constraints have encouraged public payers, such as Medicaid and Medicare, to seek the savings available under managed care programs. For managed behavioral health care firms, this movement necessitates a renewed commitment to the management of complex patient populations, including the seriously and persistently mentally ill and juvenile members of families covered by public assistance programs. A comprehensive integration with community mental health centers will be a positive step in overcoming the traditional systemic gaps between private and public mental health programs.

Additionally, a marked trend toward reintegration with the general medical health system will be seen. Although managers of behavioral health care will continue to "carve out" the financial risks of care delivery, integrated behavioral health care systems will achieve greater effectiveness by administratively "carving in" to the general medical health care system. An increasing recognition of primary care providers (PCPs) as integral members of the psychiatric and chemical dependency care delivery system is highlighting the importance of improved communications with PCPs and the need for more efficient application of the consultation-liaison function. Moreover, integration with PCPs will broaden awareness of the ability of timely psychiatric interventions to offset medical costs. Continuing cost pressures will result in expanded research into the potential of medical offset.

Developments in the managed outcome era are emphasizing the need to replace outmoded telephone and paper-based systems with sophisticated electronic communication and information systems. The administration of care delivery for more complex patient populations, the creation of deeper linkages with providers, the reintegration with the general medical system, and the implementation of more highly developed financial risk assumption techniques will require the technological capacity to electronically monitor patient intake and eligibility, maintain clinical records, and assist the clinical decision-making process. New and improved electronic communications systems will enhance the effectiveness of care delivery through more thorough and timely provider profiling and outcomes reporting.

## CURRENT OUTCOME RESEARCH NEEDS

Growing interest in outcomes management prompted a survey of ongoing mental health care outcome study efforts in early 1994 (16). More than 70 organizations answered the survey, including single-site facilities, multisite managed mental health care organizations, public departments of mental health, and outcome study firms from 23 states. Over 250 outcome projects covering approximately 150,000 people were reported and the following results were indicated (16):

- Although 69% of survey respondents reported outcome programs for inpatient services, 60% had programs for partial or day treatment services, and only 47% had programs for structured outpatient services.
- The percentages of respondents conducting group practice, intensive outpatient, and residential care outcome projects were only 44%, 40%, and 32%, respectively.
- Only 11% of the projects followed-up with patients 3–12 months after the treatment episode.

This survey represents an encouraging trend toward more widespread study and also indicates several areas for future outcome research.

The fact that outcome research still concentrates most heavily on inpatient are is due to numerous factors, including the importance of inpatient care to the treatment of the severely mentally disabled, the proportionately larger expenditures (and therefore potentially greater cost savings to be achieved through effective treatment) in the inpatient setting, a more systematic hospital maintenance of treatment records, and the potential for greater control over research conditions. However, recent trends in mental health care delivery suggest that, where possible, future researchers may be well advised to apply increased resources to alternative treatment settings. Rates of inpatient utilization continue to drop as effective treatment in other care settings is more widely applied, and more detailed outcome research geared to improving care in these settings will become increasingly important.

This survey also reflects an overall lack of adequate longitudinal study in outcomes research. Although there is a general sense of temporal variability in treatment results, hard research data are needed to provide a basis for informed clinical responses to chronic and periodic disorders and medication issues. Particularly with chronically, severely mentally ill patients, more longitudinal studies must be implemented. Short- and long-term review of the impact of hospitalization is necessary to accurately assess the presence of positive and negative changes in these patients.

Finally, outcome studies of inpatient treatment lack comparison research to account for the effects of the particular characteristics and idiosyncracies of individual treatment settings. Existing studies "can be criticized as containing the effects of specific hospital environments or admission policies, or the effects of specific cohorts within a larger, heterogeneous hospital population" (17). More frequent collaboration in studying broader and more representative patient samples is sorely needed.

## BETTER MANAGEMENT AND BETTER OUTCOMES

Integrated behavioral health care systems can overcome many restrictions in current outcome research efforts and can improve treatment outcomes. The patient populations served from the private and public sectors can provide the scope and depth of care delivery experience needed for thorough outcomes research. Programs covering millions of people in demographically and geographically diverse populations can constitute a broad research base from which datasets, unhampered by parochial limitations, can foster reliable research. Furthermore, managed behavioral health care research programs spanning a wide variety of treatment programs, settings, and modalities can remedy the current lack of comparison studies. An integrated behavioral health care program is characterized by a full continuum of care; consequently, outcome research can study the interactive dynamics of a continuum within one system, as opposed to research conducted across multiple administrative systems.

In addition, managed behavioral health care systems typically promote treatment methods that are more problem focused and goal oriented, producing more particularized and manageable patient treatment records. The availability of more organized data supports outcome research efforts, and the careful establishment and monitoring of treatment goals help to track outcomes. Some psychiatric interventions occur at periodic intervals, and the ability to identify the goals for a particular treatment time frame is important to assessing the efficacy of treatment.

Perhaps most importantly, integrated behavioral health care systems will feature electronic communication and information management systems capable of meeting the data demands of future outcome management. Outcome research will entail the processing of data on innumerable variant combinations of treatment factors. In addition to the specifics of treatment episodes and outcome studies, state-of-the-art systems will maintain and communicate data vital to the administration and improvement of outcome management, including practice parameters, standards and criteria, provider profiling information, and outcomes reporting.

As an industry, managed behavioral health care can advance the measurement of outcomes through the collection of extensive data that can track utilization and care delivery in large patient populations over extended periods of time. This longitudinally oriented outcome data can enhance research and outcome assessment.

In late 1994, AMBHA initiated an examination of a broad range of issues related to introducing better definitions and standards of quality to the behavioral health care field. The tasks involved in AMBHA's quality improvement efforts included the development of standards and formats for reporting by all parties interested in improving quality in the delivery of care; common datasets for clinical intake; and commonly used instruments and methods for measuring quality, patient satisfaction, and clinical outcome. Accomplishing these tasks will establish the standardization necessary for comparative and longitudinal studies of outcome that can be used by managed behavioral health care to deliver greater clinical value to patients.

## CONCLUSIONS

Before managed behavioral health care had a name or became a concept for discussion, concerned clinicians were attempting to deliver the best care possible to their patients. Based on acquired academic knowledge, training, and experience, responsible professionals did their utmost to attain the ultimate goal of optimal treatment outcomes. However, in the almost complete absence of reliable outcome data applicable in everyday clinical situations, the task of improving clinical expertise was often a solitary, personal mission.

Eventually, burgeoning mental health care costs forced clinicians to face further complexities in their practice. Professional responsibility to the patient had to be reconciled with the economic values of society. Although the balancing of patient care techniques with financial realities has always been an elemental function in the delivery of care, adjusting to the process of administering care within new UR and managed care reimbursement milieus was

often a source of difficulty. Many practitioners have viewed managed care as an affront to prior progress in the advancement of clinical efficacy and an unwelcome force that would stifle clinical innovation for the sake of economic gain.

Consumer and payer demands for access to affordable behavioral health care could not be ignored, and despite some controversy, managed behavioral health care is one means of addressing cost concerns while attending to quality of care. By emphasizing cost effectiveness, managed behavioral health care has responded to the market demands that outcome be worth its attendant cost. Competition is driving the mental health industry to increase the value of treatment.

As integrated behavioral health care systems become established, the needs of both consumers and payers will be met. Comprehensive data systems will provide the information necessary to make choices based on clinical quality. Advanced knowledge in clinical practice will lead to greater standardization in clinical delivery methods. Data on comparative effectiveness of different delivery systems will allow payer expenditures based on more highly informed health care purchase decisions. Greater assumption of financial risk by integrated delivery systems will foster better accountability in the provision of mental health care because incentives will reward innovations in quality.

We may never know the reasons that have brought mental health care to its current threshold. Is it irony, vision, or simply the natural progression of value-balanced approaches to the sometimes conflicting needs of the health care market? These questions may never be adequately answered, but the future now holds potential for breakthroughs in outcome management.

REFERENCES

1. Garnick DW, Hendricks AM, Dulski JD, Thorpe KE, Horgan C. Characteristics of private-sector managed care for mental health and substance

abuse treatment. Hosp Community Psychiatry 1994;45:1201–1205.

2. Geraty R, Bartlett J, Hill E, Lee F, Shusterman A, Waxman A. The impact of managed behavioral healthcare on the costs of psychiatric and chemical dependency treatment. Behav Healthcare Tomorrow 1994;3:18–30.

3. Anderson DF. Managed mental health care delivers the goods. San Francisco: William Mercer, 1989.

4. Foster Higgins. AMBHA/Foster Higgins managed behavioral healthcare quality and access survey. New York: Foster Higgins, 1994.

5. Marques C, Geraty R, Bartlett J. Quality and access in the managed behavioral healthcare industry. Alexandria: American Managed Behavioral Healthcare Association, 1994.

6. Glazer WM. What are "best practices?" Understanding the concept. Hosp Community Psychiatry 1994;45:1067–1068.

7. Wells KB, Manning WG Jr, Valdez RB. The effects of a prepaid group practice on mental health outcomes. Health Serv Res 1990;25:615–625.

8. Cole RE, Reed SK, Babigian HM, Brown SW, Fray J. A mental health capitation program. I. Patient outcomes. Hosp Community Psychiatry 1994;45:1090–1096.

9. Reed SK, Hennessy KD, Mitchell OS, Babigian HM. A mental health capitation program. II. Cost-benefit analysis. Hosp Community Psychiatry 1994;45:1097–1103.

10. Caton CLM, Gralick A. A review of issues surrounding length of psychiatric hospitalization. Hosp Community Psychiatry 1987;38:858–863.

11. Baker NJ, Giese AA. Reorganization of a private psychiatric unit to promote collaboration with managed care. Hosp Community Psychiatry 1992;43:1126–1129.

12. Goering PN, Wasylenki DA, Farkas M, Lancee WJ, Ballantyne R. What difference does case management make? Hosp Community Psychiatry 1988;39:272–276.

13. Hornstra RK, Bruce-Wolfe V, Sagduyu K, Riffle DW. The effect of intensive case management on hospitalization of patients with schizophrenia. Hosp Community Psychiatry 1993;44:844–847.

14. Dietzen LL, Bond GR. Relationship between case manager contact and outcome for frequently hospitalized psychiatric clients. Hosp Community Psychiatry 1993;44:839–843.

15. Bengen-Seltzer B. Industry analysis: overlapping of managed care and provider roles in managed behavioral health evolution. OPEN MINDS 1994;8:4–5.

16. Pallak MS. National outcomes management survey: summary report. Behav Healthcare Tomorrow 1994;3:63–69.

17. Goodrich W. Research issues in adolescent inpatient psychiatry. In: Ghuman HS, Sarles RM, eds. Handbook of adolescent inpatient psychiatric treatment. New York: Brunner/Mazel, 1994:277–292.

# CHAPTER 25

# Practice Guidelines and Outcomes Research

*John S. McIntyre, Deborah A. Zarin, Harold A. Pincus*

## INTRODUCTION

It is widely believed that practice guidelines and outcomes research will have a major impact on the delivery of mental health care over the next several decades. Not only will the consistent and widespread use of practice guidelines expedite the collection of valid outcome data, but, conversely, the data from outcomes research will be very helpful in developing more explicit, definitive practice guidelines. In this chapter, the essential link between guidelines and outcomes research will be explored.

## DEFINITION OF GUIDELINES

Practice guidelines in psychiatry can be defined as strategies for mental health care delivery that are developed to facilitate clinical decision-making and to provide patients with critical information concerning the different treatment options (1–5). These strategies are known by such terms as standards, guidelines, and options. Eddy (1) used an umbrella term, practice parameters, to include various levels of recommendations. *Standards* are recommendations that should be followed in virtually all cases; exceptions are rare and require extensive justification. *Guidelines* are strategies that should be followed in the majority of cases; exceptions are more common and require minimal justification for alternative treatment approaches. *Options* are recommendations that should be followed in those cases in which a clearly preferred strategy is not indicated. Many orga-

nizations use the term "guidelines," which best captures the level of recommendations generally included. In this chapter, guideline is used generically to include these three different levels of recommendations.

The extensive variability in the content of practice guidelines can affect their value in outcomes research. Many guidelines are developed based on clinical procedures, whereas others are based on illness or defined disorders. Some guidelines are brief, general descriptions of existing clinical practice with little or no scientific evidence to support the various recommendations, whereas others are consensus statements made by experts that are sometimes buttressed by supporting data. Fortunately, evidence-based guidelines are clearly written, contain specific recommendations, and explicitly identify the primary source of the evidence.

## DEVELOPERS OF PRACTICE GUIDELINES

Currently, four major groups are involved in developing practice guidelines: professional associations, academic centers, government agencies, and insurance companies and health maintenance organizations.

The Clinical Efficacy Assessment Project, initiated by the American College of Physicians in 1981, is perhaps the most extensive guideline endeavor undertaken by a professional association. Under the auspices of this project, a number of guidelines have been approved and published (6).

Over the past 15 years, the American College of Obstetrics and Gynecology published a number of guidelines under the title of "Technical Bulletins."

As many as 45 physician organizations have joined the Practice Parameters Forum coordinated by the American Medical Association (AMA) to discuss issues related to the development, dissemination, and assessment of guidelines. A steering committee was formed by 16 of these organizations (Table 25.1) under the banner of the Practice Parameters Partnership. One of the major tasks assigned to the partnership was to determine those attributes that would be the most valuable in the development of guidelines.

The Academic Medical Center Consortium (AMCC), consisting of 11 medical centers, the AMA, and the Rand Corporation, collaborated in a clinical appropriateness initiative. Rand and the AMCC developed appropriateness criteria for four procedures and/or illnesses: coronary artery disease, cataract removal, carotid endarterectomy, and abdominal aortic aneurysmectomy. The project called for the AMA, in collaboration with state medical societies and national medical specialty societies, to develop related practice parameters and to facilitate their dissemination. The collaborative effort included an evaluation of the effectiveness of the project in both reducing inappropriate care and promoting quality health care services.

**Table 25.1  Steering Committee**

American Academy of Family Physicians (AAFP)
American Academy of Ophthalmology (AAO)
American Academy of Orthopaedic Surgeons (AAOS)
American Academy of Pediatrics (AAP)
American College of Cardiology (ACC)
American College of Obstetricians & Gynecologists (ACOG)
American College of Physicians
American College of Radiology (ACR)
American College of Surgeons (ACS)
American Medical Association (AMA)
American Psychiatric Association (APA)
American Society of Anesthesiologists (ASA)
American Society of Internal Medicine (ASIM)
American Urological Association, Inc. (AUA)
College of American Pathologists (CAP)

The federal government has launched health care initiatives directly involving practice guidelines. In 1989, Congress established the Agency for Health Care Policy and Research. Within this agency, the Forum for Quality and Effectiveness in Health Care received a mandate to develop practice guidelines. To date, several guidelines have been published that cover the treatment of pain, benign prostatic hypertrophy, cataracts, and depression in primary care settings (7).

Although not directly involved in developing practice guidelines, state governments have shown an interest in issues related to clinical guidelines. In January 1992, in Maine, the Medical Liability Demonstration Project was initiated. Practice parameters and risk management protocols were developed for specialists in obstetrics and gynecology, emergency medicine, radiology, and anesthesiology. A result of the guideline development was that physicians who could demonstrate compliance with the practice criteria might be able to establish an affirmative defense against medical malpractice claims. Although significant opposition to this project was voiced by insurers and the association of trial lawyers, the project generated enthusiastic support from many quarters. A full report on the project is expected to be presented to the state legislature by December 1997.

A Florida statute (Chapter 408.02), entitled *Practice Parameters,* passed in 1993, created the Agency of Health Care Administration under the Office of Health Policy. The office received a mandate to "coordinate the development, endorsement, implementation, and evaluation of scientifically sound, clinically relevant practice parameters" with a goal of "decreasing unwarranted variation, improving the quality of medical care, and promoting appropriate utilization of health care resources."

Although a number of third-party payers have produced guidelines or treatment protocols for their providers, little or no evidence generally is presented to support the listed recommendations for these guidelines. Despite this drawback, many of these organizations have asked clinicians to critique the guidelines to encourage improvement in their quality and usability.

## THE EXPLOSION IN GUIDELINE DEVELOPMENT

In the last decade, over 2,000 guidelines have been written and many more are in the development stages. Several reasons can account for this increase in the creation of practice guidelines: to provide access to the latest advances in clinical practice, to foster more effective cost containment, to decrease the frequency of unnecessary clinical procedures and treatment, to produce valid outcome data, to reduce medical liability, and to provide better information on various treatment options.

It has become increasingly difficult for practitioners to remain abreast of new developments in all areas of medicine, including specialized clinical areas. For example, with regard to treatment methods, much of the information currently available on medications can be considered outdated within 5 years. Practice guidelines can provide practitioners with a clear and referenced summary of the latest advances in the field. Moreover, as the overall costs of medical care continue to rise, guidelines may help to contain these costs by encouraging a reduction in unnecessary and ineffective treatments.

Many studies have revealed the marked variation in frequency of certain clinical procedures (e.g., hysterectomy, endarterectomy) across geographic boundaries (8), indicating that thresholds for certain treatments vary from one part of the country to another. Practice guidelines may decrease some of the variations that do not appear to be related to clinically relevant issues.

Professional associations have become increasingly concerned that because of the rapid growth of managed care, sufficient scientific evidence is not being obtained to support clinical decisions concerning treatment options and practice protocols. In an effort to overcome this obstacle, the professions can take advantage of the extensive clinical experience and expertise available to their associations to develop guidelines for their own members.

The issue of malpractice has led insurance carriers, professional organizations, and clinicians to consider the potentially positive impact of widely accepted guidelines in the area of medical liability. Some have suggested that guidelines will increase the liability of clinicians; on the other hand, others have argued that a nationally accepted guideline, if well written, will lend support to those clinicians faced with malpractice actions. For example, after the American Academy of Anesthesiologists approved a set of guidelines for its members, a substantial decrease (approximately 25%) was seen in malpractice premiums for anesthesiologists (9).

Over the last few decades, the patient's involvement in clinical decision-making has increased. Practice guidelines can provide patients with organized, current information about various treatment options, including efficacy, risks, and side effects. Understandable, available guidelines can increase a patient's involvement in treatment.

## PROCESS FOR GUIDELINE DEVELOPMENT

The Institute of Medicine (IOM) has produced an excellent overview of guideline development with specific process recommendations for the preparation of high quality guidelines (10). Using the IOM report as a guide, the AMA issued a document outlining the process of guideline development, which states that practice guidelines be developed according to the following criteria: physician organizations should participate in the development, reliable methods integrating relevant research findings and appropriate clinical expertise should be used, content should be as comprehensive and as specific as possible, information should be current, and wide dissemination should be achieved.

## GUIDELINES IN PSYCHIATRY

Although generic guidelines have been promulgated for decades, guidelines developed by a defined process and with a consistent format are recent additions to the field of psychiatry. In 1851, the American Psychiatric Association (APA), then known as the Association of Medical Superintendents of American Institutes for the Insane, first approved 26 propositions on the construction of hospitals; a set of recommendations for staffing these institutions was adopted 2 years later (11). In more recent years, in an effort to advance the use of guidelines in clinical practice, the APA published a series of task force reports on benzodiazepines, laboratory tests in psychiatry, and electroconvulsive therapy (12), among others.

Other psychiatric associations also have participated in the development of guidelines. The Royal College of Psychiatry in Australia and New Zealand published a practice guideline on anxiety disorders in 1982 (13).

The U.S. Academy of Child and Adolescent Psychiatry published their first guideline on attention deficit disorder in 1991 and subsequently issued guidelines on conduct disorder, anxiety disorder, and early onset schizophrenia. The Academy currently has in progress 10 other guidelines in various stages of development and plans to publish guidelines on the psychiatric assessment of children and adolescents in 1995.

## APA GUIDELINE PROJECT

In 1989 the APA launched its formal guideline project, and the following processes for development evolved over the next several years. First, a steering committee comprising a broad representation of the membership was established to oversee the project. Second, topics for guidelines were chosen based on the following: the disorder could be considered a public health problem, development could be supported by sufficient research literature and clinical consensus, and the proposed guideline could have a positive impact on the field. Third, a work group consisting of five to six members was appointed to review the existing literature for the purpose of identifying and categorizing the relevant studies (i.e., randomized controlled trial, case report). Next, a draft guideline was prepared, and recommendations were based on the accumulated research evidence available or the strength of the clinical consensus. This first draft was reviewed by approximately 50 experts, and a second draft was subsequently prepared based on the input from this evaluation. As several additional drafts were written, an increasing number of psychiatrists were asked to participate in the reviews. In addition, input was sought from many other organizations (approximately 100 for each of the first three guidelines approved). This development process resulted in the publication of three guidelines (14–16), with six additional guidelines in various stages of development (see Table 25.2).

Developing guidelines involves a large number of practicing psychiatrists. For each of the first three guidelines published by the APA, approximately 1,000 psychiatrists reviewed the various drafts. With so many clinicians involved, difficult issues emerged. Although each guideline was evidence based, in a number of instances, the translation of recent research findings into clinical protocols was still evolving. For ex-

**Table 25.2 American Psychiatric Association Guidelines**

| Guidelines | Publication/Completion (estimated) |
|---|---|
| Eating disorders | February 1993 |
| Major depressive disorder in adults | April 1993 |
| Bipolar disorder | December 1994 |
| Substance use | Spring 1995 |
| Evaluation of adults | Spring 1995 |
| Schizophrenia | Fall 1995 |
| Nicotine dependence | Spring 1996 |
| Alzheimer's and related dementias | Spring 1996 |
| Anxiety and panic | Fall 1996 |
| Delirium | Fall 1996 |
| Mental retardation | Spring 1997 |

ample, in the development of the APA's Bipolar Guideline, considerable controversy arose over the recommendation of the use of valproate (valproic acid) as a first-line treatment for mania. Although recent studies supported this approach (17, 18), the consensus found a lack of sufficient data to support an unqualified recommendation.

## DISSEMINATION ISSUES

If practice guidelines are to achieve the goal of improved patient care, they must be written, published, and disseminated and must be available to clinicians on a regular basis. Consequently, strategies are being explored to incorporate guidelines into clinical practices and to integrate guidelines into continuing medical education programs, interactive computer programs, and formal educational programs (e.g., residency training, certification, and recertification).

In a study that investigated dissemination issues (19), the Ontario Academy of Obstetrics and Gynecology developed and strongly endorsed guidelines for the delivery of newborns whose mothers had undergone prior cesarean sections. The guidelines encouraged a trial of vaginal delivery (VBAC) if certain criteria were met. The dissemination strategy was to reach every member of the Academy by sending out a strong letter recommending the use of the guideline. Follow-up 24 months later revealed that in control and/or audit hospitals, no appreciable change was seen in practice patterns after the guideline was published—the rate of VBACs remained the same. However, after a review of a subset of the hospitals, a significant increase in the trial of labor was seen in the VBAC rates (46% and 85%). In each of these hospitals, a respected clinician designated in the study as an "opinion leader" was responsible for organizing teaching sessions to review the guideline, discuss specific examples, and answer questions. This study highlights the importance of careful consideration of dissemination strategies to en-

sure guidelines will be successful in influencing practice patterns.

## PRACTICE RESEARCH NETWORK

During the development of the first three practice guidelines, the APA recognized that feedback from clinicians would be required on a regular basis and that field testing a practice guideline would be an important part of the development process. These two stimuli led the APA to develop a Practice Research Network, which is discussed in great detail in Chapter 28.

## AN INTERDISCIPLINARY APPROACH TO DEVELOPMENT

A significant issue in the development of guidelines is the participation of key affected groups. For example, in the area of guidelines for the treatment of mental illness, the key participants would include psychiatrists, psychologists, social workers, nurses, and other therapists. Although an interdisciplinary approach is important to the development of guidelines, with the exception of government endeavors, achieving a collaborative effort of this dimension currently is very difficult. In the field of mental health, only the APA has an established process for guideline development, and these guidelines specifically state they are intended for psychiatrists only. Recently, other mental health associations have begun to consider the development of practice guidelines, and, at some future point, we may see the integration of such guidelines by the various disciplines.

## PRACTICE GUIDELINES IN OUTCOMES RESEARCH

Outcomes research is greatly enhanced by the consistency of treatments that allows for easier isolation of other variables and better methods of testing hypotheses. However, achieving such consistency has been a major problem for medicine in general and mental health in particular. Psychotherapy is a clear example in that the broad definition of the term "psychotherapy" creates considerable difficulties. In tightly controlled studies with a small number of specifically trained therapists, this problem can be minimized. In larger studies in a naturalistic setting, research is exceedingly difficult unless definitions, techniques, and practice guidelines are developed that are widely accepted and regularly and reliably used.

To achieve consistency in treatment approaches, the guidelines must be clear and the recommendations specific. Practice guidelines with vague or general recommendations can result in considerable variation in the interventions that actually occur. Outcomes research then may result in erroneous conclusions if incorrect or incomplete assumptions are made about the treatment actually delivered.

One of the major challenges in developing guidelines is to craft recommendations that are as specific as possible without excessively stretching the conclusions that are based on existing scientific data. In the development of the APA guideline on major depressive disorder, one of the difficult issues was the strength of the recommendation concerning the use and timing of antidepressant medication in patients who did not improve with psychotherapy as the only treatment. Most reviewers of the guideline argued that every patient with major depressive disorder who was treated with psychotherapy and did not begin to improve within 8 weeks should be treated with antidepressant medication. It was noted, however, that antidepressant medication may not be warranted in a number of clinical situations. After much consideration, the approved wording of the guideline states "that some patients with mild to moderate degrees of impairment may be treated with psychotherapeutic management or psychotherapy alone, provided that it is not prolonged without distinct improvement before a trial of antidepressants is initiated (unless there is a specific therapeutic contraindication)" (15).

The guideline process can highlight those areas that require further research and in so doing can help establish the outcomes research agenda. As a result of the federal government's current investment in guideline development, support for the research agenda thus identified may be increased. This is another instance in which guideline development and outcomes research can be mutually reinforcing.

## OUTCOMES RESEARCH AS INPUT FOR PRACTICE GUIDELINES

As outcomes research progresses, guidelines will become more specific and will rely more on scientific evidence. Clinical consensus may become less important as the data from outcomes studies is translated into specific treatment recommendations. Ideally, extensive outcomes research could provide the evidence-based support for practice guidelines; however, because research efforts are not always able to keep pace with all the rapid advances in technology, this goal may not be fully realized for some time. However, if outcomes research can focus on major decision-making in treatment paradigms, the validity and reliability of the guidelines can be greatly enhanced.

Further research is desperately needed in a number of areas. For example, comorbidity of illness has not been studied sufficiently. Data are lacking currently on the treatment of patients with a major depressive disorder and dysthymia (double depression) or patients diagnosed with a major depressive disorder and a personality disorder. In addition, the absence of outcomes research in the treatment of personality disorders has led to the decision by the APA Steering Committee on Practice Guidelines not to write practice guidelines for these disorders at this time.

## CONCLUSIONS

Practice guidelines are beginning to exert a major impact on the practice of medicine. Currently, a profusion of guidelines has been published, and the rate of production is rapidly increasing. Managed care companies, as well as state and federal governments, have increased spending in the development of guidelines. The AMA and medical specialty organizations also have launched major initiatives in this area. Despite this expanded activity, however, the scope and quality of these guidelines vary considerably.

Well-developed, current practice guidelines that are evidence based, clear, specific, and yet comprehensive can have a significant impact on the quality and efficacy of treatments delivered. However, because of the large gaps in our research database, outcomes research is essential to the production and assessment of such guidelines. Conversely, because outcomes studies depend on conformity of treatment protocols, practice guidelines such as those described in this chapter and their effective implementation will greatly enhance quality outcomes research.

## REFERENCES

1. Eddy D. Clinical decision making: from theory to practice: the challenge. JAMA 1990;263:287–290.
2. Woolf SH. Practice guidelines: a new reality in medicine. Arch Intern Med 1990;150:1811–1818.
3. Brook RH. Practice guidelines and practicing medicine: are they compatible? JAMA 1989;262:3027–3070.
4. Epstein AM. The outcomes movement—will it get us where we want to go? N Engl J Med 1990;323:266–270.
5. McIntyre JS, Talbott JA. Practice parameters: what they are and why they're needed. Hosp Community Psychiatry 1990;41:1103–1105.
6. American College of Physicians. Clinical efficacy reports. Philadelphia: American College of Physicians, 1987.
7. Agency for Health Care Policy and Research. Depression in primary care. Washington, DC: U.S. Department of Health and Human Services, 1993. [AHCPR Publ. No. 93-0550.]
8. Chassin M, Kosecoff J, Park E, et al. The appropriateness of selected medical and surgical procedures: relationship to geographical variations. Ann Arbor: Association for Health Services Research and Health Administration Press, 1989.
9. Stephenson G. Guidelines take the pain out of malpractice premiums for anesthesiologists. Report on Medical Guidelines and Outcomes Research 1990;7:4–6.
10. Institute of Medicine. Guidelines for clinical practice: from development to use. Washington, DC: National Academy Press, 1992.
11. Kirkbride T. On the construction, organization and general arrangement of hospitals for the insane. Philadelphia: Lindsay & Blakiston, 1854.
12. American Psychiatric Association. Task force on electroconvulsive therapy: the practice of electroconvulsive therapy. Washington, DC: American Psychiatric Association, 1990.
13. Andrews G, Armstrong MS, Brodaty H, Hall W, Harvey PR, Tennant CC, Weekes P. A methodology for preparing "ideal" treatment outlines in psychiatry. Aust N Z J Psychiatry 1982;16:153–158.
14. American Psychiatric Association. Practice guideline for eating disorders. Am J Psychiatry 1993;150:207–228.
15. American Psychiatric Association. Practice guideline for major depressive disorder in adults. Am J Psychiatry 1993;150:4.
16. American Psychiatric Association. Practice guideline for the treatment of patients with bipolar disorder. Am J Psychiatry 1994;151:12.
17. Bowden CL, Brugger AM, Swann AC, et al. Efficacy of divalproex vs. lithium and placebo in the treatment of mania. The Depakote mania study group. JAMA 1994;271:918–924.
18. Pope HG Jr, McElroy SL, Keck PE Jr, Hudson JI. Valproate in the treatment of acute mania: a placebo controlled study. Arch Gen Psychiatry 1991;48:62–68.
19. Lomas J, Enkin M, Anderson GM, Hannah WJ, Vayda E, Singer J. Opinion leaders vs. audit and feedback to implement practice guidelines. JAMA 1991;265:2202–2207.

CHAPTER 26

# The American Psychiatric Association Practice Research Network

*Deborah A. Zarin, Joyce C. West, Harold A. Pincus,*
*John S. McIntyre*

## INTRODUCTION

The American Psychiatric Association (APA) Office of Research is currently in the process of developing a national practice-based research network of psychiatrists who will collaborate to collect data and conduct clinical and health services research. The APA Practice Research Network (PRN), which is currently in the initial development and pilot testing stages, includes approximately 200 psychiatrists nationwide. Once the network is fully established it will consist of approximately 1,000 psychiatrists practicing in a variety of public and private treatment settings.

The network is being established to address the following: observations by those developing evidence-based practice guidelines and others that little data are currently available to guide psychiatrists' day-to-day clinical decision-making; concerns that randomized controlled trial data, which largely comes from tertiary settings, may not be fully generalizable to other practice settings; concerns that clinicians may be reluctant to incorporate research findings into their clinical decision-making if findings are based on patients or treatments that are dissimilar their own; and the desire among clinicians to become directly involved in the conduct of research. The PRN will serve as a "national psychiatric research laboratory" to strengthen and expand the clinical services and health services research base in psychiatry so that psychiatric treatments and outcomes of care for persons with mental disorders can be improved.

One of the primary goals of this initiative is to bridge the gap between current clinical research and the practical needs of clinicians and patients (1). The network's "observational" or "naturalistic" research design will facilitate this by assessing the effectiveness of psychiatric treatments provided in routine practice rather than the efficacy of treatments under optimal circumstances. This capability will provide an ongoing mechanism for outcomes assessment in measuring, monitoring, and providing feedback to network members on the outcomes of care (2), particularly because clinicians will be directly involved in the design and conduct of studies.

This chapter provides a general introduction to practice-based research networks and the role of these networks in conducting clinical and health services research. The APA PRN is described, including a discussion of research design, methods, and measurement issues that are being addressed to conduct practice-based clinical and health services research across a broad range of psychiatric treatment settings. The first section of this chapter provides an overview of practice-based research initiatives, describing other practice-based networks and their research contributions; the second section describes the impetus and rationale for the APA to develop a practice-based research network. The third section outlines in greater detail the APA PRN's overall research design and methods, including a discussion of network sampling, measurement, data collection, and analysis issues. Section four describes some of the methodological issues and challenges in conducting practice-based clinical effectiveness or outcomes assessment research studies.

## PRACTICE-BASED RESEARCH NETWORKS: BACKGROUND AND OVERVIEW

Practice-based research networks typically consist of a large number of clinicians who agree to collaborate to collect and report data needed to conduct a variety of research studies. They are generally ongoing research initiatives in that once the network is established, a variety of studies are conducted over time (3, 4). This offers the advantage of minimizing administrative and start-up costs associated with conducting traditional research projects.

Practice-based research networks have been used to conduct a variety of epidemiological (e.g., human immunodeficiency virus [HIV] seroprevalence), clinical services, and health services research studies as described in more detail below. Although practice-based networks primarily have been used to carry out descriptive or cross-sectional "point-in-time" studies, they are now being used to support the conduct of more sophisticated longitudinal study designs. This research includes clinical effectiveness or outcome assessment studies in which patients are followed and outcomes are assessed at multiple points over time.

Over the past three decades, investigators in other medical fields have been successful in developing practice-based research networks (5–8). Since 1967 nearly a dozen national and international medical organizations, including medical professional organizations, universities, and group practices, have developed practice-based research networks. Most of these networks have been in the fields of family practice and pediatrics (J Hickner, unpublished data, 1991) (9).

Currently, the two most active practice-based research networks in the United States are the Pediatric Research in Office Settings (PROS) network developed by the American Academy of Pediatrics and the Ambulatory Sentinel Practice Network (ASPN) developed by the American Academy of Family Physicians and the University of Colorado. The PROS network has conducted studies of gastroenteritis, vision screening (10, 11), and the onset of secondary sexual characteristics in young girls.

The ASPN network has conducted studies of the prevalence of HIV infection and the treatment of pelvic inflammatory disease (12), headaches (13, 14), spontaneous abortion (15), chest pain (16), and otitis media (17, 18). The ASPN network has generated 30 journal articles on a variety of primary care topics, and nearly all have been observational rather than intervention studies. The participating network members have not changed their behavior or clinical practice in any way to alter physician-patient interactions.

Most of the existing networks consist of clinicians who have volunteered to participate in the network or have been informally recruited by a group of peer leaders. Network members are typically not reimbursed or in other ways compensated for their time. Instead, cooperation depends on such intrinsic incentives as the opportunity to interact with peers, participate in research without major time or resource investment, and contribute to efforts that might advance the knowledge base of the field.

Most networks rely on their membership to provide input regarding the selection of research questions to be studied, to provide feedback on the feasibility of implementing study designs, and to conduct studies and collect data. The principal investigator for a specific study typically is either a member of the network or an academic investigator who collaborates with the network leadership to design and implement studies, as well as to analyze and report findings.

Networks generally use brief, paper-based data collection instruments that are completed by network clinicians and are designed to meet the needs of specific studies. Two networks, the Dartmouth Cooperative (19) and a state mental health practice-based research network in Arkansas, have used computer-based management information systems to collect detailed clinical and financial data for network studies while minimizing data reporting burden on clinicians and patients.

To supplement clinician reported data and provide follow-up, several networks have collected data from patients or patient informants. For example, the PROS and ASPN networks are jointly conducting a study that involves collecting data from the parents of pediatric patients. The PROS network also has collected data from parents for their study on the medical management and functional outcomes of asthmatic pediatric patients.

Network members are assured that their confidentiality and that of their patients will be protected. To protect patient confidentiality, most networks do not collect any data that can be used to identify patients; only the network members know the identities of patients. Standard research practices of data security are also observed (e.g., hard copies of completed data collection instruments are destroyed and data are stored under lock and key).

## IMPETUS AND RATIONALE FOR THE PRN

### Primary Purpose of the Network

The primary impetus for the development of the APA PRN was the recognition of critical gaps in the current clinical and health services research base in psychiatry. These gaps were particularly evident as the APA undertook the development of evidence-based practice guidelines (1, 20–22). Although significant research pertaining to specific disorders has been conducted, many practical questions and treatment decisions facing clinicians have not been studied.

The APA has viewed the network as a valuable opportunity to engage members in clinically meaningful research with important policy implications, particularly in light of the rapid changes in the organization, financing, delivery, and management of psychiatric care.

## Strengths and Limitations of Traditional Clinical Trials and Other Research Methods

Although randomized controlled trials provide an essential research design for establishing, with reasonable certainty, a causal relationship between an intervention and an effect, issues of statistical power and expense prompt investigators to design these trials around homogenous patient populations, a limited number of well-characterized, short term treatments, and restricted outcomes. Consequently, even the best designed traditional clinical trials generally focus on a narrowly defined set of treatments in a very limited group of patients who are seen by atypical providers in atypical treatment settings. As a result, traditional clinical trials are not easily generalized with respect to patients, treatments, providers, and settings.

Clinical trials generally use narrow subject inclusion and exclusion criteria; consequently, patients such as those with general medical or psychiatric comorbidities (e.g., substance abuse disorders), children and adolescents, or the elderly may be excluded. Unlike most treatments provided in clinical practice, treatments studied with clinical trials are generally short term, tightly controlled and monitored, and provided under ideal circumstances. Clinical trial practice settings are also atypical in primarily reflecting acute, tertiary care/academic medical settings rather than the full range of residential and community-based treatment settings. Finally, clinicians who participate in clinical trials also differ from "average" clinicians in that they are generally highly trained and carefully monitored (A Lehman, unpublished data, 1994).

Because of their narrow focus, findings from traditional clinical trials typically are limited in their relevance to clinical decision-making. Traditional clinical trials generally focus on assessing the efficacy of one treatment compared with a nontreatment control group. Some clinical trials also include one other treatment group in addition to the control group. Also, clinical trials tend to examine short-term outcomes as well as narrow symptomatic measures of outcome, excluding other outcomes that are relevant to practitioners and patients (e.g., broader measures of outcome such as measures of general health status and functional status) (2). Clinical trials are considered to be the "gold standard" for inferring causality within specific parameters (internal validity), whereas practice-based research provides more information about the expected outcomes in typical practice (external validity).

Practice-based research methods can be used to overcome many of the limitations of other commonly used traditional health services research methods, including secondary analysis of administrative datasets (e.g., clinical practice management information systems, patient medical records, or claims databases that are the administrative databases payers have developed using insurance claims), epidemiological studies, and secondary analysis of national health databases (i.e., databases developed by the federal government that are used for national reporting and monitoring purposes).

## Strengths and Limitations of Practice-Based Research Networks

The principal strengths of practice-based research methods include the ability to substantially improve the generalizability of findings for a broader range of patients, settings, and treatments; provide the capacity to study a broader range of research questions related to psychiatric patients, treatments, treatment settings, and outcomes; facilitate the conduct of a range of research designs; provide the flexibility to obtain data from a variety of perspectives, including psychiatrists, patients, and patient informants; and systematically collect and analyze clinical and health services data on an ongoing basis.

A PRN could provide the capacity to study a broader range of research questions related to psychiatric patients, treatments, treatment settings, and outcomes. For example, it could be used to describe the nature and course of mental disorders and describe psychiatric patients, treatments, and treatment settings. The study of critical target populations, including the severely mentally ill, children and adolescents, and those patients with coexisting mental and general medical disorders, could be characterized. More importantly, because the network will reflect a large patient base (approximately 96,000 patients at any point in time once fully developed), it will also facilitate studies of specific clinical problems, such as patients who have not responded to routine treatments.

The PRN could also be used to assess treatment outcomes and the relative effectiveness of alternative psychiatric treatments for different groups of patients, providing an ongoing, national outcomes assessment monitoring system. These data would be useful in identifying critical factors in matching patients to treatments. These studies would be essential for the vast majority of psychiatrists and their patients who must make clinical decisions that are not adequately guided by available clinical trials and other research data.

The network could also be used to study critical service delivery, policy, and financing issues. A large national PRN could study a range of policy issues related to the organization, financing, and delivery of psychiatric services. Because psychiatrists practicing in a wide range of public and private settings would be included, the network would have the capacity to study the interaction between systems and clinical issues and assess differences in outcomes and quality of care associated with alternative health services delivery systems. It could also be a useful tool in examining the impact of various managed care techniques on the quality, continuity, and outcomes of care.

The network design could facilitate the conduct of a range of research designs, from single point in time cross-sectional and repeated cross-sectional studies to more complex longitudinal follow-up research designs to conduct medical effectiveness studies. In addition, the network could examine outcomes of care provided to patients with similar clinical and nonclinical features to help determine which treatments might be more effective for specific categories of patients. For each of these studies, the network also could provide the flexibility to collect and analyze data from a variety of perspectives, including psychiatrists, patients, and patient informants.

The PRN approach could offer the capability of systematically collecting and analyzing clinical and health services data on an ongoing basis, providing a national monitoring system to assess changes in psychiatric patients and the practice of psychiatry. This function could be valuable in addressing many of the major gaps in the current clinical and services research base (e.g., data characterizing patients and types of treatments received by different patients).

Finally, involving clinicians in the design and implementation of research on their own patients can offer the advantage of improving the relevance and acceptance of the data generated in practice-based research networks. It can promote the integration of research findings into clinical practice. Because the network members will help select research topics, network studies generally can reflect the priority research needs of practicing clinicians.

As a primarily observational research capability, practice-based research networks share many of the limitations of other naturalistic clinical services research. For example, relying on a nonexperimental research design limits the extent to which the randomization of treatments and use of controls can be used and the extent to which "intervention"

studies can be undertaken; this limits the extent to which causal influences can be established. Naturalistic studies are limited in the ability to control or standardize interventions and treatments and are also limited in the amount of detailed information that can be collected in busy practice settings.

Although a PRN can be used to overcome the limitations of standard research designs with regard to problems of generalizability, the network cannot be used to replace clinical trials due to the limitations of PRN research in establishing internal validity that requires traditional clinical trials. Both methods, clinical trials and practice-based research, are essential, with each method complementing the deficits of the alternative approach.

## PRN RESEARCH DESIGN AND METHODS

The APA PRN will ultimately consist of 1,000 APA members representative of American psychiatry and the range of public and private psychiatric treatment settings. The network currently consists of approximately 200 APA members. Once fully established, the network will provide a nationally representative sample of psychiatrists, settings, patients, and treatments to provide statistically significant subsamples for most factors of interest. For example, the full range of psychiatric treatment settings, treatments, and patient groups will be represented in sufficient numbers so that even relatively small groups such as young children can be studied. For most network studies, a membership of this size will not be necessary; a subset of the network can be used depending on the specific research needs.

Network liaisons (psychiatrists active at the state and regional level) will work with the APA Office of Research staff to coordinate network activities at the local level. For example, the network liaisons will help to facilitate network communications, recruiting, and training on a state or regional level.

## Measurement Methods

**Core Studies.** On an annual basis, core data characterizing the network members, their practices, and patient caseloads will be collected. These data will be used to plan and assess the feasibility of specific network studies; analyze study specific findings, eliminating the need to collect this type of denominator data and basic descriptive information for each study conducted under the network; and systematically track trends and changes in the network membership, psychiatric treatment settings, patients, and treatment patterns. The network's annual core data will be developed using two data collection instruments: a core network member instrument and a core patient level instrument.

The core network member instrument will be used to characterize network members and their practices, providing data on network members' demographic characteristics, training and certification, professional activities, patient care workload,

and practice settings as well as aggregate demographic and diagnostic data on patient caseloads (Table 26.1). This instrument requires between 15 and 30 minutes to complete, depending on the complexity of the network member's practice.

The core patient level instrument will provide detailed data characterizing a sample of each network members' patients and the treatments they receive. The core patient level data will be collected on a randomly selected sample of five patients treated by each network member. The core patient level database, which has been pilot tested, will enable the network and other mental health researchers to study and analyze a wide range of issues related to psychiatric treatment patterns. They will be able to examine types and combinations of treatments provided to patients with different clinical and sociodemographic characteristics. For example, the instrument could be used to analyze the treatments (e.g., psychotropics, psychotherapies, and other so-

**Table 26.1  PRN Core Data Elements**

| Core Network Member Instrument | Core Patient Level Instrument |
| --- | --- |
| Network members' demographic characteristics | Sociodemographic characteristics of patients |
|   Age |   Age |
|   Gender |   Gender |
|   Race and ethnicity |   Race and ethnicity |
| Training |   Education level |
|   Decade graduated from medical school |   Marital status |
|   Whether international medical graduate | Insurance coverage and health plan characteristics |
|   Certification |   Source of payment |
| Professional activities |   Type of health plan |
|   Direct patient care |   Managed care interventions/constraints |
|   Teaching/supervision | Diagnostic information |
|   Research |   Principal diagnosis |
|   Consultation |   DSM-IV Axis I mental disorders |
| Patient care workload |   DSM-IV Axis II personality disorders |
|   No. of patients last typical work week |   DSM-IV Axis III general medical conditions |
|   No. of patient visits last typical work week |   DSM-IV Axis IV psychosocial and environmental |
|   No. of new patients last typical work week |     problems |
|   Number of patients seen in the last month |   DSM-IV Axis V global assessment of functioning |
| Characteristics of patients seen last typical work week |     score |
| (aggregate data) | Prior mental health treatments |
|   Age and gender | Current mental health treatments |
|   Race and ethnicity |   Setting and locus of care |
|   Setting locus and type |   Individual psychotherapy |
|   Insurance coverage and health plan |   Group, family, or couples psychotherapy |
|   Primary diagnostic category |   Psychotropics |
| |   Other somatic treatments |
| |   Other psychosocial services |
| | Future/anticipated mental health treatments |

matic or psychosocial services) provided to patients with a specific disorder or combination of disorders (such as panic disorder or major depressive disorder and substance abuse disorder). It could be used to examine variations in treatment patterns across patients within the same diagnostic categories but with different levels of severity or different health care plans. The core patient level database could also be linked with the core network member database so that a broad range of clinician characteristics and factors could be examined. Clinical patient level data provided in this detail are not readily available at this time.

**Specific Studies.** For the conduct of specific clinical services and health services, studies under the network "study-specific" instruments and measures will need to be identified or developed and refined. As study topics are developed and study variables of interest identified, existing psychiatric research instruments will be reviewed to determine whether they will meet the needs of the particular study. Section II provides examples of reliable and valid instruments that could be used by the PRN for specific clinical services research projects.

### Data Collection Methods

Initially, network data collection will be carried out using paper-based, "through-the-mail" data collection instruments that are completed by network members. As the scope of the network's data collection efforts expand and more instruments are finalized, more cost-efficient, optically scannable forms will be used. In addition, the network plans to conduct patient follow-up to collect longitudinal data from the patient perspective.

Practice-based research generally will use brief measures and instruments, particularly for clinician reported data, to obtain the quality of data necessary for the integrity of network research. In fact, collecting sufficiently detailed, reliable, and valid data from busy practicing clinicians participating in the network is one of the major challenges of practice-based research.

### THE NETWORK AND CLINICAL EFFECTIVENESS-OUTCOMES ASSESSMENT RESEARCH STUDIES

Some of the major measurement, research design, and analytic issues currently being addressed in conducting clinical effectiveness-outcome assessment studies using the network are described. Specific examples of these studies that are being planned under the network are also provided.

### Measurement Issues

The conduct of clinical effectiveness research studies using a practice-based research network requires careful attention to the psychometric measurement of diagnoses, case mix, health plan, treatments, and outcomes.

Diagnostic assessment is critical in identifying cases to be studied, because most treatment effectiveness studies will be disorder specific. The Diagnostic and Statistical Manual of Mental Disorders IV will be used as the basis for diagnostic assessment (23).

There is a need for case-mix measurement to control for intervening variables that may affect or confound outcomes. Both generic case-mix measures (e.g., socioeconomic status, age, psychiatric and general medical comorbidities) and disorder-specific measures, which take into consideration disorder-specific prognostic factors, should be examined (GR Smith, KM Rost, EP Fischer, MA Burnam, BJ Burns, unpublished data, 1994). For specific disorders, literature reviews are used to identify disorder-specific case-mix variables. The challenge, however, will be the need to develop brief measures that are practical and adequately reflect important case-mix variables.

Health plan characterization is important in delineating differences in general medical and mental health benefit coverage, constraints or limits on access to care, and service delivery components or financing arrangements that may enhance or detract from the quality of care (e.g., case management or capitation).

Treatment characterization describes the treatments provided (the independent variables in clinical effectiveness research) by network members as well as other mental health professionals who may be part of the treatment team. The different characteristics include the intensity, frequency, and duration of treatments. One major difficulty in characterizing psychiatric treatments is capturing differences in types of psychotherapy (24). Other measurement issues include accurately capturing data on treatments provided by other mental health professionals and the difficulty in controlling for the skill of the therapist.

The importance of including multiple measures of outcome (the dependent variables in effectiveness research) and incorporating multiple perspectives (clinicians as well as patients) in the conduct of outcome assessment studies has been well documented (25–28). These include the following patient measures: functional status; physical, social, and mental well being; symptoms; severity levels; adverse effects; satisfaction; and physiological measures. The critical challenges in outcome measurement include identifying brief, valid, meaningful measures of outcome as well as coordinating the collection of longitudinal patient level data in practice-based settings. Informed consent, respect for patient confidentiality, and success in following up patients is required. Assessing longitudinal outcomes necessitates the ability to track, monitor, and "follow-up" patients, as well as health care providers, and to coordinate the collection of data in remote, decentralized settings. However, this is becoming increasingly difficult given rapid changes in health care systems and problems of "provider switching" (29), in which patients change their health plans.

## EXAMPLES OF CLINICAL EFFECTIVENESS STUDIES

The PRN is conceptualized as a national laboratory for the conduct of mental health research; thus, it is available for use by network members and staff, as well as by "outside" investigators. A scientific advisory committee (technical experts, network members, and liaisons) will determine specific research priorities and, in conjunction with network members, will determine which studies to implement. The following general criteria will apply to all proposed research:

1. The topic is a significant public health, clinical, services delivery, or policy issue of importance and relevance to the field of psychiatry.
2. The research question requires a national practice-based research network and cannot more readily and cost effectively be studied using other research strategies.
3. Study of the question by the practice research network is technically and financially feasible and would not create an undue administrative burden on network members.

Examples of the studies that may be conducted with the network, which would be more difficult with a different research strategy, include studies of the treatment outcomes for major depressive disorder, bipolar disorder, and treatment-resistant schizophrenia.

For example, a depression outcomes study using the network could define the range of interventions used in routine psychiatric practice to treat major depressive disorder and could measure patient outcomes associated with various treatments.

A study of patients with bipolar disorder could characterize the patterns of use of mood stabilizers used alone and in combination in the acute and maintenance treatment of the disorder, could identify other pharmacological and psychosocial treatments used alone or in conjunction with mood stabilizers, and could assess the nature and severity of adverse treatment effects.

A study of the pharmacological treatment of treatment-resistant schizophrenia could assess the nature and severity of adverse effects from the two medications clozapine and resperidone, as well as long-term outcomes of treatments provided.

## CONCLUSIONS

A national PRN has the potential to offer a unique and powerful research capability to complement experimental approaches and other forms of traditional clinical and health services research. It also offers a significant research capability in conducting outcomes assessment studies on a national level. Key challenges will include the ability to retain a cadre of highly motivated and active network members who consistently adhere to study protocols and rigorous standards of data quality, identify and develop psychometrically validated data collection instruments that can be implemented in busy office-based practice settings, and attract and sustain ongoing funding to support the network's infrastructure and the costs of conducting specific studies.

## REFERENCES

1. Zarin DA, Pincus HA, McIntyre, JS. Practice guidelines [editorial]. Am J Psychiatry 1993; 150:175–177.
2. Davies AE, Doyle MA, Lansky D, et al. Outcomes assessment in clinical settings: a consensus statement on principles and best practices in project management. J Qual Improv 1994;20: 6–16.
3. Christoffel KK, Binns, HJ, Stockman JA, et al. Practice-based research: opportunities and obstacles. Pediatrics 1988;82(pt 2):299–406.
4. Iverson DC, Calonge N, Miller RS, Niebauer LJ, Reed FM. The development and management of a primary care research network, 1978–87. Fam Med 1988;20:177–180.
5. Charney E, Bynum R, Eldrege D. How well do patients take oral penicillin? A collaborative study in private practice. Pediatrics 1967;40: 188–195.
6. Lima J, Nazarian LF, Charney E. Compliance with short-term antimicrobial therapy: some techniques that help. Pediatrics 1976;57:383–386.
7. Nazarian LF. Research in pediatric practice. Pediatr Clin North Am 1981;28:585–599.
8. Olson AL, Klein SW, Charney E. Prevention and therapy of serious otitis medica by oral decongestant: a double-blind study in pediatric practice. Pediatrics 1978;61:679–684.
9. Green LA, Becker LA, Freeman WL, Elliott, E, Iverson DC, Reed FM. Spontaneous abortion in primary care. J Am Board Fam Pract 1988; 1:15–23.
10. Wasserman RC, Croft CA, Brotherton SE. Preschool vision screening in pediatric practice: a study from the pediatric research in office settings (PROS) network. Pediatrics 1992;89: 834–838.
11. Wasserman RC. Screening for vision problems in pediatric practice. Pediatr Rev 1992;13:4–5.
12. Freeman WL, Green LA, Becker LA. Pelvic inflammatory disease in primary care: a report from ASPN. Fam Med 1988;20:192–196.
13. Becker L, Iverson DC, Reed FM. Patients with new headache in primary-care: a report from ASPN. J Fam Pract 1988;27:41–47.
14. Becker LA, Iverson DC, Reed FM. A study of headache in North American primary care. J R Coll Gen Pract 1987;37:400–403.
15. Green LA, Becker LA, Freeman WL, Elliott E, Iverson DC, Reed FM. Spontaneous abortion in primary care: a report from ASPN. Fam Med 1988;20:197–201.
16. Rosser MW, Henderson R, Wood M, Green LA. An exploratory report of chest pain in primary care: a report from ASPN. J Am Board Fam Pract 1990;3:143–150.
17. Culpepper L, Froom J, Bridges-Webb C. Acute otitis media in adults: a report from the international primary care network. J Am Board Fam Pract 1993;6:333–339.
18. Froom J, Culpepper L, Gorb P. Diagnosis and antibiotic treatment of acute otitis media: report from international primary care network. Br Med J 1990;300:582–586.
19. Nelson EC, Kirk JW, Bise BW, et al. The cooperative information project. 1. A sentinel practice network for service and research in primary care. J Fam Pract 1981;13:641–649.
20. American Psychiatric Association Steering Committee on Practice Guidelines. Practice guidelines for major depressive disorder. Am J Psychiatry 1993;150(Suppl):4.
21. American Psychiatric Association Steering Committee on Practice Guidelines. Practice guidelines for eating disorders. Am J Psychiatry 1993;150:212–228.
22. American Psychiatric Association Steering Committee on Practice Guidelines. Practice guideline for the treatment of patients with bipolar disorder. Am J Psychiatry 1994;151 (Suppl):12.
23. American Psychiatric Association. Diagnostic and statistical manual of mental disorders. 4th ed. Washington, DC: American Psychiatric Association, 1994.
24. McNeilly, CL, Howard KI. The therapeutic procedures inventory: psychometric properties and relationship to phase of treatment. J Psychother Integr 1991;3:223–224.
25. Ciarlo JA, Brown TR, Edwards DW, et al. Assessing mental health treatment outcome measurement techniques. Washington, DC: U.S.

Government Printing Office, 1986. National Institute of Mental Health Series FN No. [DHHS Publ No. ADM-86-1301.]

26. Lohr KN. Application of health status assessment measures in clinical practice. Overview of the third conference on advances in health status assessment. Med Care 1992;30(5 Suppl): MS1–MS14.

27. Stewart AL, Ware JE, eds. Measuring functioning and well-being: the medical outcomes study approach. Durham: Duke University Press, 1992.

28. Ware JE. Measuring patient function and well-being: some lessons from the medical outcomes study. In: Heothoff K, Lohr K, eds. Effectiveness and outcomes in health care. Washington, DC: National Academy Press, 1991.

29. Wells KB, Hays RD, Burnam MA, Rogers W, Greenfield S, Ware JE. Detection of depressive disorder for patients receiving prepaid or fee-for-service care: results from the medical outcomes study. JAMA 1989;262:3298–3302.

CHAPTER 27

# The Development of Report Cards for Mental Health Care

*Barbara Dickey*

## HISTORICAL BACKGROUND

Although the 1993 Health Security Act failed to pass Congress, one particular section of the initiative caught the public's attention and, in a few cases, promoted action within the provider community. The Act called for the development of quality performance measures, including consumer report cards, to evaluate general medical care. These report cards were intended to encourage health plans to compete for customers on the basis of quality of care, as perceived by the consumer as well as the professional, and were intended to involve consumers in comparing the performance of any given health plan.

In discussing a hypothetical report card, the exact definition of such an entity is often questioned. Zimmerman (1) provided one answer: a report card is "a mechanism for collecting, analyzing, and distributing comparative performance data to all plans and consumers." To develop such a mechanism, however, requires consideration of the following factors: What information do consumers want? What health outcomes are important? What benchmarks are available for comparison of performance indicators? What methods are best for measuring outcomes?

Physicians were the first to ensure the quality of health care. Measuring the quality and reporting the outcomes of care were first advanced (without much success) in 1916 by Codman (2), a surgeon at the Massachusetts General Hospital in Boston. He published the results of his

procedures and urged his fellow surgeons to do likewise.

The involvement of consumers in the assessment of care is not a new idea. As recently as the early 1970s, comprehensive health planning legislation called for the development and implementation of state health plans. These plans were to be drawn up with the help of local providers and consumers. Today, the argument for including consumers in the development of report cards is that the usefulness of the reports will be increased if the indicators chosen for the report are meaningful to them. The more consumers are asked to pay for the cost of health care, the greater their interest in identifying the performance indicators in the quality of care.

## REVIEW OF REPORT CARDS

Report cards are in their earliest stages of development. Only a handful of proposed report cards are being developed and even fewer are actually being used. Although many ideas have been proposed in regard to what should be measured, limited financial resources and inadequate technology have forestalled the development of these ideas. Ideally, report cards should be understandable and useful to both consumers and employer purchasers, should use current data that are relatively inexpensive to obtain, should report on performance indicators that can be evaluated as good or bad, and should provide comparable valid information across plans.

Although there is no agreement about

particular performance indicators, certain categories of indicators are generally thought to capture those aspects of plan performance that concern payers and consumers. These categories include the cost of care, the access and appropriateness of care, the outcomes of care, and consumer satisfaction. Although there is general agreement about these measurement categories, the review below suggests that consensus varies as to the meaning of these indicators within categories. Providing the operational definition of each category is a challenge for those designing report cards.

## Mental Health Statistics Improvement Project (MHSIP)

MHSIP is a community of individuals, organizations, and associations actively working to improve the statistical capacity and comparability of local mental health service provider organizations within state and federal government agencies and among national mental health organizations. Last year, the MHSIP Advisory Group (funded by the Center for Mental Health Services) appointed a task force of consumers, mental health services researchers, and state mental health policy makers to develop a report card for use in the delivery of mental health care.

### Recommended Indicators

During Phase I of the project, the task force report listed 10 indicators that were defined as the "most crucial" to evaluating the performance of any plan:

- Rate of mental health expenditure;
- Rate of functional improvement;
- Availability of services beyond traditional inpatient and outpatient treatment;
- Consumer satisfaction with services;
- Consumer satisfaction with goal achievement;
- Consumer satisfaction with staff;
- Consumer ratings of outcome;
- Percent of consumers maintaining contact with their primary care provider for 1 year;

- Rate of follow-up after inpatient discharge;
- Rate of screening and follow-up treatment for depression.

Phase II of the project would identify specific measures that should be included in the report card. In addition, this phase of the project would pilot test methods of data collection and sampling. Phase III would pilot test, review, and modify the report card indicators as necessary.

## Health Plan Employer Data and Information Set (HEDIS) 2

Several years ago, anticipating the health care reform debate, the National Committee on Quality Assurance (NCQA) began the development of performance measures that would permit comparisons among health plans. Although more than 60 indicators have been included, only one is specific to mental illness. The developers did not include any indicators that directly measure outcome of treatment because they believed that outcomes measurement was not developed sufficiently. This work, referred to as HEDIS, is in its second round of development. The NCQA encourages employers and other users of HEDIS 2 to use the information internally to improve care rather than to share data across plans. NCQA cautions users to interpret information very carefully because of the limitations of the instruments and methodology.

Recommendations for indicators fall into three categories: quality of care, use of services, and member satisfaction. The report card focuses primarily on diagnoses other than mental health care, but one diagnosis, major affective disorder, is included. A single indicator is provided for plan performance comparison on the treatment of major affective disorders: percent of consumers receiving a follow-up visit within 30 days of hospital discharge.

In addition to this indicator, HEDIS 2 recommends that the following questions about access to mental health services be included in the report card: Compared to the plan standard, what is the actual telephone access to providers and what are the actual waiting times for a visit? How does a patient access a provider outside the normal operating hours of the plan? What is the plan doing to encourage access to care?

### Hospital-Based Initiatives

Chapter 4 describes the use of report cards in hospitals, under the rubic of quality assurance. Similar efforts are underway at McLean Hospital in Belmont, Massachusetts. Providing treatment programs with individualized report cards is proving to be a very effective mechanism for continuous quality improvement (CQI) activities.

### DISCUSSION

The development of report card activities has slowed somewhat since the failure of the Health Security Act. Nevertheless, early attempts to provide comparative information have found support among staff responsible for two different internal functions: marketing and CQI. The enthusiasm for report cards by the former may be waning as difficulties arise in making reports simple, understandable, and useful. This diminished enthusiasm by those in marketing may be offset by the growing acceptance of report cards by those who carry out CQI activities. Report cards will not become a reality, however, until a number of major challenges have been met.

### Benefits and Limitations of Report Cards

Activities related to the development and implementation of report cards have already proven to be valuable to some providers of care. These efforts have resulted in increased attention to consumer satisfaction, to improved quality of care, and to treatment directed toward specific goals and outcomes important to consumers. It is too soon to say whether these activities will be permanently integrated into mental health care on a widespread basis, but, to date, the most direct beneficiary of these activities has been staff responsible for CQI. Although marketing may benefit from the collection of satisfaction and outcome data (for internal consumption), the leap to report cards that can compare data across plans is still in the planning stage.

### Feasibility Questions

During the developmental stage of report cards, a number of questions have been raised that address the issue of their feasibility. Specifically, five questions have emerged and are discussed below.

1. *Which performance indicators best distinguish "good" plans from plans that are "not so good?"* Not only is there a lack of consensus about what indicators to include in a report card, but even the definition of quality is elusive. Perhaps one of the most vexing problems is how to define indicators so that there is consensus about their positive or negative values. For example, days of hospitalization per 1,000 members per year is relatively easy to calculate, but the level of agreement concerning the meaning of rates is difficult to determine. What is too high? What is too low?

A report card represents only a sample of the overall behavior of a health plan. Moreover, mental health indicators may be vulnerable to manipulation by plan managers to gain marketing advantage. For instance, suicide rates can be manipulated by reducing the number of adolescents or elderly in the plan. The potential for this maneuvering is significantly reduced by the use of multiple indicators. Using multiple measures may also provide a corrective to the assumption that "more is always better" (e.g., higher expenditures per enrollee means better services).

2. *What data collection strategies are most cost efficient?* The goal of minimizing the costs of collecting, maintaining, analyzing, and reporting information should be weighed against the benefits to the members of the plan and the internal information requirements of CQI. Existing needs for large-scale data systems and consumer surveys for internal management often overlap with those needs useful for report cards.

However, these data, whether reported to others or used internally, are not collected easily or inexpensively. Primary data (e.g., data collected directly from consumers or providers) are the most labor intensive, but even the reanalysis of secondary administrative data (e.g., benefit claims data) is time consuming and complicated.

Because current measures for assessing outcomes of mental health services are in their infancy, setting overly high reliability and validity standards will delay development of a report card that includes all key domains. Important variables, such as consumer satisfaction, should not be excluded because they have not been sufficiently tested. On the other hand, measures that have high reporting reliability, such as suicide rates, should not always be assumed to be negative indicators of performance unless the data can be risk adjusted.

Because evidence indicates that consumers tend to respond positively to surveys, questions should be asked about both consumer satisfaction and dissatisfaction. Evidence that ratings of satisfaction correlate with respondents' emotional state at the time of survey should not have a significant effect on comparisons of average satisfaction ratings among plans.

3. *What methods of risk adjustment can be used to make fair comparisons across plans?* Many factors, other than plan effectiveness, may cause differences in reported indicators. Of these, the age, sex, and health status of plan members are probably the most important. A plan that encourages young healthy employed families to join is likely to appear far more effective than a plan with older, sicker, and poorer members. Some plans may specialize in certain types of complicated cases and may be unfairly penalized by a report card that does not take this into account. Unfortunately, using techniques for making data more equivalent, such as risk adjustments, are complicated and do not always entirely remove these systematic differences. Nevertheless, consumers will need to be mindful that comparisons can only be made

when there is information about the context in which care is delivered. This might include the general makeup of the membership, whether the plan serves a predominately rural area or one in which rates of poverty or unemployment are high.

4. *What format provides the optimal amount of information without overwhelming consumers and purchasers of care?* Suggestions about format range from consumer report "circles" to sophisticated online databases that can be queried by consumers or purchasers of care. The latter certainly can accommodate more specialized information, but access to that information may be limited by consumers' knowledge of computers and how to access the information.

Despite these limitations, a consumer could obtain additional information beyond "global ratings of satisfaction" to determine how other individuals with similar backgrounds, gender, or problems rated services. Developing a written report card that would be accessible to most consumers and, at the same time, would respond to detailed questions might prove very difficult. Few consumers have the sophistication or the interest to wade through a volume of detailed statistics to sort out answers to such questions. However, if computer software could be developed to make such inquiries easier, a more extensive database could form the basis of a detailed report card. This approach would require some agreement on uniform standards for data collection and reporting.

5. *How can the information used in report cards be verified?* Last year the General Accounting Office (GOA) issued a report reviewing efforts to measure quality of care (3). One chapter was devoted to the need for independent verification of information. The GOA report pointed out the lack of consensus about who should undertake such verification and what information should be included. Without such verification, however, consumers may see the development of report cards that are more advertising than they are perfor-

mance indicators. There is also concern that issuing data before it can be verified might have unintended adverse consequences, such as plans avoiding enrollment of the sickest patients to ensure the appearance of better performance.

## CONCLUSIONS

The idea of rating health plans has captured the imagination of consumers and providers alike. Even if health care reform does not move in the direction of managed competition as envisioned by the Clinton Administration, developing a rating scheme that permits comparisons across health plans is a logical and important step. Whether such comparisons will lead to improvements in the quality of care delivered has not yet been determined, but the effort to develop reports cards may draw more attention to the needs and the quality of treatment of patients. At a time when providers are in a quandary as to the myriad changes being proposed in the organization and financing of health care, a focus on patient care could help to shift attention and resources toward consumer needs and expectations.

*Acknowledgments.* We acknowledge the following members of the MHSIP Task Force who contributed to a section of this chapter: John A. Hornik, Ph.D., New York State Office of Mental Health (Chair); Bill Brown, Consumer Affairs Coordinator, Catawba Mental Health; Colette Croze, M.S.W., National Association of State Mental Health Program Directors; Vijay Ganju, Ph.D., Texas Department of Mental Health; David W. Hilton, Office of Consumer Affairs, New Hampshire Division of Mental Health; Carolyn Kaufmann, Ph.D., Western Psychiatric Institute and Clinic; Richard C. Lippincott, M.D., Mental Health & Development Disability Services Division; Tanya Temkin, Center for Self-Help Research; and Ron Manderscheid, Ph.D., Center for Mental Health Services, Substance Abuse Mental Health Services Administration, U.S. Department of Health and Human services.

## REFERENCES

1. Zimmerman D. Grading the graders: using "report cards" to enhance the quality of care under health care reform. 1993. National Health Policy Form Issue Brief 642 (February).
2. Palmer RH, Donabedian A, Povar GJ. Striving for quality in health care. Ann Arbor, MI: Health Administration Press, 1991.
3. Health care reform: report cards are useful but significant issues need to be addressed. Washington, DC: U.S. General Accounting Office, 1994.

# CHAPTER 28

# Measurement Sensitivity in Clinical Mental Health Services Research: Recommendation for the Future[a]

*Ann A. Hohmann*

## INTRODUCTION

Mental health services research is one of the most rapidly expanding fields of federally funded health research. Two factors are strongly influencing the acceleration in interest and funding: public concern about mental health treatment effectiveness, as evidenced in the health care reform discussions, and the passage in 1992 of the Alcohol, Drug Abuse and Mental Health Administration Reorganization Act, P.L. 102-321, that moved the National Institute of Mental Health (NIMH) to the National Institutes of Health (NIH). That Act also directed the Institute to spend not less than 15% of its appropriation on health services research.

With these expansions in interest and funding, it is easy to lose sight of the need for basic research on the instruments used to assess treatment effectiveness. Typically, investigators have used whatever instruments are available that seem to cover the conceptual domains they wish to measure. However, a combination of administrative and scientific factors necessitate more serious consideration to the validity of the measurement strategies and instruments currently used.

Preceding the increased interest in mental health treatment effectiveness and increased funding for health services research, the NIH issued strict guidelines requiring inclusion of women and members of minority populations in all the research funded by the NIH. This policy has been strengthened significantly since it was first issued (1). An assessment of gender and minority issues is now an explicit part of the review of every application that is submitted to the NIH, and no application may receive funding unless it contains adequate or appropriate representation of both genders and minority populations.

Scientifically, data produced from effectiveness studies in which large-scale system changes were made and evaluated have found no significant effect of those system changes in improving outcomes (2) (L Bickman, PR Guthrie, EM Foster, et al., unpublished data, 1994). However, more circumscribed studies examining targeted service delivery conditions and changes have shown provocative and interesting effects (3, 4).

Thus, for a combination of reasons, it is time to consider the nature of our methodological research and the interpretation of the data we collect. Currently, we lack information about the differential psychometric properties for many population groups of the instruments currently in use. This chapter explores the issues that need to be considered in the basic methodological research that must occur for these measures to be useful tools in assessing the effectiveness of mental health services.

[a]Participants in the National Institute of Mental Health sponsored meeting convened to draft the recommendations presented in this chapter include Ronald Angel, Ph.D., Glorisa Canino, Ph.D., Judith A. Cook, Ph.D., James C. Coyne, Ph.D., Robert Drake, Ph.D., Anthony Lehman, M.D., M.S.P.H., Norweeta Milburn, Ph.D., Kathryn M. Rost, Ph.D., and David Williams, Ph.D.

NIMH began to address these issues in the strategic research plan in mental health services research (5). Part of that plan focused on the measurement of clinical mental health services outcomes and used a framework to define the domains of outcome measurement: clinical, rehabilitation, humanistic and/or quality of life, and public welfare and/or legal (6). NIMH commissioned papers reviewing the research measures and their known psychometric properties in each of the four domains (7) (EA McGlynn, unpublished data, 1992; JA Cook, unpublished data, 1992; JQ Lafond, unpublished data, 1992). These papers became the foundation for a 1993 meeting of nine services research investigators during which the validity of outcomes instruments was discussed from several perspectives: gender; ethnic, racial, or cultural minorities; persons with severe mental disorders; persons with co-occurring substance abuse disorders; rural populations; homeless populations; and persons with mental disorders seen in primary care or general health care settings. A synthesis of those discussions follows.

**Measurement Issues**

The measurement of patient or client outcomes in health services or mental health services research is a difficult task. To understand fully what the outcomes are, many aspects of a person's life must be assessed. However, measurement of mental health services outcomes is especially difficult for persons who suffer from severe mental disorders.

Each of the specific groups covered in this chapter present unique challenges to outcomes measurement. There are several dominant issues to be considered in the measurement of outcomes for all individuals receiving mental health services. These issues include the need for multidimensional measurement; multiple perspectives or informants; measurement of preferences or utilities; standardized measurement; longitudinal assessments; inclusion of cost data; and an understanding the data requirements of science, clinical practice, and policy (8).

For specific subpopulations, such as ethnic, racial, or cultural minorities and homeless or rural populations, two other issues are of particular importance: an individual's sociocultural, economic, personal, and clinical context and the methods of assessment.

**Context**

Outcomes must be assessed in the context in which they occur. When the context is ignored, invalid and inappropriate measures may be used or potentially valid measures may be misinterpreted, leading to invalid and, at the very least, useless conclusions. Outside of the treatment setting, the contexts that need to be taken into account in assessing outcomes include (a) individual clinical condition; (b) community and cultural norms regarding pathology, mental illness, and expected behaviors and outcomes; (c) current economic and environmental conditions; and (d) individual goals and expectations for outcomes. Although each context represents a distinct influence on outcomes, they are not mutually exclusive. It should not be forgotten that another critical context in assessing outcomes is that in which an individual receives treatment. Treatment consistency and quality and the patient-clinician relationship are crucial to understanding whether and why an intervention was successful and for whom. Measures of treatment process are necessary and should be considered in every study of treatment effectiveness.

**Clinical Conditions.** Foremost we must consider the individual's physical and mental condition. For persons with mental illness, and those with substance abuse disorders, for example, their cognitive functioning may be impaired to such an extent that the validity of the responses to assessments may be low. The severity of the psychiatric illness may also affect the reliability and validity of their responses (9).

**Community and Cultural Norms.** Community and cultural norms may have a significant impact at both the individual and community levels (10> (L Bickman, PR Guthrie, EM Foster et al., unpublished data, 1994). At the individual level, the expression of symptoms, whether somatic or psychological, is likely to be influenced by cultural expectations. Thus, in the clinical assessment of symptoms, it is important to be sensitive to the community norms regarding pathology. For example, an individual's report of hearing voices needs to be assessed in the context of that person's cultural milieu and religious beliefs.

Expression of symptoms may not only be culture based but gender based as well. The cultural and gender acceptability of psychological versus somatic symptoms also needs to be considered. This increased sensitivity to the influence of culture on symptom expression is reflected in the *Diagnostic and Statistical Manual for Mental Disorder,* 4th ed. (11).

Cultural, community, and social network expectations can also help define what outcomes are appropriate for an individual with a mental disorder. For example, community expectations can affect which social skills are important and what types of housing are considered necessary and desirable. In rural areas, many of the independent living and social skills that may be important in large urban settings may not be as relevant. Similarly, instruments assessing housing assume that independent living is an important goal; for many minority communities and for those in rural areas, such independence may be a form of social isolation.

At the community level, expectations for behavior can affect a community's reaction to psychiatric symptoms and therefore affect critical outcome dimensions, such as rates of rehospitalization. For example, community and family tolerance of bizarre behavior, perceptions of dangerousness, and gender-based expectations of behavior can affect the probability that a person with positive psychotic symptoms will be incarcerated, victimized, involuntarily hospitalized, treated in an emergency room, or

will fail to receive treatment or become homeless. This has special importance for minority populations.

Community patterns of dealing with minority populations need to be considered when assessing outcomes for severely disabled persons who are nonwhite. If members of minority groups within a community are more likely to be questioned by police, arrested, and incarcerated or to be victimized, then it is reasonable to assume the same will be true for persons with severe menatl disorders who are members of minority groups.

**Current Economic and Environmental Conditions.** The economic conditions of a community are important influences on vocational, housing, and quality of life outcomes. The rate of unemployment, the types of jobs available, the degree of gender and racial bias in hiring, the norms relating to the gender appropriateness of certain jobs, and the relative abundance or scarcity of those jobs will affect vocational outcome assessment. For example, the inability to find a job in a setting where 50% of the nondisabled, same-age, same-gender cohort is unemployed has a very different measuring than the inability to find a job when the unemployment rate for the community cohort is 7%. In addition, a focus only on "mainstream" avenues of employment may lead to a bias in actual employment estimates; some settings are likely to have thriving underground economies that may provide a substantial, though unreported, source of work and income for many members of a community.

Ability to acquire housing will also be affected by the community conditions. Independent housing is less available, or nonexistent, in many areas of the country, particularly rural areas. The availability of group housing is also affected by community zoning ordinances and the degree of public resistance to particular types of housing.

Current economic conditions of a community can affect a person's perceived quality of life. The economic conditions and location of a community help to determine the range of leisure activities that are available, the quality of housing available, the amounts of economic stress felt by an individual or family, the amount of crime, perceived safety, and availability of illegal drugs.

**Goals and Expectations for Outcomes.** Each person being treated in the mental health system holds a different set of preferences regarding clinical, social, vocational, educational, housing, quality of life, and legal outcomes. In other words, each person feels differently about what he or she wants from mental health treatment. These preferences function much like a paradigm does; each person's set of preferences affects how he or she perceives treatment progress. These preferences are likely to be strongly influenced by gender, age, length and severity of illness, diagnosis or diagnoses, cognitive functioning, current levels of self-esteem or self-efficacy, size and extent of social networks, cultural or subcultural norms, and location of residence (e.g., urban versus rural).

Within each person's preference set, the elements of that set are not all equal. Each person places a different value on clinical, social, vocational, and other outcomes; they are not equally important. Therefore, the ordering or weighting of the elements will also differ across individuals. This conceptualization of outcomes is fundamental to utility analyses within clinical decision analysis (12).

Preference sets can affect a clinical trial in two ways: they can influence whether an intervention is truly efficacious or effective for an individual and whether the measurement of that effect is valid. The likelihood of success of a particular intervention is dependent on the fit between the focus of the intervention and the ordering of the elements of the preference set. For example, if an intervention focuses on improving vocational outcomes and the individual is homeless, success is unlikely because the most salient issue in this person's life has

not been addressed. Two major issues relating to present sets should be considered in assessing the validity of measures in a clinical trial: the inclusion of all elements in the preference sets of the persons in the study and the inclusion of relative utilities of or preferences for the elements in those sets.

First, if the assessment of outcomes of a particular intervention fails to include elements that are very high in an individual's preference set, it is likely that the outcomes assessment will misestimate the degree of success of the intervention. For example, in an assessment of a clinical treatment trial, the investigators have chosen to measure change in psychiatric symptoms over time as the primary outcome.

Second, even if all the relevant elements in the population's preference sets have been assessed, if we do not assess how important different outcomes are relative to each other, that is, the ordering of the elements in the preference set, we are likely to misestimate the effect of the intervention. For example, consider the following case. In a longitudinal, effectiveness trial for a new antidepressant medication, we are using a quality of life assessment instrument that includes a section on religious involvement. At the baseline assessment, subject A and B both score 0 on the subscale, indicating the lowest possible involvement. At a 6-month follow-up, their scores are still 0. From the numbers, we could assume that the quality of their lives, relative to religious involvement, was identical. However, what the numbers do not show us is that subject A is an atheist and that subject B had entered the priesthood as a young man, though chose later to marry, and the current lack of religious involvement and/or desire to be connected to a religious institution is destroying his sense of self. Therefore, unless we know what the ordering is of the elements within an individual's preference set, our simplistic numerical categorization of his or her outcome on some dimension may completely misrepresent the true state.

Ideally, to understand outcomes for each individual in a clinical trial, we need to measure three things for each outcome domain: current state, the desired state, and the subjective importance of that state. So, in other words, if one of the goals of treatment is to reduce the amount of emotional conflict a patient has with family members, we would need to know how much conflict there is at the beginning of the trial, how much of a reduction in conflict the patient hoped to achieve, and how important a reduction in family conflict would be, relative to other treatment goals. This assessment can be represented mathematically as follows:

$$(\text{desired state} - \text{current state}) \times \text{preference weight}.$$

With such an assessment, the researcher is not imposing his or her own preferences or biases about what the patient ought to achieve or feel as a result of treatment. For members of minority groups and other subpopulations about whom we know very little, this approach could be an important step toward understanding what works, for whom, and under what circumstances.

## Methods of Assessment

The manner in which outcome measures are structured, administered, and combined for analysis may also have an important impact on the validity of the assessment.

**Structure.** The structural characteristics of a battery of outcome measures can affect not only the validity of assessment but also whether an individual will be able or willing to complete the assessment. The language, reading or comprehension level, and idioms (such as "feeling blue") should match those of the respondents. There must also be a match between the level of the psychiatric sophistication of the questions asked and a respondent's willingness to perceive his or her problems as psychologically or psychiatrically based.

Even if the assessment is completely understandable and acceptable to respondents, the length of the instrument or battery of instruments can affect the validity of the assessment. Finally, the instrument should be appropriate for the expected prevalence of disorder in the study population, and it should avoid ceiling and floor effects. For example, if an instrument is designed to screen for a disorder in a population that is severely disabled, using such an instrument in a primary care population would produce a false estimate of prevalence and would miss more subtle indicators of distress. The reverse would also be true. In both cases, the type and severity of symptoms in the instrument would be inappropriate to the study population.

**Administration.** How, when, where, and by whom an assessment is conducted are all important factors that can affect the validity of the conclusions drawn (13). Each factor is independently important. First, the manner in which questions are asked or presented can affect the ability of some persons to provide information (14). For example, with cultural or ethnic groups for whom direct eye contact is a sign of disrespect, a face-to-face interview is likely to engender a great deal of anxiety; therefore, the validity of the responses would be suspect. For some groups, and for some types of information, paper-and-pencil tests may be far superior in eliciting valid responses, particularly if the assessment includes questions on sensitive topics such as illegal behavior or culturally taboo feelings or behaviors. Another method that may improve the validity of responses is to use an interviewer with whom the respondent can identify, such as someone from the same racial group, the same gender, or (in the case of a homeless respondent) someone who was formerly homeless.

Second, the timing of assessments may affect the validity of the conclusions drawn. For example, a person diagnosed with schizophrenia who also has a co-occurring substance abuse disorder may have a completely different "recovery" timetable than someone suffering from schizophrenia alone. Because of this difference, changes in clinical, rehabilitation, and quality of life outcomes may occur at different rates. Although individuals suffering from schizophrenia and substance abuse may attain, on average, the same levels of symptom reduction, social and vocational skills, and perceived quality of life as those suffering from schizophrenia alone, they may do so at a much slower rate. In fact, changes in quality of life may not be evident for at least 2 or 3 years. Outcome assessments should be made longitudinally, and the realistic treatment and functional recovery trajectories of the population(s) being studied should be considered in making conclusions about treatment effectiveness.

Third, the location in which assessments are conducted is critically important. Differences in interview conditions, such as time of day, noise of the location, number and relationship of people who could potentially overhear the interviews or see questionnaire responses, and perceived safety of the location, should all be considered when conducting assessments.

Fourth, the number and type of informant, in addition to the respondent, should be carefully considered. In the assessment of children and adolescents it is becoming standard procedure to obtain more than one perspective on a child's symptoms and functioning. Although there is increasing acknowledgement that the same strategy must be used in the assessment of adults, particularly of those most severely impaired (15), the relative importance given to those assessments should receive careful attention. This is particularly true for assessments of quality of life and goals for rehabilitation and functioning in which significant differences may exist between the clinician's perspective and that of the client or patient. These differences may be magnified if a cultural or gender gap exists between the clinician and the client.

**Analysis.** Sensitivity to the effects of such factors as culture, language, severity of illness, co-occurring disorders, and gender needs to be extended beyond measurement consideration. How the chosen measures are analyzed or combined can also affect the validity of the assessment. Although convenient for simple statistical re-porting of the data, summary measures, including diagnostic and overall quality of life assessments, can conceal more than they reveal. To understand the meaning of a respondent's answers and to examine carefully what works, for whom, and under what circumstances, a thoughtful approach to the data is necessary. For example, if a particular group has a higher than expected prevalence of disorder, it is important to examine how particular symptoms, or clusters of symptoms, are related to functioning. Similarly, if a group's average composite quality of life score is lower than the norm, it is important to determine what aspect of life being affected and then to analyze and interpret that component in the context of their social networks, economic opportunities of the area, housing and financial situations, resistance of the community to group homes, and other factors. The interactions of these factors should also be considered.

## RECOMMENDATIONS FOR MEASUREMENT RESEARCH

The conceptual issues raised in this chapter suggest a number of immediate research issues that should be addressed if the field is to move forward. The issues fall into two major categories: instrument development and instrument refinement, testing, or modification.

### Instrument Development

Instruments for all gender and cultural groups are needed in a wide variety of areas. These instruments should

- Serve as brief screens for psychosis;
- Assess substance abuse, with high sensitivity and specificity, for persons who also have a severe mental disorder;
- Be appropriately sensitive and specific for the level of symptoms experienced by persons seeking care from primary care physicians;
- Measure the negative, as well as the positive, aspects of support;
- Measure the reciprocity of that support;
- Assess low level skills (e.g., making and

keeping appointments or negotiating the social service bureaucracies) and not just high level skills (e.g., job performance);

- Incorporate behavioral measures of social skills;
- Measure an individual's quality of life expectations, as well as current state;
- Distinguish situational mood from fundamental quality of life issues;
- Measure patient preferences for various treatments and outcomes and measure how clinicians cope with those preference to determine whether these differ by gender, ethnic or cultural group, severity of disorder, co-occurring disorder, or homeless status;
- Measure victimization, specific to the severe mental illness population, perceived vulnerability to various forms of victimization, and the ability of mentally disordered individuals to obtain help when threatened;
- Measure dangerousness by focusing on behavior that causes physical harm or creates a reasonable fear of such harm and not behaviors that offend social norms;
- Measure the intensity of the treatment received so that, for example, rural-urban comparisons can be made.

## Instrument Refinement

Virtually all instruments in use require further psychometric testing, particularly among ethnic and cultural minority groups, women, and persons who are homeless and/or have co-occurring substance abuse disorders. The validity of the assessment methods and the effect of differences in response styles and item recall need to be evaluated for all of these groups. Finally, normative data for disadvantaged groups are needed for the rehabilitation, quality of life, and functioning measures so that they can be used as comparison data for similarly disadvantaged groups suffering from severe mental disorders. These data will allow us to separate the effects of social disadvantage from disability on treatment outcomes and to evaluate the interaction between the two.

## CONCLUSIONS

As the field of services research matures, challenging measurement issues will require careful consideration. Fundamental issues relating to the nature and consequences of disorder will need to be addressed. Should assessment packages be generic or disorder specific? Should a core set of measures applicable across groups and disorders be available, as well as other sets that are disorder and/or culture, setting, or gender specific? Should thresholds for defining disorder and "normal" be set by functioning, based on culture, socioeconomic status, rural location, and/or homeless status? Are diagnostic or behavioral measures better predictors of longterm outcome? Does the predictive validity vary by group (cultural, homeless, primary care patients)? These questions, and many more, need to be addressed in the coming years.

## REFERENCES

1. Department of Health and Human Services. NIH Guidelines on the inclusion of women and minorities as subjects in clinical research. Federal Register 1994;59:14508–14513.
2. Goldman HH, Morrissey JP, Ridgely MS. Evaluating the Robert Wood Johnson Foundation Program on chronic mental illness. Milbank Q 1994;72:37–47.
3. Dozier M, Cue KL, Barnett L. Clinicians as caregivers: role of attachment organization in treatment. J Consult Clin Psychol 1994;62:793–800.
4. Glisson C. The effect of services coordination teams on outcomes for children in state custody. Admin Soc Work 1994;18:1–23.
5. National Institute of Mental Health. Caring for people with severe mental disorders: a national plan of research to improve services. Washington, DC: U.S. Government Printing Office, 1991. [DHHS Publ. No. (ADM)91-1762.]
6. Hargreaves WA, Shumway M. Effectiveness of mental health services for the severely mentally ill. In: Taube CA, Mechanic D, Hohmann AA, eds. The future of mental health services research. Washington, DC: U.S. Government Printing Office, 1989. [DHHS Publ. No. (ADM)89-1600.]
7. Lehman AF. Measures of quality of life among persons with severe and persistent mental dis-

orders. Soc Psychiatry Psychiatr Epidemiol (in press).

8. Attkisson C, Cook J, Karno M, et al. Clinical services research. Schizophr Bull 1992;18:561–626.

9. Drake RE, McHugh GJ, Biesanz JC. The test-retest relability of standardized instruments among homeless persons with substance abuse disorder. J Stud Alcohol 1995:56:161–167.

10. Reid PT. The real problem in the study of culture. Am Psychol 1994;49:524–525.

11. American Psychiatric Association. Diagnostic and statistical manual of mental disorders. 4th ed. Washington, DC: American Psychiatric Association, 1994.

12. Weinstein MC, Fineberg HV. Clinical Decision Analysis. Philadelphia: WB Saunders, 1980.

13. Milburn NG, Gary LE, Booth JA, Brown DR. Conducting epidemiologic research in a minority community: methodological considerations. J Comm Psychol 1994;19:3–12.

14. Babor TF, Stephens RS, Marlatt GA. Verbal report methods in clinical research on alcoholism: response bias and its minimization. J Stud Alcohol 1987;48:410–424.

15. Drake RE, Alterman AL, Rosenberg SR. Detection of substance abuse disorders in severely mentally ill patients. Community Ment Health J 1993;29:175–192.

## APPENDIX A

# Summary of Instruments, Authors, and Respondents

| OUTCOMES ASSESSMENT IN CLINICAL PRACTICE | | | | |
|---|---|---|---|---|
| **INSTRUMENT** | **AUTHOR** | **RESPONDENT** | | |
| | | *Clinician* | *Patient* | *Family* |
| ***Global Well Being*** | | | | |
| SF-36 | *Ware* | | X | |
| QOLI | *Lehman* | | X | |
| ***Functioning and Symptoms*** | | | | |
| GAF | *Spitzer et al.* | X | | |
| BASIS-32 | *Eisen* | | X | |
| ASI** | *McLellan et al.* | | X | |
| DOM** | *Smith et al.* | X | X | |
| SAOM** | *Smith et al.* | X | X | |
| CBCL | *Achenbach* | X | X | X* |
| ***Symptom-based*** | | | | |
| SCL-90-R®/BSI® | *Derogatis* | | X | |
| BDI™ | *Beck* | | X | |
| BPRS | *Overall, Gorham* | X | X | |
| EDI-2 | *Garner* | | X | |
| SATS** | *Drake et al.* | X | | |
| ***Functioning-based*** | | | | |
| LSP | *Parker et al.* | X | | |
| AUS/DUS | *Drake et al.* | X | | |
| FBIS/SF | *Tessler, Gamache* | | | X |
| ***Satisfaction*** | | | | |
| CSQ | *Attkisson* | | X | |
| SSS-30 | *Greenfield, Attkisson* | | X | |
| ***Service Use*** | | | | |
| TSR | *McLellan et al* | | X | |

\* teachers or other observers
\*\* report by clinician, but based on all sources of report

# Examples of Specific Instruments

| The MOS 36-Item Short-Form Health Survey, *See Chapter 8* |
|---|

# Rand 36-Item Health Survey 1.0
# Questionnaire Items

1. In general, would you say your health is:

**(circle one number)**

Excellent ................................. 1

Very good ............................... 2

Good ...................................... 3

Fair........................................ 4

Poor ...................................... 5

2. Compared to one year ago, how would you rate your health in general now?

**(circle one number)**

Much better now than one year ago................ 1

Somewhat better now than one year ago........ 2

About the same................................................ 3

Somewhat worse now than one year ago ......... 4

Much worse now than one year ago ................ 5

The following items are about activities you might do during a typical day. Does your health now limit you in these activities? If so, how much?

**(circle one number on each line)**

|  | *Yes, Limited a Lot* | *Yes, Limited a Little* | *No, Not Limited at All* |
|---|---|---|---|
| 3. Vigorous activities, such as running, lifting heavy objects, participating in strenuous sports........................................ | 1 | 2 | 3 |
| 4. Moderate activities, such as moving a table, pushing a vacuum cleaner, bowling, or playing golf.................................... | 1 | 2 | 3 |
| 5. Lifting or carrying groceries .............................................. | 1 | 2 | 3 |
| 6. Climbing several flights of stairs .................................... | 1 | 2 | 3 |
| 7. Climbing one flight of stairs ............................................ | 1 | 2 | 3 |
| 8. Bending, kneeling, or stooping ........................................ | 1 | 2 | 3 |
| 9. Walking more than a mile ............................................... | 1 | 2 | 3 |
| 10. Walking several blocks.................................................... | 1 | 2 | 3 |
| 11. Walking one block ........................................................... | 1 | 2 | 3 |
| 12. Bathing or dressing yourself........................................... | 1 | 2 | 3 |

During the past 4 weeks, have you had any of the following problems with your work or other regular daily activities as a result of your physical health?

**(circle one number on each line)**

| | *Yes* | *No* |
|---|---|---|
| 13. Cut down the amount of time you spent on work or other activities............................................................ | 1 | 2 |
| 14. Accomplished less than you would like............................................ | 1 | 2 |
| 15. Were limited in the kind of work or other activities ...................... | 1 | 2 |
| 16. Had difficulty performing the work or other activities (for example, it took extra effort)...................................................... | 1 | 2 |

During the past 4 weeks, have you had any of the following problems with your work or other regular daily activities as a result of any emotional problems (such as feeling depressed or anxious)?

**(circle one number on each line)**

| | *Yes* | *No* |
|---|---|---|
| 17. Cut down the amount of time you spent on work or other activities ...................................................................... | 1 | 2 |
| 18. Accomplished less than you would like............................................. | 1 | 2 |
| 19. Didn't do work or other activities as carefully as usual................. | 1 | 2 |

20. During the past 4 weeks, to what extent has your physical health or emotional problems interfered with your normal social activities with family, friends, neighbors, or groups?

**(circle one number)**

Not at all................................... 1

Slightly...................................... 2

Moderately................................ 3

Quite a bit................................. 4

Extremely ................................. 5

21. How much bodily pain have you had during the past 4 weeks?

**(circle one number)**

None......................................... 1

Very mild ................................. 2

Mild.......................................... 3

Moderate................................... 4

Severe ...................................... 5

Very severe ............................... 6

22. During the past 4 weeks, how much did pain interfere with your normal work (including both work outside the home and housework)?

**(circle one number)**

Not at all................................... 1

A little bit.................................. 2

Moderately................................ 3

Quite a bit................................. 4

Extremely ................................. 5

These questions are about how you feel and how things have been with you during the past 4 weeks. For each question, please give the one answer that comes closest to the way you have been feeling.

How much of the time during the past 4 weeks . . .

**(circle one number on each line)**

| | All of the Time | Most of the Time | A Good Bit of the Time | Some of the Time | A Little of the Time | None of the Time |
|---|---|---|---|---|---|---|
| 23. Did you feel full of pep? ............................ | 1 | 2 | 3 | 4 | 5 | 6 |
| 24. Have you been a very nervous person?.... | 1 | 2 | 3 | 4 | 5 | 6 |
| 25. Have you felt so down in the dumps that nothing could cheer you up?............. | 1 | 2 | 3 | 4 | 5 | 6 |
| 26. Have you felt calm and peaceful?............ | 1 | 2 | 3 | 4 | 5 | 6 |
| 27. Did you have a lot of energy? ................... | 1 | 2 | 3 | 4 | 5 | 6 |
| 28. Have you felt downhearted and blue? ..... | 1 | 2 | 3 | 4 | 5 | 6 |
| 29. Did you feel worn out? .............................. | 1 | 2 | 3 | 4 | 5 | 6 |
| 30. Have you been a happy person?............... | 1 | 2 | 3 | 4 | 5 | 6 |
| 31. Did you feel tired?..................................... | 1 | 2 | 3 | 4 | 5 | 6 |

32. During the past 4 weeks, how much of the time has your physical health or emotional problems interfered with your social activities (like visiting with friends, relatives, etc.)?

**(circle one number)**

All of the time.......................... 1

Most of the time ..................... 2

Some of the time..................... 3

A little of the time .................. 4

None of the time ..................... 5

How TRUE or FALSE is *each* of the following statements for you?

**(circle one number on each line)**

| | Definitely True | Mostly True | Don't Know | Mostly False | Definitely False |
|---|---|---|---|---|---|
| 33. I seem to get sick a little easier than other people ................................................ | 1 | 2 | 3 | 4 | 5 |
| 34. I am as healthy as anybody I know......................... | 1 | 2 | 3 | 4 | 5 |
| 35. I expect my health to get worse............................... | 1 | 2 | 3 | 4 | 5 |
| 36. My health is excellent............................................. | 1 | 2 | 3 | 4 | 5 |

BASIS 32

### BEHAVIOR AND SYMPTOM IDENTIFICATION SCALE

NAME _____ I.D.# _____ Date _____

---

#### INSTRUCTIONS

Below is a list of problems and areas of life functioning in which some people experience difficulties. Using the scale below, WRITE IN THE BOX THE NUMBER that best describes THE DEGREE OF DIFFICULTY YOU HAVE BEEN EXPERIENCING IN EACH AREA DURING THE PAST WEEK.

    0   no difficulty
    1   a little
    2   moderate
    3   quite a bit
    4   extreme

Please respond to each item. Do not leave any blank. If there is an area that you consider to be inapplicable, indicate that it is NO DIFFICULTY ("0").

<u>Example</u>

To what extent are you experiencing
difficulty in the area of <u>FRIENDSHIPS</u>:    ☐ 2

---

TO WHAT EXTENT ARE YOU EXPERIENCING
DIFFICULTY IN THE AREA OF:

1.  MANAGING DAY-TO-DAY LIFE (e.g., getting
    places on time, handling money, making          ☐
    every day decisions)

2.  HOUSEHOLD RESPONSIBILITIES (e.g., shop-
    ping, cooking, laundry, keeping room             ☐
    clean, other chores)

3.  WORK (e.g., completing tasks, performance
    level, finding/keeping a job)                    ☐

4.  SCHOOL (e.g., academic performance,
    completing assignments, attendance)              ☐

WRITE THE NUMBER IN THE BOX

0  no difficulty
1  a little
2  moderate
3  quite a bit
4  extreme

TO WHAT EXTENT ARE YOUR EXPERIENCING
DIFFICULTY IN THE AREA OF:

5.  LEISURE TIME OR RECREATIONAL ACTIVITIES ☐

6.  ADJUSTING TO MAJOR LIFE STRESSES (e.g.,
separation, divorce, moving, new job,
new school, a death) ☐

7.  RELATIONSHIPS WITH FAMILY MEMERS ☐

8.  GETTING ALONG WITH PEOPLE OUTSIDE OF THE
FAMILY ☐

9.  ISOLATION OR FEELINGS OF LONELINESS ☐

10.  BEING ABLE TO FEEL CLOSE TO OTHERS ☐

11.  BEING REALISTIC ABOUT YOURSELF OR OTHERS ☐

12.  RECOGNIZING AND EXPRESSING EMOTIONS
APPROPRIATELY ☐

13.  DEVELOPING INDEPENDENCE, AUTONOMY ☐

14.  GOALS OR DIRECTION IN LIFE ☐

15.  LACK OF SELF-CONFIDENCE, FEELING BAD
ABOUT YOURSELF ☐

16.  APATHY, LACK OF INTEREST IN THINGS ☐

17.  DEPRESSION, HOPELESSNESS ☐

18.  SUICIDAL FEELINGS OR BEHAVIOR ☐

19.  PHYSICAL SYMPTOMS (e.g., headaches,
aches & pains, sleep disturbance,
stomach aches, dizziness) ☐

WRITE THE NUMBER IN THE BOX

0 no difficulty
1 a little
2 moderate
3 quite a bit
4 extreme

TO WHAT EXTENT ARE YOUR EXPERIENCING
DIFFICULTY IN THE AREA OF:

20. FEAR, ANXIETY OR PANIC ☐

21. CONFUSION, CONCENTRATION< MEMORY ☐

22. DISTURBING OR UNREAL THOUGHTS OR BELIEFS ☐

23. HEARING VOICES, SEEING THINGS ☐

24. MANIC, BIZARRE BEHAVIOR ☐

25. MOOD SWINGS, UNSTABLE MOODS ☐

26. UNCONTROLLABLE, COMPULSIVE BEHAVIOR
(e.g., eating disorder, hand-washing,
huring yourself)
SPECIFY_____ ☐

27. SEXUAL ACTIVITY OR PREOCCUPATION ☐

28. DRINKING ALCOHOLIC BEVERAGES ☐

29. TAKING ILLEGAL DRUGS, MISUSING DRUGS ☐

30. CONTROLLING TEMPER, OUTBURSTS OF ANGER
VIOLENCE ☐

31. IMPULSIVE, ILLEGAL OR RECKLESS BEHAVIOR ☐

32. FEELING SATISFACTION WITH YOUR LIFE ☐

## The Addiction Severity Index, *See Chapter 10*

DATE ___/___/___                                    ID_____

Now, I need to ask you a series of questions about your alcohol and drug use. Remember, all your answers are confidential.

(PROBE: Do you administer your medications yourself, or do you take them from a nurse at the shelter or at your home? Do you take any other drugs other than those given to you?)

I. **INSTRUCTIONS:** In this section below, ask the following questions for each substance.

a) In the past **30 days,** how many days have you used_____?

b) Do you usually_____?

**(Route of Administration in Order of Severity)**

eat or drink?............................................................................................ Oral = 1
snort or sniff?........................................................................................... Nasal = 2
smoke?...................................................................................................... Smoking = 3
shoot?........................................................................................................ Non-IV = 4
................................................................................................................... or IV = 5

Note: 1) The *usual* and *most recent* route of administration should be recorded.
2) If multiple routes, code most serious.
3) Prescribed medication should be counted under the generic category.

|  | 30 days | Adminis. Route |
|---|---|---|
| 1. Alcohol—*any use at all* | __ __ (1d) | _____ (1r) |
| 2. Alcohol—*to intoxication* (Prompt: feeling light-headed, dizzy, high) | __ __ (2d) | _____ (2r) |
| 3. Heroin *(Smack, horse)* | __ __ (3d) | _____ (3r) |
| 4. Methadone | __ __ (4d) | _____ (4r) |
| 5. Other opiates/analgesics *(morphine/dreamer junk, demerol, darvon/darvoset, Codeine/school boy, Percodan, Dilaudid, Talwin)* | __ __ (5d) | _____ (5r) |
| 6. Barbiturates — Sedatives *(seconals/reds/red devils, Nembutal, tuinals/Rainbows, Veronal, phenobarbital, yellow jackets, Purple Hearts)* | __ __ (6d) | _____ (6r) |
| 7. Other sedatives/tranquilizers or hypnotics *(Valium, Librium, Xanax, Quaaludes/ludes/supers, Cloripin)* | __ __ (7d) | _____ (7r) |
| 8. Cocaine/crack/coca leaves | __ __ (8d) | _____ (8r) |

9. Amphetamines, Stimulants
(*bennies, speed, uppers, speedball, dexies, pep pill, crank, crystal, monster pep pill, moth, black beauties*)

   \_\_ \_\_ (9d)   \_\_\_\_ (9r)

10. Marijuana
(*pot, reefer, hashish, cannabis*)

   \_\_ \_\_ (10d)   \_\_\_\_ (10r)

11. Hallucinogens
(*LSD, acid / purple haze, mescaline / MESC / cactus, PCP / angel dust / supra w / marijuana, peyote*)

   \_\_ \_\_ (11d)   \_\_\_\_ (11r)

12. Inhalants
(*nitrous oxide / whippets, glue, amyl nitrate / mush / lockeroom, Poppers / Snappers, gasoline, paint, nail polish remover*)

   \_\_ \_\_ (12d)   \_\_\_\_ (12r)

13. Any drug at all *not including alcohol*

   \_\_ \_\_ (13d)   \_\_\_\_ (13r)

14. More than one substance per day, *including alcohol*

   \_\_\_ (14)

15. **For interviewer:**
Which substance do you think has been the client's
**major problem for the past 30 days?**

   \_\_ \_\_ (15)

(If interviewer cannot determine, then ask the client:
*Which substance is your biggest problem?*)
   Coding:

| | |
|---|---|
| 00 No alcohol | 07 Cocaine/crack |
| 01 Alcohol | 08 Amphetamines |
| 02 Heroin | 09 Cannabis |
| 03 Methadone | 10 Hallucinogens |
| 04 Other opiates/analgesics | 11 Inhalants |
| 05 Barbiturates | 12 Alcohol and drug |
| 06 Other sedatives/hypnotics/tranquilizers | 13 Polydrug |

16. **If answer to 15 is dual addiction of alcohol and drug,** which is the drug other
than alcohol? (Use codes 02-11 listed above)

   \_\_ \_\_ (16)

17. **If the answer to 15 is polydrug,** what are the two most problematic drugs?
(Use codes 02-11 listed above)

   \_\_ \_\_ (17a)   \_\_ \_\_ (17b)

18. How long was your last period of voluntary abstinence from
(this major substance)? (000 Never abstinent)
(Note: Round up to nearest month.
Periods of hospitalization or incarceration are not counted.
Periods of abstinence during which the patient was taking
Methadone, Antabuse, or Naltrexone as an outpatient are included.)

   \_\_ \_\_ \_\_months (18)

19. How long ago did this abstinence end? (000 Still abstinent)
(Note: Round up to nearest month.)

   \_\_ \_\_ \_\_ (19)

20. Over the past **30 days,** how much money have you spent on alcohol?
(Note: Enter only the money spent, not the street value.
Round up to the nearest dollar.)

   \_\_ \_\_ \_\_ \_\_ dollars (20)

21. Over the past **30 days,** how much money have you spent on drugs?
(Note: Enter only the money spent, not the street value.
Round up to the nearest dollar.)

   \_\_ \_\_ \_\_ \_\_ dollars (21)

22. Over the past **30 days,** how many days have you been treated in an
outpatient setting for alcohol or drugs?                                    _ _ days (22)
(Note: Include AA, NA, CA meetings, Antabuse, methadone maintenance.
Attend at least 3 sessions to qualify.)

23. In the past **30 days,** how many days have you experienced alcohol problems,
including a craving for alcohol, adverse effects from alcohol, withdrawal
symptoms from alcohol, or the desire but inability to stop drinking?        _ _ days (23)
Do not include inability to find alcohol.

Using the rating scale below for the following questions . . .

24. In the past **30 days,** how troubled or bothered have you been by alcohol problems?    ___ (24)

25. In the past **30 days,** how troubled or bothered have you been by drug problems?       ___ (25)

26. How important to you is additional treatment for alcohol problems now?                  ___ (26)
*(Rate specific need for substance abuse treatment, not general therapy)*

27. How important to you is additional treatment for drug problems now?                     ___ (27)
*(Rate specific need for substance abuse treatment, not general therapy.)*

    0 = Not at all                                                      ___ (R)
    1 = Slightly
    2 = Moderately
    3 = Considerably
    4 = Extremely

## The Treatment Service Review, *See Chapter 10*

Name: _____    Date: _____

Interviewer:_____    Pt. I.D. #: _____

Treatment Week #:_____ _____    Program #: _____

How many days in the past week have you attended this program? _____

### *TREATMENT SERVICES REVIEW (2/1/89)*

Please record services (provided or referred) by the treatment program (IN-PROG)
separately from those provided by other sources (OUT-PROG)

*MEDICAL PROBLEMS:* How many days in the past week have you:

1. experienced significant *physical medical* problems?

| | IN-PROG | OUT-PROG |
|---|---|---|
| 2. been hospitalized for *physical medical* problems? | _____ | _____ |
| 3. received medication for a medical problem? | _____ | _____ |

How many times in the past week have you:

| | IN-PROG | OUT-PROG |
|---|---|---|
| 4. seen a physician for medical care? | _\|_ | |
| 5. seen a nurse, nurse practitioner, or physician's assistant for medical care? | _\|_ | _\|_ |
| 6. had a significant discussion pertinent to your medical problems: individual session? | _\|_ | _\|_ |
| group session? | _\|_ | _\|_ |

*EMPLOYMENT AND SUPPORT PROBLEMS:* How many days in the past week have you:

1. been paid for working?

| | IN-PROG | OUT-PROG |
|---|---|---|
| 2. been in school or training? | _____ | _____ |

How many times in the past week have you:

| | IN-PROG | OUT-PROG |
|---|---|---|
| 3. seen someone regarding employment opportunities, training or education: employment specialist? | _\|_ | _\|_ |
| counselor/social worker? | _\|_ | _\|_ |
| 4. seen someone regarding unemployment compensation, welfare, social security, housing or other income: benefits specialist? | _\|_ | _\|_ |
| counselor/social worker? | _\|_ | _\|_ |
| 5. had a significant discussion pertinent to your employment/support problem: individual session? | _\|_ | _\|_ |
| group session? | _\|_ | _\|_ |

*ALCOHOL PROBLEMS:* How many days in the past week have you:

1. drunk any alcohol?
2. drunk any alcohol to the point of intoxication (note definition)?

| | IN-PROG | OUT-PROG |
|---|---|---|
| 3. been in inpatient treatment for an alcohol problem? | _____ | _____ |
| 4. received medication to help you to detoxify from alcohol? | _____ | _____ |
| 5. received medication to *prevent* you from drinking? | _____ | _____ |
| 6. received a blood alcohol test (e.g., breathalyzer)? | _____ | _____ |

How many times in the past week have you:

| | IN-PROG | OUT-PROG |
|---|---|---|
| 7. attended an alcohol education session? | _\|_ | _\|_ |
| 8. attended an AA or 12 step meeting? | _\|_ | _\|_ |
| 9. attended an alcohol relapse prevention meeting? | _\|_ | _\|_ |
| 10. had a significant discussion pertinent to your alcohol problem: individual session? | _\|_ | _\|_ |
| group session? | _\|_ | _\|_ |

*DRUG PROBLEMS:* How many days in the past week have you:
1. used any illicit drug?

|  | IN-PROG | OUT-PROG |
|---|---|---|

2. been in inpatient treatment for a drug problem?
3. received medication to help you detoxify/come off a drug?
4. received medication to maintain/stabilize your drug use?
5. received medication to block the effects of drugs?
6. received a urinalysis, or other test for drug use?
    How many times in the past week have you:
7. attended a drug education session?
8. attended a session of NA or CA?
9. attended a drug relapse prevention group or session?
10. had a significant discussion pertinent to your drug problem:
    individual session?
    group session?

*LEGAL PROBLEMS:* How many days in the past week have you:
1. been incarcerated?
2. engaged in illegal activities for profit?
    How many times in the past week have:          IN-PROG    OUT-PROG
3. the courts, criminal justice system, probation/parole office been
    contacted regarding your legal problem (either by patient or program)?
4. you had a significant discussion pertinent to your legal problems:
    individual session?
    group session?

*FAMILY PROBLEMS:* How many days in the past week have you:
1. experienced significant family/social problems?
2. experienced significant loneliness and/or boredom?
    How many times in the past week have you:          IN-PROG    OUT-PROG
3. had a significant discussion pertinent to your *family* problems
    with family present:
    family specialist?
    counselor/social worker?
4. had a significant discussion pertinent to your *family* problems
    without family present:
    family specialist?
    counselor/social worker?

*PSYCHOLOGICAL / EMOTIONAL PROBLEMS:*
    How many days in the past week have you:
1. experienced significant emotional problems?

|  | IN-PROG | OUT-PROG |
|---|---|---|

2. been hospitalized for an emotional or psychological problem?
3. received testing for psychological or emotional problems?
4. received medication for your psychological or emotional problems?
    How many times in the past week have you:
5. received a session in which you *practiced* a form of relaxation training,
    biofeedback or meditation:
    psych specialist?
    counselor/social worker?
6. received a session in which you *practiced* a form of behavior modification
    (e.g., role play, rehearsal, psychodrama, etc.):
    psych specialist?
    counselor/social worker?
7. had a significant discussion pertinent to your psychological or
    emotional problems:
    psych specialist?
    counselor/social worker?

## Global Assessment of Functioning Scale, *See Chapter 11*

### Global Assessment of Functioning Scale (GAF Scale)

Consider psychological, social, and occupational functioning on a hypothetical continuum of mental health-illness. Do not include impairment in functioning due to physical (or environmental) limitations.

**Note:** Use intermediate codes when appropriate, e.g., 45, 68, 72.

**Code**

90
|
81
80

Absent or minimal symptoms (e.g., mild anxiety before an exam), good functioning in all areas, interested and involved in a wide range of activities, socially effective, generally satisfied with life, no more than everyday problems or concerns (e.g., an occasional argument with family members).

|
71
70

If symptoms are present, they are transient and expectable reactions to psychosocial stressors (e.g., difficulty concentrating after family argument); no more than slight impairment in social, occupational, or school functioning (e.g., temporarily falling behind in school work).

|
61
60

Some mild symptoms (e.g., depressed mood and mild insomnia) OR some difficulty in social, occupational, or school functioning (e.g., occasional truancy, or theft within the household), but generally functioning pretty well, has some meaningful interpersonal relationships.

|
51
50

Moderate symptoms (e.g., flat affect and circumstantial speech, occasional panic attacks) OR moderate difficulty in social, occupational, or school functioning (e.g., few friends, conflicts with co-workers).

|
41
40

Serious symptoms (e.g., suicidal ideation, severe obsessional rituals, frequent shoplifting) OR any serious impairment in social, occupational, or school functioning (e.g., no friends, unable to keep a job).

|
|
31
30

Some impairment in reality testing or communication (e.g., speech is at times illogical, obscure, or irrelevant) OR major impairment in several areas, such as work or school, family relations, judgment, thinking, or mood (e.g., depressed man avoids friends, neglects family, and is unable to work; child frequently beats up younger children, is defiant at home, and is failing at school).

|
21
20

Behavior is considerably influenced by delusions or hallucinations OR serious impairment in communication or judgment (e.g., sometimes incoherent, acts grossly inappropriately, suicidal preoccupation) OR inability to function in almost all areas (e.g., stays in bed all day; no job, home, or friends).

|
11
10

Some danger of hurting self or others (e.g., suicide attempts without clear expectation of death, frequently violent, manic excitement) OR occasionally fails to maintain minimal personal hygiene (e.g., smears feces) OR gross impairment in communication (e.g., largely incoherent or mute).

|
1

Persistent danger of severely hurting self or others (e.g., recurrent violence) OR persistent inability to maintain minimal personal hygiene OR serious suicidal act with clear expectation of death.

0     Inadequate information.

**Depression Outcomes Module,** *See Chapter 13*

Depression Outcomes Module:
# Patient Baseline Assessment (Form 8.1)

Name _____    Clinician_____

ID#_____    Site _____

Date Completed _____

INSTRUCTIONS:

This survey asks for your views about your feelings and your health. This information will be kept confidential and will help your doctors keep track of how you feel.

Answer every question by circling the appropriate number, 1, 2, 3, etc., checking off the appropriate answer, or writing a number where indicated. If you are unsure about how to answer a question, please give the best answer you can and make a comment in the **left margin**.

1. Do you have or have you had any of the following medical conditions?

**(circle one number on each line)**

|  | YES | NO |
|---|---|---|
| a. Anemia | 1 | 2 |
| b. Arthritis or any kind of rheumatism | 1 | 2 |
| c. Asthma | 1 | 2 |
| d. Bronchitis | 1 | 2 |
| e. Cancer | 1 | 2 |
| f. Cataracts | 1 | 2 |
| g. Diabetes | 1 | 2 |
| h. Gall bladder trouble | 1 | 2 |
| i. Heart disease | 1 | 2 |
| j. High blood pressure | 1 | 2 |
| k. Kidney trouble | 1 | 2 |
| l. Lung disease | 1 | 2 |
| m. Migraine headaches | 1 | 2 |
| n. Repeated bladder disorders | 1 | 2 |
| o. Repeated seizures | 1 | 2 |
| p. Repeated stomach problems | 1 | 2 |
| q. Repeated trouble with neck, back, or spine | 1 | 2 |
| r. Stroke | 1 | 2 |
| s. Tuberculosis | 1 | 2 |
| t. Ulcer | 1 | 2 |

2. Have you ever spent any time as a patient in a hospital for mental or emotional problems? ............ 1    2

3. Do any blood relatives (mother, father, sisters, or brothers) have a history of problems with depression or alcoholism? ............ 1    2

4. How old were you the first time you had a period when you felt sad, blue, or depressed for **2 weeks or more**?

      \_\_\_\_less than 12 years old
      \_\_\_\_12 - 18 years old
      \_\_\_\_19 - 35 years old
      \_\_\_\_36 - 64 years old
      \_\_\_\_65 years or older

5. Before the current episode, how many different times in your life have you had a period when you felt sad, blue, or depressed for **at least 2 weeks**?

      \_\_\_\_0
      \_\_\_\_1
      \_\_\_\_2
      \_\_\_\_3
      \_\_\_\_4 or more
      \_\_\_\_I have always felt sad

|  | YES | NO |
|---|---|---|
| 6. Did this current period of feeling sad occur just after someone close to you had died? | 1 | 2 |

7. How many people do you feel you can tell just about anything to, people you can count on for understanding or support? .............. \_\_\_\_people
(If none, enter 0)

**(circle one)**

|  | YES | NO |
|---|---|---|
| 8. **During the past 2 years,** have you felt depressed or sad **most days?** | 1 | 2 |
| 9. **During the past 2 years,** was there a period of **2 months or more** when you did **not** feel depressed or sad most days? | 1 | 2 |

**The following questions ask you how you have been feeling during the past 4 weeks.**

10. **During the past 4 weeks,** how many days did your physical health or emotional problems keep you in bed **all or most of the day? (Your answer may range from 0 to 28 days.)** .............. \_\_\_\_days
(If none, enter 0)

11. **During the past 4 weeks,** how many days did you cut down on the things you usually do for **one-half day or more** because of your physical health or emotional problems? **(Your answer may range from 0 to 28 days. Do not include days already counted in Question 10.)** .............. \_\_\_\_days
(If none, enter 0)

**(circle one)**

|  | YES | NO |
|---|---|---|
| 12. **During the past 4 weeks,** did you work at any time at a job or business not counting work around the house? | 1 | 2 |

(If no, skip to Question 14)

13. **During the past 4 weeks,** how many days did you miss more than half of the day from your job or business because of illness or injury? **(Your answer may range from 0 to 28 days.)** .............. \_\_\_\_days
(If none, enter 0)

14. **During the past 4 weeks,** to what extent did emotional problems interfere with your social activities?

|  | (circle one) |
|---|---|
| Not At All | 1 |
| Slightly | 2 |
| Moderately | 3 |
| Quite a Bit | 4 |
| Extremely | 5 |

The following questions ask you about your daily living. Questions 15-17 are about your use of alcoholic beverages.

|  | (circle one) | |
|---|---|---|
|  | **YES** | **NO** |
| 15. Did you ever think that you were an excessive drinker? | 1 | 2 |

16. Have you ever drunk as much as a fifth of liquor in one day? That would be about 20 drinks, or 3 bottles of wine, or as much as 3 six-packs of beer in one day

| | |
|---|---|
| Yes, more than once | 1 |
| Yes, but only once | 2 |
| No | 3 |

|  | (circle one) | |
|---|---|---|
|  | **YES** | **NO** |
| 17. Has there ever been a period of 2 weeks when every day you were drinking 7 or more beers, 7 or more drinks, or 7 or more glasses of wine? | 1 | 2 |

Questions 18-20 are about any experiences you have had with the drugs and other substances listed below.

a. **Marijuana** (hashish, pot, grass)
b. **Stimulants** (speed, amphetamines, crystal, methamphetamines)
c. **Sedatives** (barbiturates, sleeping pills, Quaaludes, Xanax, tranquilizers, Valium, Librium, red devils)
d. **Cocaine** (coke, crack)
e. **Heroin**
f. **Opiates** (Other than heroin: codeine, demerol, morphine, Methadone, Darvon, opium)
g. **Psychedelics** (LSD, Mescaline, peyote, psilocybin, mushrooms, DMT)
h. **PCP**
i. **Inhalants** (glue, toluene, gasoline, paint)
j. **Other** (nitrous oxide, amyl nitrite)

|  | (circle one) | |
|---|---|---|
|  | **YES** | **NO** |
| 18. Have you ever used one of these drugs on your own more than 5 times in your life? "On your own," means to get high or without a prescription, or more than was prescribed **(If yes, circle drugs above. If no, skip to Question 21.)** | 1 | 2 |
| 19. Did you ever find you needed larger amounts of these drugs to get an effect, or that you could no longer get high on the amount you used to use? | 1 | 2 |
| 20. Did you ever have any emotional or psychological problems from using drugs—like feeling crazy or paranoid or depressed, or uninterested in things? | 1 | 2 |

The following questions ask you about how you have been feeling in the past 4 weeks?

21. How often **in the past 4 weeks** have you felt depressed, blue, or low in
    spirits most of the day?                                                   **(circle one)**
    - Not at all ........................................................................ 1
    - 1 to 3 days a week ........................................................ 2
    - Most days a week .......................................................... 3
    - Nearly every day for at least 2 weeks .......................... 4

22. How often **in the past 4 weeks** did you have days in which you experienced
    little or no pleasure in most of your activities?
    - Not at all ........................................................................ 1
    - 1 to 3 days a week ........................................................ 2
    - Most days a week .......................................................... 3
    - Nearly every day for at least 2 weeks .......................... 4

23. How often **in the past 4 weeks** has your appetite been either less than usual
    or greater than usual?
    - Not at all ........................................................................ 1
    - 1 to 3 days a week ........................................................ 2
    - Most days a week .......................................................... 3
    - Nearly every day for at least 2 weeks .......................... 4

24. **In the past 4 weeks,** have you gained or lost weight without trying to?
    - No .................................................................................. 1
    - Yes, a little weight ........................................................ 2
    - Yes, some weight .......................................................... 3
    - Yes, a lot of weight ...................................................... 4

25. How often **in the past 4 weeks** have you had difficulty sleeping or trouble
    with sleeping too much?
    - Not at all ........................................................................ 1
    - 1 to 3 days a week ........................................................ 2
    - Most days a week .......................................................... 3
    - Nearly every day for at least 2 weeks .......................... 4

26. **In the past 4 weeks,** has your physical activity been slowed down or
    speeded up so much that people who know you could notice?
    - No .................................................................................. 1
    - Yes, a little slowed or speeded up .............................. 2
    - Yes, somewhat slowed or speeded up ........................ 3
    - Yes, very slowed or speeded up .................................. 4

27. **In the past 4 weeks,** have you often felt more tired out or less energetic
    than usual?
    - No .................................................................................. 1
    - Yes, a little tired out .................................................... 2
    - Yes, somewhat tired out ............................................... 3
    - Yes, very tired out ........................................................ 4

28. How often **in the past 4 weeks** have you felt worthless or been bothered
    by feelings of guilt?
    - Not at all ........................................................................ 1
    - 1 to 3 days a week ........................................................ 2
    - Most days a week .......................................................... 3
    - Nearly every day for at least 2 weeks .......................... 4

29. **In the past 4 weeks,** have you often had trouble thinking, concentrating,
    ............................................................or making decisions?
    - No .................................................................................. 1
    - Yes, a little trouble thinking ........................................ 2
    - Yes, some trouble thinking .......................................... 3
    - Yes, a lot of trouble thinking ...................................... 4

30. How often have you thought about death or suicide **in the past 4 weeks**?

|                                              | (circle one) |
|----------------------------------------------|:---:|
| Not at all                                   | 1 |
| 1 to 3 days a week                           | 2 |
| Most days a week                             | 3 |
| Nearly every day for at least 2 weeks        | 4 |

31. **In the past 4 weeks,** have you thought a lot about a specific way to commit suicide?

|       |   |
|-------|:---:|
| No    | 1 |
| Yes   | 2 |

32. In general, would you say your health is:

|             |   |
|-------------|:---:|
| Excellent   | 1 |
| Very good   | 2 |
| Good        | 3 |
| Fair        | 4 |
| Poor        | 5 |

33. **Compared to one year ago,** how would you rate your health in general now?

|                                         |   |
|-----------------------------------------|:---:|
| Much better now than one year ago       | 1 |
| Somewhat better now than one year ago   | 2 |
| About the same                          | 3 |
| Somewhat worse now than one year ago    | 4 |
| Much worse now than one year ago        | 5 |

The following items are about activities you might do during a typical day. Does your health now limit you in these activities? If so, how much?

|  | (circle one number on each line) | | |
|---|:---:|:---:|:---:|
|  | Yes, limited a lot | Yes, limited a little | No, not limited at all |
| 34. Vigorous activities, such as running, lifting heavy objects, participating in strenuous sports | 1 | 2 | 3 |
| 35. Moderate activities, such as moving a table, pushing a vacuum cleaner, bowling, or playing golf | 1 | 2 | 3 |
| 36. Lifting or carrying groceries | 1 | 2 | 3 |
| 37. Climbing several flights of stairs | 1 | 2 | 3 |
| 38. Climbing one flight of stairs | 1 | 2 | 3 |
| 39. Bending, kneeling, or stooping | 1 | 2 | 3 |
| 40. Walking more than a mile | 1 | 2 | 3 |
| 41. Walking several blocks | 1 | 2 | 3 |
| 42. Walking one block | 1 | 2 | 3 |
| 43. Bathing or dressing yourself | 1 | 2 | 3 |

**During the past 4 weeks,** have you had any of the following problems with your work or other regular daily activities as a result of your physical health?

|  | **YES** | **NO** |
|---|:---:|:---:|
| 44. Cut down the amount of time you spent on work or other activities ............... | 1 | 2 |
| 45. Accomplished less than you would like ............................................... | 1 | 2 |
| 46. Were limited in the kind of work or other activities ........................................ | 1 | 2 |
| 47. Had difficulty performing the work or other activities (for example, it took extra effort) ...................................................................................... | 1 | 2 |

*(circle one number on each line)*

**During the past 4 weeks,** have you had any of the following problems with your work or other regular daily activities as a result of any emotional problems (such as feeling depressed or anxious)?

|  | **YES** | **NO** |
|---|:---:|:---:|
| 48. Cut down the amount of time you spent on work or other activities ............... | 1 | 2 |
| 49. Accomplished less than you would like ............................................... | 1 | 2 |
| 50. Didn't do work or other activities as carefully as usual ..................................... | 1 | 2 |

*(circle one number on each line)*

51. **During the past 4 weeks,** to what extent has your physical health or emotional problems interfered with your normal social activities with family, friends, neighbors, or groups?

*(circle one number)*

| | |
|---|:---:|
| Not at all ................................................................................. | 1 |
| Slightly .................................................................................... | 2 |
| Moderately .............................................................................. | 3 |
| Quite a bit ............................................................................... | 4 |
| Extremely ................................................................................ | 5 |

52. How much bodily pain have you had during the past 4 weeks?

*(circle one number)*

| | |
|---|:---:|
| None ........................................................................................ | 1 |
| Very mild ................................................................................ | 2 |
| Mild ........................................................................................ | 3 |
| Moderate ................................................................................. | 4 |
| Severe ..................................................................................... | 5 |
| Very severe ............................................................................. | 6 |

53. **During the past 4 weeks,** how much did pain interfere with your normal work (including both work outside the home and housework)?

*(circle one number)*

| | |
|---|:---:|
| Not at all ................................................................................. | 1 |
| A little bit ............................................................................... | 2 |
| Moderately .............................................................................. | 3 |
| Quite a bit ............................................................................... | 4 |
| Extremely ................................................................................ | 5 |

These questions are about how you feel and how things have been with you **during the past 4 weeks.** For each question, please give the one answer that comes closest to the way you have been feeling.

How much of the time **during the past 4 weeks.** . . .

**(Circle one number on each line)**

| | All of the time | Most of the time | A good bit of the time | Some of the time | A little of the time | None of the time |
|---|---|---|---|---|---|---|
| 54. Did you feel full of pep? | 1 | 2 | 3 | 4 | 5 | 6 |
| 55. Have you been a very nervous person? | 1 | 2 | 3 | 4 | 5 | 6 |
| 56. Have you felt so down in the dumps that nothing could cheer you up? | 1 | 2 | 3 | 4 | 5 | 6 |
| 57. Have you felt calm and peaceful? | 1 | 2 | 3 | 4 | 5 | 6 |
| 58. Did you have a lot of energy? | 1 | 2 | 3 | 4 | 5 | 6 |
| 59. Have you felt downhearted and blue? | 1 | 2 | 3 | 4 | 5 | 6 |
| 60. Did you feel worn out? | 1 | 2 | 3 | 4 | 5 | 6 |
| 61. Have you been a happy person? | 1 | 2 | 3 | 4 | 5 | 6 |
| 62. Did you feel tired? | 1 | 2 | 3 | 4 | 5 | 6 |

63. **During the past 4 weeks,** how much of the time has your **physical health or emotional problems** interfered with your social activities (like visiting with friends, relatives, etc.)?

**(Circle one number)**

| | |
|---|---|
| All of the time | 1 |
| Most of the time | 2 |
| Some of the time | 3 |
| A little of the time | 4 |
| None of the time | 5 |

How TRUE or FALSE is *each* of the following statements for you?

**(Circle one number on each line)**

| | Definitely true | Mostly true | Don't know | Mostly false | Definitely false |
|---|---|---|---|---|---|
| 64. I seem to get sick a little easier than other people. | 1 | 2 | 3 | 4 | 5 |
| 65. I am as healthy as anybody I know. | 1 | 2 | 3 | 4 | 5 |
| 66. I expect my health to get worse. | 1 | 2 | 3 | 4 | 5 |
| 67. My health is excellent. | 1 | 2 | 3 | 4 | 5 |

Please answer YES or NO for each question by circling "1" or "2" on each line.

|  | YES | NO |
|---|---|---|
| 68. In the past year, have you had 2 weeks or more during which you felt sad, blue, or depressed; or when you lost all interest or pleasure in things that you usually cared about or enjoyed? | 1 | 2 |
| 69. Have you had 2 years or more in your life when you felt depressed or sad most days, even if you felt okay sometimes? | 1 | 2 |
| 70. Have you felt depressed or sad much of the time in the past year? | 1 | 2 |

71. What is your birth date? _____/_____/_____
                         Month        Day          Year

For the following questions, please **circle one number**.

72. What is your sex?
Male ................................................................................................ 1
Female ............................................................................................. 2

73. Which of the following best describes your racial background?
American Indian or Alaskan Native ........................................... 1
Asian/Oriental or Pacific Islander ............................................. 2
Black/African-American .............................................................. 3
White/Caucasian ......................................................................... 4
Other ............................................................................................ 5

74. Are you of Spanish or Hispanic origin or ancestry?
Yes ................................................................................................ 1
No ................................................................................................. 2

75. Which of the following best describes your current marital status?
Married ........................................................................................ 1
Widowed ....................................................................................... 2
Separated ..................................................................................... 3
Divorced ....................................................................................... 4
Never married ............................................................................. 5

76. What is the highest grade you completed in school?
8th grade or less .......................................................................... 1
Some high school ......................................................................... 2
High school graduate .................................................................. 3
Some college ................................................................................ 4
College graduate .......................................................................... 5
Any post-graduate work .............................................................. 6

77. How many people **other than yourself** live in your household?
(fill in the blanks)
Number of adults: ........................................................................ _____
Number of children: .................................................................... _____

78. Which of the following categories best describes your household's total income before taxes last year? Please include income from all sources such as salaries and wages, Social Security, retirement income, investments, and other sources.
Less than $20,000 ....................................................................... 1
$20,000 - $39,999 ........................................................................ 2
$40,000 - $59,999 ........................................................................ 3
$60,000 - $79,999 ........................................................................ 4
$80,000 or more .......................................................................... 5

79. What is your zip code? _____

80. Who completed this form?

| | |
|---|---|
| I filled it out with no help | 1 |
| I filled it out with help from family or friends | 2 |
| I filled it out with help from a health care provider | 3 |
| Family or friends | 4 |
| Health care provider | 5 |

| **Depression Outcomes Module,** *See Chapter 13* |
|---|

## Depression Outcomes Module:
# Clinician Baseline Assessment (Form 8.2)

Name _____     Clinician_____

ID#_____     Site _____

Date Completed _____

1. Does the patient currently have (check one):

    a. _____ Major Depression (Single Episode or Recurrent)
    b. _____ Dysthymia
    c. _____ Major Depression superimposed upon Dysthymia
    d. _____ No Major Depression or Dysthymia

2. Does this patient:                                    **(circle one number on each line)**

|  | **YES** | **NO** |
|---|---|---|
| a. read and write English?............................................................................ | 1 | 2 |
| b. have sufficient cognitive function to report about the last 6 months?......... | 1 | 2 |

When evaluating the following symptoms, please do not include symptoms due to physical conditions, medication, or drug/alcohol use.

During the past 2 weeks, has the patient experienced nearly every day:    **YES    NO**

| | **YES** | **NO** |
|---|---|---|
| 3. **Depressed mood** most of the day by their own report or the report of others?............................................................................................................. | 1 | 2 |
| 4. Markedly **diminished interest** or pleasure in all, or almost all, activities most of the day?......................................................................................... | 1 | 2 |
| 5. **Decrease or increase in appetite** or significant weight loss or weight gain when not dieting?....................................................................................... | 1 | 2 |
| 6. **Insomnia or hypersomnia?** ................................................................... | 1 | 2 |
| 7. **Psychomotor agitation or retardation** by their own report or the report of others?............................................................................................................. | 1 | 2 |
| 8. **Fatigue** or loss of energy? ..................................................................... | 1 | 2 |
| 9. Feelings of **worthlessness** or excessive or inappropriate guilt? ..................... | 1 | 2 |
| 10. **Diminished ability to think** or concentrate, or indecisiveness?.................... | 1 | 2 |
| 11. Recurrent **thoughts of death,** recurrent suicidal ideation with or without a specific plan, or a suicide attempt?................................................................. | 1 | 2 |

Please give your clinical opinion about other possible causes for the depressed mood.

12. Has an **organic factor** initiated and maintained the depression? ................

    1. [   ] **YES**
    2. [   ] **NO**
    3. [   ] **UNSURE**

13. Is the depression a **normal reaction to the death** of a loved one? ...............

    1. [   ] **YES**
    2. [   ] **NO**
    3. [   ] **UNSURE**

14. Does the patient have Schizophrenia, Schizophreniform Disorder, Delusional Disorder, or Psychotic Disorders? ....................................................

    1. [   ] **YES**
    2. [   ] **NO**
    3. [   ] **UNSURE**

Has the patient ever demonstrated:

**(circle one)**

| | YES | NO |
|---|---|---|
| 15. a pattern of **drug abuse** that interferes with health, relationships, or work? | 1 | 2 |
| 16. a pattern of **alcohol use** that interferes with health, relationships, or work? | 1 | 2 |
| 17. a **manic episode**? | 1 | 2 |
| 18. **delusions** or **hallucinations** without mood symptoms? | 1 | 2 |

19. Please check which, if any, of the following drugs the patient has regularly taken during the month before the visit. If the patient is taking **none** of these drugs, please check the appropriate box at the end of the list.

    a. _____ reserpine
    b. _____ anabolic steroids (testosterone)
    c. _____ glucocorticoids (cortisone, dexamethesone, hydrocortisone, prednisone, triamcinolone)
    d. _____ none of the above drugs

20. What medications for emotional problems are currently prescribed for the patient? Check below if no drugs prescribed.

_____ None

| DRUG NAME | DOSAGE (mg/day) | DATE STARTED |
|---|---|---|
| A. **Tricyclics** | | |
| 1. Amitriptyline (Elavil, Endep) | | |
| 2. Clomipramine (Anafranil) | | |
| 3. Desipramine (Norpramin, Petofrane) | | |
| 4. Doxepin (Adapin, Sinequan) | | |
| 5. Imipramine (Janimine, Tofranil) | | |
| 6. Nortriptyline (Aventyl, Pamelor) | | |
| 7. Protriptyline (Vivactil) | | |
| 8. Trimipramine (Surmontil) | | |
| B. **Heterocyclics** | | |
| 9. Amoxapine (Asendin) | | |
| 10. Bupropion (Wellbutrin) | | |
| 11. Maprotiline (Ludiomil) | | |
| 12. Trazodone (Desyrel) | | |
| C. **Selective Serotonin Reuptake Inhibitors (SSRIs)** | | |
| 13. Fluoxetine (Prozac) | | |
| 14. Paroxetine (Paxil) | | |
| 15. Sertraline (Zoloft) | | |
| D. **Monoamine Oxidase Inhibitors (MAOIs)** | | |
| 16. Isocarboxazid (Marplan) | | |
| 17. Phenelzine (Nardil) | | |
| 18. Tranylcypromine (Parnate) | | |
| 19. Other (specify) _____ | | |

**Depression Outcomes Module,** *See Chapter 13*

Depression Outcomes Module:
# Patient Follow-Up Assessment (Form 8.3)

Name _____    Clinician_____

ID#_____    Site _____

Date Completed _____

**INSTRUCTIONS:**

This survey asks for your views about your feelings and your health. This information will be kept confidential and will help your doctors keep track of how you feel.

Answer every question by circling the appropriate number, 1,2,3, etc., checking off the appropriate answer, or writing a number where indicated. If you are unsure about how to answer a question, please give the best answer you can and make a comment in the **left margin.**

1.  **During the past 4 weeks,** how many days did your physical health or emotional problems keep you in bed **all or most of the day?** **(Your answer may range from 0 to 28 days.)** ............................................    _____days
    (If none, enter 0)

2.  **During the past 4 weeks,** how many days did you cut down on the things you usually do for **one-half day or more** because of your physical health or emotional problems? **(Your answer may range from 0 to 28 days. Do not include days already counted in Question 1.)** ........................................    _____days
    (If none, enter 0)

    **(circle one)**
    **YES    NO**

3.  **During the past 4 weeks,** did you work at any time at a job or business not counting work around the house?    1       2
    (If no, skip to
    Question 5)

4.  **During the past 4 weeks,** how many days did you miss more than half of the day from your job or business because of illness or injury? **(Your answer may range from 0 to 28 days.)** ...........................................    _____days
    (If none, enter 0)

5.  **During the past 4 weeks,** to what extent did emotional problems interfere with your social activities?

    **(circle one)**

    Not At All....................................................................................    1
    Slightly........................................................................................    2
    Moderately...................................................................................    3
    Quite a Bit ..................................................................................    4
    Extremely ...................................................................................    5

The following questions ask you about how you have been feeling in the past 4 weeks.

6. How often **in the past 4 weeks** have you felt depressed, blue, or in low
spirits for most of the day? **(circle one)**
Not at all ............................................................................................ 1
1 to 3 days a week .............................................................................. 2
Most days a week ............................................................................... 3
Nearly every day for at least 2 weeks .............................................. 4

7. How often **in the past 4 weeks** did you have days in which you experienced
little or no pleasure in most of your activities?
Not at all ............................................................................................ 1
1 to 3 days a week .............................................................................. 2
Most days a week ............................................................................... 3
Nearly every day for at least 2 weeks .............................................. 4

8. How often **in the past 4 weeks** has your appetite been either less than
usual or greater than usual?
Not at all ............................................................................................ 1
1 to 3 days a week .............................................................................. 2
Most days a week ............................................................................... 3
Nearly every day for at least 2 weeks .............................................. 4

9. **In the past 4 weeks,** have you gained or lost weight without trying to?
No ...................................................................................................... 1
Yes, a little weight............................................................................. 2
Yes, some weight ............................................................................... 3
Yes, a lot of weight ........................................................................... 4

10. How often **in the past 4 weeks** have you had difficulty sleeping or trouble
with sleeping too much?
Not at all ............................................................................................ 1
1 to 3 days a week .............................................................................. 2
Most days a week ............................................................................... 3
Nearly every day for at least 2 weeks .............................................. 4

11. **In the past 4 weeks,** has your physical activity been slowed down or
speeded up so much that people who know you could notice? ................
No ...................................................................................................... 1
Yes, a little slowed or speeded up.................................................... 2
Yes, somewhat slowed or speeded up.............................................. 3
Yes, very slowed or speeded up ....................................................... 4

12. **In the past 4 weeks,** have you often felt more tired out or less energetic
than usual?
No ...................................................................................................... 1
Yes, a little tired out ......................................................................... 2
Yes, somewhat tired out.................................................................... 3
Yes, very tired out ............................................................................ 4

13. How often **in the past 4 week**s have you felt worthless or been bothered
by feelings of guilt?
Not at all ............................................................................................ 1
1 to 3 days a week .............................................................................. 2
Most days a week ............................................................................... 3
Nearly every day for at least 2 weeks .............................................. 4

14. **In the past 4 weeks,** have you often had trouble thinking, concentrating, or making decisions? **(circle one)**

    No ............................................................................................................ 1
    Yes, a little trouble thinking .................................................................. 2
    Yes, some trouble thinking ..................................................................... 3
    Yes, a lot of trouble thinking ................................................................. 4

15. How often have you thought about death or suicide **in the past 4 weeks**?

    Not at all .................................................................................................. 1
    1 to 3 days a week ................................................................................... 2
    Most days a week .................................................................................... 3
    Nearly every day for at least 2 weeks ................................................... 4

16. **In the past 4 weeks,** have you thought a lot about a specific way to commit suicide?

    No ............................................................................................................ 1
    Yes ........................................................................................................... 2

17. **In the past 4 months,** have you had a period of **one month** or more when you felt almost or completely back to your usual self? That is, a period when you were not depressed?

    No ............................................................ 1   (If no, skip to Question 19)
    Yes .......................................................... 2
    Have always been depressed ................. 3   (If always depressed, skip to Question 19)

18. How many weeks did that period of feeling almost or completely back to your usual self last? ...................................................................................... _____ weeks

The remaining questions ask you about services that you received during the past 4 months that were NOT provided by (insert name of health care system) or that were NOT paid for by (insert name of insurer). If you did not use any services that were NOT provided by (insert name of health care system) or NOT paid for by (insert name of insurer), check here ☐ and skip to Question 31.

|  | **(circle one)** | |
| --- | --- | --- |
|  | **YES** | **NO** |

19. **During the past 4 months** did you talk to a doctor (other than a mental health professional) about depression or any emotional problems?     1     2
    (If no, skip to Question 22)

20. How many of these visits have you had **during the past 4 months**? ............ _____ visits

21. In how many of these visits did you receive psychotherapy/counseling **during the past 4 months**? ............................................................................ _____ visits

|  | **YES** | **NO** |
| --- | --- | --- |

22. Did you talk to a mental health professional about depression or any emotional problem **during the past 4 months**?     1     2
    (If no, skip to Question 25)

23. How many of these visits have you had **during the past 4 months**? ............ _____ visits

24. In how many of these visits did you receive psychotherapy/counseling **during the past 4 months**? ............................................................................ _____ visits

|  | (circle one) |  |
|  | YES | NO |

25. Were you admitted into the hospital for depression or emotional problems **during the past 4 months**?

YES 1   NO 2
(If no, skip to Question 28)

26. How many times were you admitted to the hospital for depression and/or emotional problems **during the past 4 months**?.............................................. _____admissions

27. How many nights did you spend in the hospital for depression and/or emotional problems in total **during the past 4 months**?................................. _____nights

|  | YES | NO |

28. Did you receive treatment at an Emergency Room because of depression or emotional problems **during the past 4 months**?

YES 1   NO 2

29. Did you participate in a partial hospitalization/day treatment program for depression **during the past 4 months**?

YES 1   NO 2

30. Did you receive electroconvulsive shock therapy for depression **during the past 4 months**?

YES 1   NO 2

31. Did your doctor prescribe medication for your depression **during the past 4 months**?

YES 1   NO 2
(If no, skip to Question 34)

32. Please read down the list of drugs in the following table. In the left hand column, circle NOW if you are currently taking the drug. Circle BEFORE if you have taken the drug sometime in the past 4 months, but are **not** taking it now.

For each drug you circle, please tell us

- dosage (how much of the drug in milligrams you took each time you took it)
- frequency (how often you took the drug)
- starting date (the first day during the current episode of depression that you started taking the drug)
- stopping date (the last day you took the drug if you have stopped taking it)

in the right hand columns. If you circled NOW, leave the stopping date column blank. You can often find information about your medication on the pill bottle label.

If the doctor prescribed one or more of these medications, but you did not take any of them, please check the box at the end of the list.

| | | DRUG NAME | DOSAGE (mg) | FREQUENCY | STARTING DATE | STOPPING DATE |
|---|---|---|---|---|---|---|
| | | A. **Tricyclics** | | | | |
| NOW | BEFORE | 1. Amitriptyline (Elavil, Endep) | | | | |
| NOW | BEFORE | 2. Clomipramine (Anafranil) | | | | |
| NOW | BEFORE | 3. Desipramine (Norpramin, Petofrane) | | | | |
| NOW | BEFORE | 4. Doxepin (Adapin, Sinequan) | | | | |
| NOW | BEFORE | 5. Imipramine (Janimine, Tofranil) | | | | |
| NOW | BEFORE | 6. Nortriptyline (Aventyl, Pamelor) | | | | |
| NOW | BEFORE | 7. Protriptyline (Vivactil) | | | | |
| NOW | BEFORE | 8. Trimipramine (Surmontil) | | | | |
| | | B. **Heterocyclics** | | | | |
| NOW | BEFORE | 9. Amoxapine (Asendin) | | | | |
| NOW | BEFORE | 10. Bupropion (Wellbutrin) | | | | |
| NOW | BEFORE | 11. Maprotiline (Ludiomil) | | | | |
| NOW | BEFORE | 12. Trazodone (Desyrel) | | | | |
| | | C. **Selective Serotonin Reuptake Inhibitors (SSRIs)** | | | | |
| NOW | BEFORE | 13. Fluoxetine (Prozac) | | | | |
| NOW | BEFORE | 14. Paroxetine (Paxil) | | | | |
| NOW | BEFORE | 15. Sertraline (Zoloft) | | | | |
| | | D. **Monoamine Oxidase Inhibitors (MAOIs)** | | | | |
| NOW | BEFORE | 16. Isocarboxazid (Marplan) | | | | |
| NOW | BEFORE | 17. Phenelzine (Nardil) | | | | |
| NOW | BEFORE | 18. Tranylcypromine (Parnate) | | | | |
| NOW | BEFORE | 19. Other (specify) _____ | | | | |

[  ] Medicines were prescribed by doctor, but not taken.

33. **During the past 4 weeks,** how often did you follow your doctor's instructions regarding medication for your depression?

|  | **(circle one)** |
|---|---|
| Every day | 1 |
| Nearly every day | 2 |
| Three or four times a week | 3 |
| Once or twice a week | 4 |
| Not at all | 5 |
| Not prescribed in past four weeks | 6 |

34. **During the past 4 weeks**, how often was each of the following statements true for you?

**(circle one number on each line)**

| Statement | None of the time | A little of the time | Some of the time | A good bit of the time | Most of the time | All of the time |
|---|---|---|---|---|---|---|
| a. I had a hard time doing what the doctor suggested I do . . . | 1 | 2 | 3 | 4 | 5 | 6 |
| b. I followed my doctor's suggestions exactly . . . | 1 | 2 | 3 | 4 | 5 | 6 |
| c. I was unable to do what was necessary to follow my doctor's treatment plans . . . | 1 | 2 | 3 | 4 | 5 | 6 |
| d. I found it easy to do the things my doctor suggested I do . . . | 1 | 2 | 3 | 4 | 5 | 6 |
| e. Generally speaking, I was able to do what the doctor told me . . . | 1 | 2 | 3 | 4 | 5 | 6 |

35. In general, would you say your health is:

|  | **(circle one)** |
|---|---|
| Excellent | 1 |
| Very good | 2 |
| Good | 3 |
| Fair | 4 |
| Poor | 5 |

36. Compared to one year ago, how would you rate your health in general now?

|  | **(circle one)** |
|---|---|
| Much better now than one year ago | 1 |
| Somewhat better now than one year ago | 2 |
| About the same | 3 |
| Somewhat worse now than one year ago | 4 |
| Much worse now than one year ago | 5 |

The following items are about activities you might do during a typical day.
Does your health now limit you in these activities? If so, how much?

| | Yes, limited a lot | Yes, limited a little | No, not limited at all |
|---|:---:|:---:|:---:|
| 37. Vigorous activities, such as running, lifting heavy objects, participating in strenuous sports | 1 | 2 | 3 |
| 38. Moderate activities, such as moving a table, pushing a vacuum cleaner, bowling, or playing golf | 1 | 2 | 3 |
| 39. Lifting or carrying groceries | 1 | 2 | 3 |
| 40. Climbing several flights of stairs | 1 | 2 | 3 |
| 41. Climbing one flight of stairs | 1 | 2 | 3 |
| 42. Bending, kneeling, or stooping | 1 | 2 | 3 |
| 43. Walking more than a mile | 1 | 2 | 3 |
| 44. Walking several blocks | 1 | 2 | 3 |
| 45. Walking one block | 1 | 2 | 3 |
| 46. Bathing or dressing yourself | 1 | 2 | 3 |

*(circle one number on each line)*

**During the past 4 weeks,** have you had any of the following problems with
your work or other regular daily activities as a result of your physical health?

| | YES | NO |
|---|:---:|:---:|
| 47. Cut down the amount of time you spent on work or other activities | 1 | 2 |
| 48. Accomplished less than you would like | 1 | 2 |
| 49. Were limited in the kind of work or other activities | 1 | 2 |
| 50. Had difficulty performing the work or other activities (for example, it took extra effort) | 1 | 2 |

*(circle one number on each line)*

**During the past 4 weeks,** have you had any of the following problems with
your work or other regular daily activities as a result of any emotional problems
(such as feeling depressed or anxious)?

| | YES | NO |
|---|:---:|:---:|
| 51. Cut down the amount of time you spent on work or other activities | 1 | 2 |
| 52. Accomplished less than you would like | 1 | 2 |
| 53. Didn't do work or other activities as carefully as usual | 1 | 2 |

*(circle one number on each line)*

54. **During the past 4 weeks,** to what extent has your physical health or emotional problems interfered with your normal social activities with family, friends, neighbors, or groups?

| | (circle one number) |
|---|---|
| Not at all | 1 |
| Slightly | 2 |
| Moderately | 3 |
| Quite a bit | 4 |
| Extremely | 5 |

55. How much bodily pain have you had during **the past 4 weeks**?

| | (circle one number) |
|---|---|
| None | 1 |
| Very mild | 2 |
| Mild | 3 |
| Moderate | 4 |
| Severe | 5 |
| Very severe | 6 |

56. **During the past 4 weeks,** how much did pain interfere with your normal work (including both work outside the home and housework)?

| | (circle one number) |
|---|---|
| Not at all | 1 |
| A little bit | 2 |
| Moderately | 3 |
| Quite a bit | 4 |
| Extremely | 5 |

These questions are about how you feel and how things have been with you **during the past 4 weeks.** For each question, please give the one answer that comes closest to the way you have been feeling.

How much of the time **during the past 4 weeks**. . . .

(circle one number on each line)

| | All of the time | Most of the time | A good bit of the time | Some of the time | A little of the time | None of the time |
|---|---|---|---|---|---|---|
| 57. Did you feel full of pep? | 1 | 2 | 3 | 4 | 5 | 6 |
| 58. Have you been a very nervous person? | 1 | 2 | 3 | 4 | 5 | 6 |
| 59. Have you felt so down in the dumps that nothing could cheer you up? | 1 | 2 | 3 | 4 | 5 | 6 |
| 60. Have you felt calm and peaceful? | 1 | 2 | 3 | 4 | 5 | 6 |
| 61. Did you have a lot of energy? | 1 | 2 | 3 | 4 | 5 | 6 |
| 62. Have you felt downhearted and blue? | 1 | 2 | 3 | 4 | 5 | 6 |
| 63. Did you feel worn out? | 1 | 2 | 3 | 4 | 5 | 6 |
| 64. Have you been a happy person? | 1 | 2 | 3 | 4 | 5 | 6 |
| 65. Did you feel tired? | 1 | 2 | 3 | 4 | 5 | 6 |

66. **During the past 4 weeks,** how much of the time has your **physical health or emotional problems** interfered with your social activities (like visiting with friends, relatives, etc.)?

**(circle one number)**

| | |
|---|---|
| All of the time................................................................................................ | 1 |
| Most of the time............................................................................................. | 2 |
| Some of the time............................................................................................. | 3 |
| A little of the time .......................................................................................... | 4 |
| None of the time ............................................................................................. | 5 |

How TRUE or FALSE is *each* of the following statements for you?

**(circle one number on each line)**

| | Definitely true | Mostly true | Don't know | Mostly false | Definitely false |
|---|---|---|---|---|---|
| 67. I seem to get sick a little easier than other people | 1 | 2 | 3 | 4 | 5 |
| 68. I am as healthy as anybody I know | 1 | 2 | 3 | 4 | 5 |
| 69. I expect my health to get worse. | 1 | 2 | 3 | 4 | 5 |
| 70. My health is excellent. | 1 | 2 | 3 | 4 | 5 |

Please answer YES or NO for each question by circling "1" or "2" on each line.

| | YES | NO |
|---|---|---|
| 71. In the past year, have you had 2 weeks or more during which you felt sad, blue, or depressed; or when you lost all interest or pleasure in things that you usually cared about or enjoyed?.......................................... | 1 | 2 |
| 72. Have you had 2 years or more in your life when you felt depressed or sad most days, even if you felt okay sometimes?...................................................... | 1 | 2 |
| 73. Have you felt depressed or sad much of the time in the past year? .................. | 1 | 2 |

74. What is your birth date? _____/_____/_____
                               Month      Day      Year

For the following questions, please **circle one number**.

75. What is your sex?

| | |
|---|---|
| Male........................................................................................................ | 1 |
| Female..................................................................................................... | 2 |

76. Which of the following best describes your racial background?

| | |
|---|---|
| American Indian or Alaskan Native ...................................................... | 1 |
| Asian/Oriental or Pacific Islander............................................................ | 2 |
| Black/African-American............................................................................. | 3 |
| White/Caucasian ....................................................................................... | 4 |
| Other........................................................................................................... | 5 |

77. Are you of Spanish or Hispanic origin or ancestry?

| | |
|---|---|
| Yes.............................................................................................................. | 1 |
| No................................................................................................................ | 2 |

78. Which of the following best describes your current marital status?

| | |
|---|---|
| Married ...................................................................................................... | 1 |
| Widowed..................................................................................................... | 2 |
| Separated................................................................................................... | 3 |
| Divorced ..................................................................................................... | 4 |
| Never married ........................................................................................... | 5 |

79. What is the highest grade you completed in school?

| | |
|---|---|
| 8th grade or less | 1 |
| Some high school | 2 |
| High school graduate | 3 |
| Some college | 4 |
| College graduate | 5 |
| Any post-graduate work | 6 |

80. How many people **other than yourself** live in your household?
    (fill in the blanks)

| | |
|---|---|
| Number of adults: | _____ |
| Number of children: | _____ |

81. Which of the following categories best describes your household's total income before taxes last year? Please include income from all sources such as salaries and wages, Social Security, retirement income, investments, and other sources.

| | |
|---|---|
| Less than $20,000 | 1 |
| $20,000 - $39,999 | 2 |
| $40,000 - $59,999 | 3 |
| $60,000 - $79,999 | 4 |
| $80,000 or more | 5 |

82. What is your zip code? _____

83. Who completed this form?

| | |
|---|---|
| I filled it out with no help | 1 |
| I filled it out with help from family or friends | 2 |
| I filled it out with help from a health care provider | 3 |
| Family or friends | 4 |
| Health care provider | 5 |

---

**Depression Outcomes Module,** *See Chapter 13*

---

Depression Outcomes Module:
# Medical Record Review (Form 8.4)

---

Name _____     Clinician_____

ID#_____     Site _____

Date Completed _____     Date of Initial Assessment/Last Follow-up _____

All of the following questions refer to the interval between date of initial visit/last follow-up, and date of completion recorded above.

Please indicate:

1. the number of outpatient visits the patient has had in the general
   medicine setting for depression ......................................................... _____visits
   [ ] N/A

2. the number of psychotherapy/counseling sessions the patient has had in
   a mental health setting for depression............................................... _____visits

3. what type of therapy the patient received from mental health professionals
   **(circle all that apply)**
   Individual .............................................................................................     1
   Group .....................................................................................................     2
   Both Individual and Group...................................................................     3
   Unspecified ...........................................................................................     4

4. the number of visits the patient has made in the mental health setting for
   medication checks only (do not count psychotherapy/counseling sessions) ...... _____visits

5. the number of hospital admissions for depression ............................................ _____admissions

6. the total length of stay for all hospital admissions for depression .................... _____nights

7. the number of electroconvulsive treatments for depression .............................. _____treatments

8. the number of days patient participated in a partial hospitalization/day
   treatment program for depression.................................................................... _____days

9. the number of emergency room visits for depression ........................................ _____visits

10. Was the patient prescribed any psychotropic medications? .............................. **YES     NO**
    (If no, skip
    to Question 11)

Please complete the following table for all psychotropic drugs prescribed. Circle the drug prescribed. If the drug has been discontinued, but exact stop date is not known, mark D/C in stopping date column.

| DRUG NAME | THERAPEUTIC DOSAGE RANGE (mg/day) | DOSAGE (mg) | FREQUENCY | STARTING DATE | STOPPING DATE |
|---|---|---|---|---|---|
| A. **Tricyclics** | | | | | |
| 1. Amitriptyline (Elavil, Endep) | 75-300 | | | | |
| 2. Clomipramine (Anafranil) | 75-300 | | | | |
| 3. Desipramine (Norpramin, Petofrane) | 75-300 | | | | |
| 4. Doxepin (Adapin, Sinequan) | 75-300 | | | | |
| 5. Imipramine (Janimine, Tofranil) | 75-300 | | | | |
| 6. Nortriptyline (Aventyl, Pamelor) | 40-200 | | | | |
| 7. Protriptyline (Vivactil) | 40-200 | | | | |
| 8. Trimipramine (Surmontil) | 75-300 | | | | |
| B. **Heterocyclics** | | | | | |
| 9. Amoxapine (Asendin) | 100-600 | | | | |
| 10. Bupropion (Wellbutrin) | 225-450 | | | | |
| 11. Maprotiline (Ludiomil) | 100-225 | | | | |
| 12. Trazodone (Desyrel) | 150-600 | | | | |
| C. **Selective Serotonin Reuptake Inhibitors (SSRIs)** | | | | | |
| 13. Fluoxetine (Prozac) | 10-40 | | | | |
| 14. Paroxetine (Paxil) | 20-50 | | | | |
| 15. Sertraline (Zoloft) | 50-150 | | | | |
| D. **Monoamine Oxidase Inhibitors (MAOIs)** | | | | | |
| 16. Isocarboxazid (Marplan) | 30-50 | | | | |
| 17. Phenelzine (Nardil) | 45-90 | | | | |
| 18. Tranylcypromine (Parnate) | 20-60 | | | | |
| 19. Other (specify) _____ | | | | | |

11.	If the patient is deceased, please state the cause of death.
	[ ] Suicide
	[ ] Accident
	[ ] Other (please specify)_____
	[ ] Not deceased

---

**Substance Abuse Outcomes Module,** *See Chapter 14*

---

## Substance Abuse Outcomes Module:
# Patient Baseline Assessment

---

Name _____    Clinician_____

ID#_____    Site _____

Date Completed _____/_____/_____
                 Month     Day      Year

**Mode of Collection**

| | |
|---|---|
| Self-administered ........................................................................................ | 1 |
| Personal Interview ...................................................................................... | 2 |
| Telephone Interview ................................................................................... | 3 |
| Mail............................................................................................................... | 4 |
| Other............................................................................................................. | 5 |

**INSTRUCTIONS:** This survey asks for your views about your health. This information will help keep track of how you feel and how well you are able to do your usual activities.

Answer every question by marking the answer as indicated. If you are unsure about how to answer a question, please give the best answer you can.

1. In general, would you say your health is:

                                                                           **(circle one)**

| | |
|---|---|
| Excellent ...................................................................................................... | 1 |
| Very Good ................................................................................................... | 2 |
| Good ............................................................................................................. | 3 |
| Fair................................................................................................................ | 4 |
| Poor .............................................................................................................. | 5 |

2. **Compared to one year ago,** how would you rate your health in general **now**?

                                                                           **(circle one)**

| | |
|---|---|
| Much better now than one year ago........................................................ | 1 |
| Somewhat better now than one year ago................................................. | 2 |
| About the same........................................................................................... | 3 |
| Somewhat worse now than one year ago ................................................. | 4 |
| Much worse now than one year ago ........................................................ | 5 |

3. The following items are about activities you might do during a typical day. Does **your health now limit you** in these activities? If so, how much?

(circle one number on each line)

| ACTIVITIES | Yes, Limited A Lot | Yes, Limited A Little | No, Not Limited At All |
|---|:---:|:---:|:---:|
| a. **Vigorous activities,** such as running, lifting heavy objects, participating in strenuous sports | 1 | 2 | 3 |
| b. **Moderate activities,** such as moving a table, pushing a vacuum cleaner, bowling, or playing golf | 1 | 2 | 3 |
| c. Lifting or carrying groceries | 1 | 2 | 3 |
| d. Climbing **several** flights of stairs | 1 | 2 | 3 |
| e. Climbing **one** flight of stairs | 1 | 2 | 3 |
| f. Bending, kneeling, or stooping | 1 | 2 | 3 |
| g. Walking **more than a mile** | 1 | 2 | 3 |
| h. Walking **several blocks** | 1 | 2 | 3 |
| i. Walking **one block** | 1 | 2 | 3 |
| j. Bathing or dressing yourself | 1 | 2 | 3 |

The following questions ask about problems and experiences during the **past 4 weeks.** Remember, **past 4 weeks** means in the **4 weeks before** entering treatment this time.

4. **During the past 4 weeks,** have you had any of the following problems with your work or other regular daily activities **as a result of your physical health?**

(circle one number on each line)

| | YES | NO |
|---|:---:|:---:|
| a. Cut down on the **amount of time** you spent on work or other activities | 1 | 2 |
| b. **Accomplished less** than you would like | 1 | 2 |
| c. Were limited in the **kind** of work or other activities | 1 | 2 |
| d. Had **difficulty** performing the work or other activities (for example, it took extra effort) | 1 | 2 |

5. **During the past 4 weeks,** have you had any of the following problems with your work or other regular daily activities **as a result of any emotional problems** (such as feeling depressed or anxious)?

(circle one number on each line)

| | YES | NO |
|---|:---:|:---:|
| a. Cut down on the **amount of time** you spent on work or other activities | 1 | 2 |
| b. **Accomplished less** than you would like | 1 | 2 |
| c. Didn't do work or other activities as **carefully** as usual | 1 | 2 |

6. **During the past 4 weeks,** to what extent has your physical health or emotional problems interfered with your normal social activities with family, friends, neighbors, or groups?

|  | (circle one) |
|---|---|
| Not at all | 1 |
| Slightly | 2 |
| Moderately | 3 |
| Quite a bit | 4 |
| Extremely | 5 |

7. How much **bodily** pain have you had **during the past 4 weeks**?

|  | (circle one) |
|---|---|
| None | 1 |
| Very mild | 2 |
| Mild | 3 |
| Moderate | 4 |
| Severe | 5 |
| Very Severe | 6 |

8. **During the past 4 weeks,** how much did **pain** interfere with your normal work (including both work outside the home and housework)?

|  | (circle one) |
|---|---|
| Not at all | 1 |
| A little bit | 2 |
| Moderately | 3 |
| Quite a bit | 4 |
| Extremely | 5 |

9. These questions are about how you feel and how things have been with you **during the past 4 weeks.** For each question, please give the one answer that comes closest to the way you have been feeling. How much of the time during the **past 4 weeks . . .**

**(circle one number on each line)**

|  | All of the Time | Most of the Time | A Good Bit of the Time | Some of the Time | A Little of the Time | None of the Time |
|---|---|---|---|---|---|---|
| a. Did you feel full of pep? | 1 | 2 | 3 | 4 | 5 | 6 |
| b. Have you been a very nervous person? | 1 | 2 | 3 | 4 | 5 | 6 |
| c. Have you felt so down in the dumps that nothing could cheer you up? | 1 | 2 | 3 | 4 | 5 | 6 |
| d. Have you felt calm and peaceful? | 1 | 2 | 3 | 4 | 5 | 6 |
| e. Did you have a lot of energy? | 1 | 2 | 3 | 4 | 5 | 6 |
| f. Have you felt downhearted and blue? | 1 | 2 | 3 | 4 | 5 | 6 |
| g. Did you feel worn out? | 1 | 2 | 3 | 4 | 5 | 6 |
| h. Have you been a happy person? | 1 | 2 | 3 | 4 | 5 | 6 |
| i. Did you feel tired? | 1 | 2 | 3 | 4 | 5 | 6 |

10. During the **past 4 weeks,** how much of the time has your **physical health
    or emotional problems** interfered with your social activities (like visiting
    with friends, relatives, etc.)?

    |  | (circle one) |
    |---|:---:|
    | All of the time | 1 |
    | Most of the time | 2 |
    | Some of the time | 3 |
    | A little of the time | 4 |
    | None of the time | 5 |

11. How **TRUE** OR **FALSE** is *each* of the following statements for you?

    **(circle one number on each line)**

    |  | Definitely True | Mostly True | Don't Know | Mostly False | Definitely False |
    |---|:---:|:---:|:---:|:---:|:---:|
    | a. I seem to get sick a little easier than other people | 1 | 2 | 3 | 4 | 5 |
    | b. I am as healthy as anybody I know | 1 | 2 | 3 | 4 | 5 |
    | c. I expect my health to get worse | 1 | 2 | 3 | 4 | 5 |
    | d. My health is excellent | 1 | 2 | 3 | 4 | 5 |

12. **In the past year,** have you ever had a period of **2 weeks or more** during
    which you felt sad, blue or depressed; or when you lost all interest or
    pleasure in things that you usually cared about or enjoyed?

    |  | (circle one) |
    |---|:---:|
    | Yes | 1 |
    | No | 2 |

13. Have you had **2 years or more** in your life when you felt depressed or sad
    most days even if you felt okay sometimes?

    |  | (circle one) |
    |---|:---:|
    | Yes | 1 |
    | No | 2 |

14. Have you felt depressed or sad much of the time **in the past year**?

    |  | (circle one) |
    |---|:---:|
    | Yes | 1 |
    | No | 2 |

15. Do you have or have you had any of the following medical conditions?

**(circle one number on each line)**

|   | | YES | NO |
|---|---|---|---|
| a. | Anemia | 1 | 2 |
| b. | Arthritis or any kind of rheumatism | 1 | 2 |
| c. | Asthma | 1 | 2 |
| d. | Bronchitis | 1 | 2 |
| e. | Cancer | 1 | 2 |
| f. | Cataracts | 1 | 2 |
| g. | Diabetes | 1 | 2 |
| h. | Gall bladder trouble | 1 | 2 |
| i. | Heart disease | 1 | 2 |
| j. | High blood pressure | 1 | 2 |
| k. | Kidney trouble | 1 | 2 |
| l. | Lung disease | 1 | 2 |
| m. | Migraine headaches | 1 | 2 |
| n. | Repeated bladder disorders | 1 | 2 |
| o. | Repeated seizures | 1 | 2 |
| p. | Repeated stomach problems | 1 | 2 |
| q. | Repeated trouble with neck, back, or spine | 1 | 2 |
| r. | Stroke | 1 | 2 |
| s. | Tuberculosis | 1 | 2 |
| t. | Ulcer | 1 | 2 |

16. **During the past 4 weeks,** how many days did your physical health or emotional problems keep you in bed **all or most of the day**? **(Your answer may range from 0-28 days.)** ............................................... _____days
(If none, enter 0)

17. **During the past 4 weeks,** how many days did you cut down on things you usually do for **one-half day or more** because of physical health or emotional problems. NOT counting days spent ion bed? **(Your answer may range from 0-28 days. Do not include days already counted in Question 16.)** ............................................... _____days
(If none, enter 0)

**(circle one)**
YES     NO

18. **During the past four weeks,** did you work at any time at a job or business not counting work around the house? ................................... 1     2
(If no, skip to Question 20.)

19. **During the past 4 weeks,** how many days did you miss more than half of the day from your job or business because of illness or injury? **(Your answer may range from 0 to 28 days.)** ............................................... _____days
(If none, enter 0)

20. **During the past 4 weeks,** how many days did you fail to do what was expected of you at work, school, or home **because of drinking or drug use? (Your answer may range from 0 to 28 days.)** .................................. _____days
(If none, enter 0)

The following list describes behaviors often seen in children.
Please indicate whether you had experienced any of them **before you were 15 years old.**

**(circle one number on each line)**

| | YES | NO |
|---|---|---|
| 21. Did you frequently get into trouble with the teacher or principal for misbehaving in school? | 1 | 2 |
| 22. Did you ever skip school or play hooky as much as 5 days a year in at least 2 school years, not counting your last year in school? | 1 | 2 |
| 23. Did you tell a lot of lies when you were a child or teenager? | 1 | 2 |
| 24. Did you more than once swipe things from stores or from other children or steal from your parent or from anyone else? | 1 | 2 |
| 25. Did you ever rob or mug anyone or snatch a purse or threaten to hurt anyone if they didn't give you money or jewelry? | 1 | 2 |
| 26. Were you ever expelled or suspended from school? | 1 | 2 |

The following questions ask you about problems you may have had **since you were 18 years old.**

**(circle one number on each line)**

| | YES | NO |
|---|---|---|
| 27. Has there ever been a period when you had no regular place to live, for at least a month or so? | 1 | 2 |
| 28. Have you had at least 4 traffic tickets in your life for speeding or running a light or causing an accident? | 1 | 2 |
| 29. Have you thought that you lied pretty often since you have been an adult? | 1 | 2 |
| 30. Have you ever been in more than one fight that came to swapping blows, other than fights with your partner? | 1 | 2 |
| 31. Did you ever hold 3 or more different jobs within a 5 year period? | 1 | 2 |
| 32. Have you ever traveled around for a month or more without having any arrangements ahead of time and not knowing how long you were going to stay or where you were going to work? | 1 | 2 |
| 33. Did you ever hit or throw things at your partner first on more than one occasion? | 1 | 2 |
| 34. Have you ever been arrested for anything other than traffic violations? | 1 | 2 |
| 35. Did you ever walk out on your partner either permanently or for at least several weeks? | 1 | 2 |
| 36. Have you ever spanked or hit any child hard enough so that he or she had bruises, had to stay in bed or see a doctor? | 1 | 2 |
| 37. On any job you have had since you were 18, were you late or absent an average of 3 days a month or more? | 1 | 2 |
| 38. Have you quit a job 3 times or more before you already had another job lined up? | 1 | 2 |

The following questions ask about your legal status.

**(circle one number on each line)**

| | YES | NO |
|---|---|---|
| 39. Are you **now** on **probation or parole**? | 1 | 2 |
| 40. Did the court or a criminal justice office **order** you to come for treatment this time? | 1 | 2 |

41. How many times **during the past 6 months** have people suggested you get treatment for your drinking problem or drug use?

**(circle one)**

| | |
|---|---|
| About daily............................................................................................. | 1 |
| 2-4 times a week.................................................................................... | 2 |
| About once a week................................................................................ | 3 |
| About once every 2 weeks ................................................................... | 4 |
| Around once a month ........................................................................... | 5 |
| 2-5 times in the past 6 months........................................................... | 6 |
| Once in the past 6 months .................................................................. | 7 |
| Never........................................................................................................ | 8 |

42. How many times **during the past 6 months** have people commented positively when you had not been drinking or using drugs recently?

| | |
|---|---|
| About daily............................................................................................. | 1 |
| 2-4 times a week.................................................................................... | 2 |
| About once a week................................................................................ | 3 |
| About once every 2 weeks ................................................................... | 4 |
| Around once a month ........................................................................... | 5 |
| 2-5 times in the past 6 months........................................................... | 6 |
| Once in the past 6 months .................................................................. | 7 |
| Never........................................................................................................ | 8 |

43. How many times **during the past 6 months** have people done something for you to show they approve when you have not been drinking or using drugs recently?

**(circle one)**

| | |
|---|---|
| About daily............................................................................................. | 1 |
| 2-4 times a week.................................................................................... | 2 |
| About once a week................................................................................ | 3 |
| About once every 2 weeks ................................................................... | 4 |
| Around once a month ........................................................................... | 5 |
| 2-5 times in the past 6 months........................................................... | 6 |
| Once in the past 6 months .................................................................. | 7 |
| Never........................................................................................................ | 8 |

**(circle one)**

| | YES | NO |
|---|---|---|
| 44. Do you live with anyone who **currently** has an alcohol or drug problem?................................................................................................ | 1 | 2 |

45. For each of the following statements, please think about your **current** relationships with friends, family members, co-workers, neighbors, and others. **For each statement circle the number that best describes your current relationships.** For example, if a statement is very true of your relationships, circle number 4 (strongly agree). If it is not at all true, circle number 1 (strongly disagree).

**(circle one number on each line)**

|  | Strongly Disagree | Disagree | Agree | Strongly Agree |
|---|---|---|---|---|
| a. There are people I can have a good time with. | 1 | 2 | 3 | 4 |
| b. There is someone I can talk to about important decisions in my life. | 1 | 2 | 3 | 4 |
| c. There are people who recognize my abilities. | 1 | 2 | 3 | 4 |
| d. There are people who show they love or care for me. | 1 | 2 | 3 | 4 |
| e. There are people who I can count on in an emergency. | 1 | 2 | 3 | 4 |
| f. There are people who give me encouragement to deal with my drug or alcohol problems. | 1 | 2 | 3 | 4 |

46. **Not including the treatment program you are currently in,** how many times have you received formal treatment for alcohol and drug problems? (Do not include self-help groups like Alcoholics Anonymous [AA] or Narcotics Anonymous [NA].)

**(circle one)**

| | |
|---|---|
| Not at all | 0 |
| Once | 1 |
| Twice | 2 |
| Three times | 3 |
| Four or more times | 4 |

**(circle one)**
**YES        NO**

47. Have you ever attended a **self-help group** like Alcoholics Anonymous (AA) or Narcotics Anonymous (NA) **before you came here this time?** ............. 1        2
(If no, skip to Question 49)

48. If yes, how many years have you attended a self-help group? **(If less than one year or none, enter 0.)** .......................................

_____
(Number of years)

49. Has either your **natural** mother or father had a **serious drinking or drug problem**?

**(circle one)**

| | |
|---|---|
| Yes | 1 |
| No | 2 |
| Uncertain | 3 |

**REMEMBER**—None of the information you give us regarding drugs taken or alcohol consumed will be reported to anyone connected with your treatment, family or friends, or law enforcement agencies.

A DRINK means a can or bottle of beer, a glass of wine, a wine cooler, or a shot of hard liquor (like scotch, gin, vodka), including a mixed drink.

| BEER (12 oz.) | = | WINE (4 oz.) | = | WINE COOLERS (4 oz.) | = | MIXED DRINK (with 1 shot) |
|---|---|---|---|---|---|---|

(circle one)

|  | YES | NO |
|---|---|---|
| 50. **During the past 6 months,** have you had any alcohol to drink?.................... | 1 | 2 |

51. **During the past 4 weeks,** how many days have you had any alcohol to drink? (**Your answer may range from 0 to 28 days.**)................................... _____days

52. **During the past 4 weeks,** on the days that you drank, how much did you usually drink?.............................................................................................. _____drinks

53. **During the past 4 weeks,** how many heavy drinking days have you had? Heavy drinking means 6 drinks or more in one day. (**Your answer may range from 0 to 28 days.**) .............................................................. _____days

54. **During the past 4 weeks,** on the days you drank heavily, how much did you usually drink?............................................................................................. _____drinks

55. How does your **DRINKING AND DRUG USE in the 4 weeks before you came here this time** compare to your **DRINKING AND DRUG USE during the past 6 months**?

(circle one)

| Much less ........................................................................................... | 1 |
|---|---|
| Less .................................................................................................... | 2 |
| About the same................................................................................... | 3 |
| More ................................................................................................... | 4 |
| Much more .......................................................................................... | 5 |

56. Please indicate which of the following drugs you have used **on your own** more than five times in your life. "On your own" means to get high, or without a prescription, or more than was prescribed.

**(circle one number on each line)**

|  | YES | NO |
|---|---|---|
| a. marijuana or hash (grass, pot, ganja) | 1 | 2 |
| b. cocaine or crack (rock, coca leaves, blow, snow) | 1 | 2 |
| c. heroin (skag, speedballs) | 1 | 2 |
| d. hallucinogens (like LSD, PCP, sherms, acid, TKO, DMT) | 1 | 2 |
| e. inhalants (whippets, glue, amyl nitrite, poppers) | 1 | 2 |
| f. methadone **prescribed to you** | 1 | 2 |
| g. methadone **prescribed to others** | 1 | 2 |
| h. other opiates and analgesics **prescribed to you** (morphine, demerol) | 1 | 2 |
| i. other opiates and analgesics **prescribed to others or street drugs** | 1 | 2 |
| j. barbiturates **prescribed to you** (reds, yellows, downers) | 1 | 2 |
| k. barbiturates **prescribed to others or street drugs** | 1 | 2 |
| l. other sedatives, hypnotics, or tranquilizers, **prescribed to you** (Zanax, Librium, Valium, Quaaludes, Halcion) | 1 | 2 |
| m. other sedatives, hypnotics, or tranquilizers, **prescribed to others or street drugs** | 1 | 2 |
| n. amphetamines **prescribed to you** (black beauties, crank, bennies, speed, crystal) | 1 | 2 |
| o. amphetamines **prescribed to others or street drugs** | 1 | 2 |

57. Please indicate how many days you have used each of the following drugs **on your own** in the 4 weeks before coming into treatment this time. **(Each answer may range from 0 - 28.)**

| | **(Number of days used in the past 4 weeks)** **(Each answer may range from 0-28)** |
|---|---|
| a.  marijuana or hash (grass, pot, ganja) | _____ Number of days used in past 4 weeks |
| b.  cocaine or crack (rock, coca leaves, blow, snow) | _____ Number of days used in past 4 weeks |
| c.  heroin (skag, speedballs) | _____ Number of days used in past 4 weeks |
| d.  hallucinogens (like LSD, PCP, sherms, acid, TKO, DMT) | _____ Number of days used in past 4 weeks |
| e.  inhalants (whippets, glue, amyl nitrite, popper) | _____ Number of days used in past 4 weeks |
| f.  methadone **prescribed to you** | _____ Number of days used in past 4 weeks |
| g.  methadone **prescribed to others** | _____ Number of days used in past 4 weeks |
| h.  other opiates and analgesics **prescribed to you** (morphine, demerol) | _____ Number of days used in past 4 weeks |
| i.  other opiates and analgesics **prescribed to others or street drugs** | _____ Number of days used in past 4 weeks |
| j.  barbiturates **prescribed to you** (reds, yellows, downers) | _____ Number of days used in past 4 weeks |
| k.  barbiturates **prescribed to others or street drugs** | _____ Number of days used in past 4 weeks |
| l.  other sedatives, hypnotics, or tranquilizers, **prescribed to you** (Zanax, Librium, Valium, Quaaludes, Halcion) | _____ Number of days used in past 4 weeks |
| m.  other sedatives, hypnotics, or tranquilizers, **prescribed to others or street drugs** | _____ Number of days used in past 4 weeks |
| n.  amphetamines **prescribed to you** (black beauties, crank, bennies, speed, crystal) | _____ Number of days used in past 4 weeks |
| o.  amphetamines **prescribed to others or street drugs** | _____ Number of days used in past 4 weeks |

58. **In the 4 weeks before you came here this time,** how many days did you use more than one drug a day? COUNT ALCOHOL AS A DRUG, BUT DO **NOT** INCLUDE DRUGS PRESCRIBED TO YOU TAKEN AS YOUR DOCTOR RECOMMENDED.
    **(Your answer may range from 0-28.)** ........................................................... _____days
    (If none, enter 0)

59. At what age did you first begin drinking or using drugs regularly? ................. _____years old

60. Which **one** of the following is your **biggest** problem now?

**(circle one number)**

| | |
|---|---|
| Alcohol.................................................................................................. | 01 |
| Marijuana or hash (grass, pot, ganja)...................................................... | 02 |
| Cocaine or crack (rock, coca leaves, blow, snow)..................................... | 03 |
| Hallucinogens (LSD, PCP, sherms, acid, TKO, DMT)............................ | 04 |
| Inhalants (whippets, glue, amyl nitrite, poppers)................................... | 05 |
| Heroin (skag, speedballs)....................................................................... | 06 |
| Methadone............................................................................................. | 07 |
| Other opiates/analgesics (morphine, demerol)....................................... | 08 |
| Barbiturates (reds, yellows, downers)..................................................... | 09 |
| Other sedatives, hypnotics, or tranquilizers (Zanax, Librium, Valium, Quaaludes, Halcion)................................................................ | 10 |
| Amphetamines (black beauties, crank, bennies)...................................... | 11 |

Please indicate if each of the following statements have been true for you in the **PAST 6 MONTHS.** For those statements that are true for you in the **PAST 6 MONTHS** please indicate if it was primarily to alcohol, drugs other than alcohol or both.

| | Was this true in the **PAST 6 MONTHS?** | | | Was this due primarily to alcohol, drugs or both? | | |
|---|---|---|---|---|---|---|
| | No | Yes | | Alcohol | Drugs | Both |
| 61. I was arrested, questioned or warned by the police as a result of using alcohol or drugs. | No | Yes | If Yes → | 1 | 2 | 3 |
| 62. I neglected family or friends for two or more days in a row as a result of alcohol or drugs. | No | Yes | If Yes → | 1 | 2 | 3 |
| 63. My alcohol or drug use caused arguments or fights with others. | No | Yes | If Yes → | 1 | 2 | 3 |
| 64. I used alcohol or drugs the first thing when I got up in the morning. | No | Yes | If Yes → | 1 | 2 | 3 |
| 65. I used alcohol or drugs before going to a party to make sure I had enough. | No | Yes | If Yes → | 1 | 2 | 3 |
| 66. After several hours without alcohol or drugs, I had to get more to "fortify" myself. | No | Yes | If Yes → | 1 | 2 | 3 |
| 67. I needed more and more alcohol or drugs to get the same effect as before. | No | Yes | If Yes → | 1 | 2 | 3 |
| 68. I found I was getting less effect from using the same amount of drugs or alcohol. | No | Yes | If Yes → | 1 | 2 | 3 |
| 69. Stopping or cutting down on my alcohol or drugs made me sick (vomiting, cramps, head spinning, the shakes) or gave me withdrawal symptoms. | No | Yes | If Yes → | 1 | 2 | 3 |
| 70. I used alcohol or drugs to keep from having withdrawal symptoms. | No | Yes | If Yes → | 1 | 2 | 3 |
| 71. I used alcohol or drugs to get rid of a hangover or the shakes. | No | Yes | If Yes → | 1 | 2 | 3 |
| 72. Without realizing it, I ended up using more alcohol or drugs than I planned. | No | Yes | If Yes → | 1 | 2 | 3 |

| | Was this true in the PAST 6 MONTHS? | | | Was this due primarily to alcohol, drugs or both? | | |
|---|---|---|---|---|---|---|
| | No | Yes | | Alcohol | Drugs | Both |
| 73. Once I started using alcohol or drugs it was difficult for me to stop before becoming "drunk or wasted." | No | Yes | If Yes → | 1 | 2 | 3 |
| 74. I kept on using alcohol or drugs even after I promised myself not to. | No | Yes | If Yes → | 1 | 2 | 3 |
| 75. I found it difficult to stop using alcohol or drugs, even for a single day. | No | Yes | If Yes → | 1 | 2 | 3 |
| 76. I tried to cut down on alcohol or drugs but couldn't. | No | Yes | If Yes → | 1 | 2 | 3 |
| 77. I spent a great deal of time getting, using, or getting over the effects of alcohol or drugs. | No | Yes | If Yes → | 1 | 2 | 3 |
| 78. I gave up or cut way back on important activities in order to use alcohol or drugs (activities like sports, work, or associating with friends or relatives). | No | Yes | If Yes → | 1 | 2 | 3 |
| 79. I had difficulty doing my work, inside and outside the house, because of physical problems resulting from alcohol or drug use. | No | Yes | If Yes → | 1 | 2 | 3 |
| 80. I continued using alcohol or drugs even though they caused repeated problems (like problems with my health, emotional or mental state, family or friends, school, or the law). | No | Yes | If Yes → | 1 | 2 | 3 |
| 81. I continued to use alcohol or drugs in dangerous situations, like driving a car, operating a machine. | No | Yes | If Yes → | 1 | 2 | 3 |
| 82. My family has objected strongly to my alcohol or drug use. | No | Yes | If Yes → | 1 | 2 | 3 |
| 83. My friends, doctor, or clergyman have objected strongly to my alcohol or drug use. | No | Yes | If Yes → | 1 | 2 | 3 |
| 84. My boss or people at work or school have objected strongly to my alcohol or drug use. | No | Yes | If Yes → | 1 | 2 | 3 |
| 85. I got into physical fights while using alcohol or drugs. | No | Yes | If Yes → | 1 | 2 | 3 |

86. Here are a number of events that people who use alcohol or drugs sometimes experience. Read each one carefully, and indicate **how often** each one has happened to you **DURING THE 4 WEEKS BEFORE ENTERING TREATMENT THIS TIME** by circling the appropriate number (0 = Never, 1 = Once or a few times, 2 = Once or twice a week, 3 = Daily or almost daily, etc.). **If an item does not apply to you, circle zero (0).**

During the **4 weeks prior to entering treatment this time,** about how often has this happened to you?

**(circle one number on each line)**

|  | Never | Once or a few times | Once or twice a week | Daily or almost daily |
|---|:---:|:---:|:---:|:---:|
| a. I have been unhappy because of my drinking or use of drugs. | 0 | 1 | 2 | 3 |
| b. Because of my drinking or use of drugs, I have not eaten properly. | 0 | 1 | 2 | 3 |
| c. I have failed to do what is expected of me because of my drinking or use of drugs. | 0 | 1 | 2 | 3 |
| d. I have felt guilty or ashamed because of drinking or drug use. | 0 | 1 | 2 | 3 |
| e. I have taken foolish risks when I have been drinking or using drugs. | 0 | 1 | 2 | 3 |
| f. When drinking or using drugs, I have done impulsive things that I regretted later. | 0 | 1 | 2 | 3 |
| g. My physical health has been harmed by my drinking or use of drugs. | 0 | 1 | 2 | 3 |
| h. I have had money problems because of my drinking or use of drugs. | 0 | 1 | 2 | 3 |
| i. My physical appearance has been harmed by my drinking or use of drugs. | 0 | 1 | 2 | 3 |
| j. My family has been hurt by my drinking or use of drugs. | 0 | 1 | 2 | 3 |
| k. A friendship or close relationship has been damaged by my drinking or use of drugs. | 0 | 1 | 2 | 3 |
| l. My drinking or use of drugs has gotten in the way of my growth as a person. | 0 | 1 | 2 | 3 |
| m. My drinking or use of drugs has damaged my social life, popularity, or reputation. | 0 | 1 | 2 | 3 |
| n. I have spent too much time or lost a lot of money because of my drinking or use of drugs. | 0 | 1 | 2 | 3 |
| o. I have had an accident while drinking or using drugs. | 0 | 1 | 2 | 3 |

These next questions are about you and your background.

87. What is your birth date?.................................................................  _____/_____/_____

Month    Day        Year

88. What is your sex?

(circle one)

Male ......................................................................................... 1
Female ..................................................................................... 2

89. Which of the following best describes your racial background?

(circle one)

American Indian or Alaskan Native ...................................... 1
Asian/Oriental or Pacific Islander........................................ 2
Black/African-American......................................................... 3
White/Caucasian .................................................................... 4
Other........................................................................................ 5

90. Are you of Spanish or Hispanic origin or ancestry?

(circle one)

Yes........................................................................................... 1
No ............................................................................................ 2

91. Which of the following best describes your current marital status?

(circle one)

Married ................................................................................... 1
Widowed.................................................................................. 2
Separated................................................................................ 3
Divorced ................................................................................. 4
Never married ........................................................................ 5

92. What is the highest grade you completed in school?

(circle one)

8th grade or less .................................................................... 1
Some high school ................................................................... 2
High school graduate ............................................................ 3
Some college........................................................................... 4
College graduate..................................................................... 5
Any post-graduate work......................................................... 6

93. How many people *other than yourself* live in your household?
(fill in the blanks)
        Number of adults:...........................................................  _____
        Number of children: ......................................................  _____

94. Which of the following categories best describes your household's total
income before taxes last year? Please include income from all sources such
as salaries and wages, Social Security, retirement income, investments,
and other sources.

(circle one)

Less than $20,000 ................................................................. 1
$20,000 - $39,999.................................................................. 2
$40,000 - $59,999.................................................................. 3
$60,000 - $79,999.................................................................. 4
$80,000 or more ..................................................................... 5

95. What is your zip code? _____

| | (circle one) | |
|---|---|---|
| | **YES** | **NO** |

96. **In the past 6 months,** were you . . .
   a. enrolled in any vocational or technical schools?........................................ 1     2
   b. enrolled in any college or other school? ...................................................... 1     2
   c. received any job training?............................................................................... 1     2

97. How many months out of the last 5 years have you been without a job? Do not count months you were retired, in school full time, a housewife, or physically too ill to work ................................................................. _____months

98. In the past 6 months, how many **weeks** were you employed? ......................... _____weeks
(If none, enter 0 and skip to Question 99)

   a. If employed in the past 6 months, how many **hours per week** did you usually work? ..................................................................................... _____hours/week
(If none, enter 0)

   b. If employed in the past 6 months, what was your **average hourly wage**? ............................................................................................... _____wage \$\_\_.00

   c. If employed in the past 6 months, how many sick days did you take due to problems using alcohol or drugs?............................................... _____sick days
due to alcohol or drugs
(If none, enter 0)

   d. If employed in the past 6 months, how many sick days have you taken for other reasons?........................................................................... _____sick days
due to other reasons
(If none, enter 0)

| | (circle one) | |
|---|---|---|
| | **YES** | **NO** |

   e. If employed in the past 6 months, were you employed in the **month** before entering this program? ..................................................................... 1     2

   f. If employed in the past 6 months, were you employed **when you entered this program**? ........................................................................... 1     2
(If no, skip to Question 99)

   g. If employed before you entered this program do you plan to return to this job?....................................................................................................... 1     2

99. If unemployed, what is the **main** reason you are not currently employed? (If employed, skip to Question 101)

| | (circle one) |
|---|---|
| Student ............................................................................................ | 1 |
| Poor health or disabled ............................................................... | 2 |
| Retired ............................................................................................ | 3 |
| Homemaker .................................................................................... | 4 |
| Laid off............................................................................................ | 5 |
| Jail................................................................................................... | 6 |
| Other (please specify)................................................................... | 7 |

100. If unemployed, how long have you been without steady or regular work?

**(circle one)**

| | |
|---|---|
| Less than one month.................................................................................. | 1 |
| Less than 3 months................................................................................... | 2 |
| 4 to 6 months........................................................................................... | 3 |
| 7 to 9 months........................................................................................... | 4 |
| 10 to 12 months....................................................................................... | 5 |
| More than a year...................................................................................... | 6 |

101. What is your occupation or line of work? If you have been unemployed, what was your last job?

_____

_____

102. What occupation, trade or skill are you most qualified to perform?

_____

_____

103. Please circle the number for the phrase that **best** describes your usual
employment pattern **over the past 3 years:**

**(circle one)**

| | |
|---|---|
| Full-time (35 hours per week or more)....................................... | 01 |
| Regular part-time (regular but less than 35 hours per week)................ | 02 |
| Irregular part-time (irregular day work)................................... | 03 |
| Regularly self-employed.................................................... | 04 |
| Irregularly self-employed (panhandling, recycling) ........................ | 05 |
| Vocational training program/supported employment ........................... | 06 |
| Military service........................................................... | 07 |
| Student ................................................................... | 08 |
| Retired/disability........................................................ | 09 |
| Unemployed................................................................. | 10 |
| In controlled environment (for example jail)............................... | 11 |
| Homemaker (chose to stay at home) ......................................... | 12 |

104. Do you have a valid driver's license?

**(circle one)**

| | |
|---|---|
| Yes....................................................................................................... | 1 |
| No........................................................................................................ | 2 |

105. Do you have an automobile available for your use?

**(circle one)**

| | |
|---|---|
| Yes....................................................................................................... | 1 |
| No........................................................................................................ | 2 |

106. Which category **best** describes your living situation **before you came** for treatment this time?

**(circle one)**

| | |
|---|---|
| A house or apartment ............................................................... | 1 |
| A rooming house or hotel .......................................................... | 2 |
| A halfway house or group home .................................................... | 3 |
| A hospital or other inpatient treatment facility................................. | 4 |
| In jail or prison................................................................. | 5 |
| A shelter or domiciliary ......................................................... | 6 |
| On the streets, in a park, a car or a vacant building ............................ | 7 |

107. What type of residence was typical for you **in the past 6 months**?

|  | (circle one) |
|---|---|
| A house or apartment | 1 |
| A rooming house or hotel | 2 |
| A halfway house or group home | 3 |
| A hospital or other inpatient treatment facility | 4 |
| In jail or prison | 5 |
| A shelter or domiciliary | 6 |
| On the street, in a park, a car, or a vacant building | 7 |

108. **In the past 6 months** how many times have you moved?

|  | (circle one) |
|---|---|
| None | 1 |
| Once | 2 |
| Two to five times | 3 |
| More than five times | 4 |

109. **In the 4 weeks before you came here this time,** please indicate if you received money from any of the following sources. (For those marked **YES,** please indicate if this made up most of your support).

|  | Received money from this source | | *IF YES,* Did this make up most of your support? | |
|---|---|---|---|---|
|  | NO | YES | NO | YES |
| Employment | ___ | ___]→ If yes → | ___ | ___ |
| Investments | ___ | ___]→ If yes → | ___ | ___ |
| Unemployment Compensation | ___ | ___]→ If yes → | ___ | ___ |
| Public Assistance including welfare, food stamps | ___ | ___]→ If yes → | ___ | ___ |
| Pension benefits or social security (Including SSI, VA benefits, worker's compensation, pensions for disability and retirement) | ___ | ___]→ If yes → | ___ | ___ |
| Mate, family or friends | ___ | ___]→ If yes → | ___ | ___ |
| Other(for example: tax returns, donating blood, selling drugs, prostitution, and pan handling, recycling) | ___ | ___]→ If yes → | ___ | ___ |

110. Who completed this form?

|  | (circle one) |
|---|---|
| I filled it out with no help | 1 |
| I filled it out with help from family or friends | 2 |
| I filled it out with help from a health care provider | 3 |
| Family or friends | 4 |
| Health care provider | 5 |

---

**Substance Abuse Outcomes Module,** *See Chapter 14*

---

Substance Abuse Outcomes Module:
# Clinician Baseline Assessment

---

Name _____     Clinician_____

ID#_____     Site _____

Date Completed _____/_____/_____
                Month     Day      Year

|  | **(circle one number on each line)** | |
|---|---|---|
| 1. Does this patient: | **YES** | **NO** |
|   a. read and write English?................................................. | 1 | 2 |
|   b. have sufficient cognitive function to report about the last 6 months?........ | 1 | 2 |
|   c. currently have psychotic episodes? ................................. | 1 | 2 |

|  | **(circle one)** |
|---|---|
| 2. Does the patient: | |
|   abuse alcohol ................................................................ | 1 |
|   show dependence on alcohol ........................................ | 2 |
|   neither ........................................................................... | 3 |

|  | **(circle one)** |
|---|---|
| 3. Does the patient: | |
|   abuse drugs (other than alcohol)................................. | 1 |
|   show dependence on drugs (other than alcohol)......... | 2 |
|   neither ........................................................................... | 3 |

4. Does the patient show a maladaptive pattern of substance use, leading to
clinically significant impairment or distress, as manifested by one (or more)
of the following, occurring at any time in the same 12-month period:

|  | **(circle one number on each line)** | |
|---|---|---|
|  | **YES** | **NO** |
|   I. tolerance, as defined by either of the following: | | |
|     a. a need for markedly increased amounts of the substance to achieve intoxication or desired effect............................. | 1 | 2 |
|     b. markedly diminished effect with continued use of the same amount of the substance ................................. | 1 | 2 |
|   II. withdrawal, as manifested by either of the following: | | |
|     a. the characteristic withdrawal syndrome for the substance .............. | 1 | 2 |
|     b. the same (or a closely related) substance is taken to relieve or avoid withdrawal symptoms ................................. | 1 | 2 |
|   III. the substance is often taken in larger amounts or over a longer period than was intended ................................. | 1 | 2 |
|   IV. there is a persistent desire or unsuccessful efforts to cut down or control substance use ................................. | 1 | 2 |
|   V. a great deal of time is spent in activities necessary to obtain the substance (e.g., visiting multiple doctors or driving long distances), use the substance (e.g., chain-smoking), or recover from its effects....... | 1 | 2 |
|   VI. important social, occupational, or recreational activities are given up or reduced because of substance abuse ................................. | 1 | 2 |

**(circle one number on each line)**

| | YES | NO |
|---|---|---|
| VII. the substance use is continued despite knowledge of having a persistent or recurrent physical or psychological problem that is likely to have been caused or exacerbated by the substance (e.g., current cocaine use despite recognition of cocaine-induced depression, or continued drinking despite recognition that an ulcer was made worse by alcohol consumption) ..................... | 1 | 2 |
| VIII. recurrent substance use resulting in a failure to fulfill major role obligations at work, school, or home (e.g., repeated absences or poor work performance related to substance use; substance-related absences, suspensions, or expulsions from school; neglect of children or household) ............................................... | 1 | 2 |
| IX. recurrent substance use in situations in which it is physically hazardous (e.g., driving an automobile or operating a machine when impaired by substance use)........................................... | 1 | 2 |
| X. recurrent substance-related legal problems (e.g., arrests for substance-related disorderly conduct)...................................... | 1 | 2 |
| XI. continued substance use despite having persistent or recurrent social or interpersonal problems caused or exacerbated by the effects of the substance (e.g., arguments with spouse about consequences of intoxication, physical fights)................................................. | 1 | 2 |

5. Which of the following substances is most problematic for this patient?

**(circle one)**

| | YES | NO |
|---|---|---|
| a. Alcohol ......................................................... | 1 | 2 |
| b. Marijuana or hash (grass, pot, ganja)............................. | 1 | 2 |
| c. Cocaine or crack (rock, coca leaves, blow, snow).................... | 1 | 2 |
| d. Heroin (skag, speedballs)........................................ | 1 | 2 |
| e. Hallucinogens (like LSD, PCP, sherms, acid, TKO, DMT)............... | 1 | 2 |
| f. Inhalants (whippets, glue, amyl nitrite, popper) ..................... | 1 | 2 |
| g. Methadone **prescribed to patient**................................ | 1 | 2 |
| h. Methadone **prescribed to others** ................................ | 1 | 2 |
| i. Other opiates and analgesics **prescribed to patient** (morphine, demerol)........................................................ | 1 | 2 |
| j. Other opiates and analgesics **prescribed to others or street drugs**...... | 1 | 2 |
| k. Barbiturates **prescribed to patient** (reds, yellows, downers)................... | 1 | 2 |
| l. Barbiturates **prescribed to others or street drugs**............................ | 1 | 2 |
| m. Other sedatives, hypnotics, or tranquilizers **prescribed to patient** (Zanax, Librium, Valium, Quaaludes, Halcion) ......................... | 1 | 2 |
| n. Other sedatives, hypnotics, or tranquilizers **prescribed to others or street drugs**................................................. | 1 | 2 |
| o. Amphetamines **prescribed to patient** (black beauties, crank, bennies, speed, crystal)............................................. | 1 | 2 |
| p. Amphetamines **prescribed to others or street drugs**........................... | 1 | 2 |

6. Does the patient have signs or symptoms of the following conditions?

**(circle one number on each line)**

| | YES | NO |
|---|---|---|
| a. Hepatitis, cirrhosis, or liver disease ............................. | 1 | 2 |
| b. Delirium tremens (DT's) or seizures............................... | 1 | 2 |
| c. Gait abnormalities, hand or tongue tremors, other neuropathies .............. | 1 | 2 |
| d. Cognitive deficits or organic brain syndrome........................... | 1 | 2 |
| e. Gastritis, esophagitis, ulcers, or pancreatitis......................... | 1 | 2 |
| f. Abnormal skin vascularization ................................... | 1 | 2 |
| g. Mucous membrane changes in conjunctiva or oral cavity ........................... | 1 | 2 |

7. Do you have any indication patient has used drugs or alcohol today (e.g., alcohol on his/her breath during the visit)? ............................................. 1     2

8. If the patient is pregnant, which trimester is she? **(circle one)**

First..................................................................................................... 1

Second................................................................................................ 2

Third .................................................................................................. 3

Not pregnant ..................................................................................... 4

Not applicable.................................................................................... 5

9. What setting are you treating this patient in? **(circle one)**

General medical setting...................................................................... 1 skip to 10

General mental health setting ........................................................... 2 skip to 10

Other .................................................................................................. 3 skip to 10

(specify)_____

Specialized alcohol and other drug (AOD) treatment setting          4 (If yes, answer
                                                                       Question 9a.)

9a. If specialized AOD treatment setting, specify one of the following.

Inpatient unit                                                                           1 (If yes, answer
                                                                       Question 9b.)

Non-residential treatment program for AOD problem ................... 2 skip to 10

Partial hospitalization/day treatment for AOD problems ............. 3 skip to 10

Other .................................................................................................. 4 skip to 10

(specify)_____

9b. If inpatient unit, specify one of the following.

Free-standing chemical dependency unit......................................... 1

Hospital-based chemical dependency unit........................................ 2

General psychiatry unit....................................................................... 3

Detox only............................................................................................ 4

10. What kind of treatment did you recommend to the patient at today's visit?

**(circle all that apply)**

| | YES | NO |
|---|---|---|
| a. Told patient to stop or cut down.................................................. | 1 | 2 |
| b. Antabuse......................................................................................... | 1 | 2 |
| c. Psychotropic medication .............................................................. | 1 | 2 |
| (specify)_____ | | |
| d. Family psychotherapy................................................................... | 1 | 2 |
| e. Group psychotherapy..................................................................... | 1 | 2 |
| f. Therapy with certified AOD counselor ........................................ | 1 | 2 |
| g. Individual psychotherapy ............................................................. | 1 | 2 |
| h. Other............................................................................................... | 1 | 2 |
| (specify)_____ | | |

11. What type of referrals did you recommend to the patient?

**(circle all that apply)**

| | YES | NO |
|---|---|---|
| a. Inpatient unit................................................................................ | 1 | 2 |
| b. Non-residential treatment program for AOD problems ............. | 1 | 2 |
| c. Partial hospitalization/day treatment for AOD problems .......... | 1 | 2 |
| d. Alcoholics Anonymous ................................................................. | 1 | 2 |
| e. Narcotics Anonymous ................................................................... | 1 | 2 |
| f. Cocaine Anonymous...................................................................... | 1 | 2 |
| g. 12 step program ............................................................................ | 1 | 2 |
| h. Job training ................................................................................... | 1 | 2 |
| i. Nutritional counseling.................................................................. | 1 | 2 |
| j. Social agencies (assistance with income or housing)................. | 1 | 2 |
| k. Other............................................................................................... | 1 | 2 |
| (specify)_____ | | |

12. If referral to inpatient unit, specify one of the following.

|  |  | (circle one) |
|---|---|:---:|
| a. | Free-standing chemical dependency unit | 1 |
| b. | Hospital-based chemical dependency unit | 2 |
| c. | General psychiatry unit | 3 |
| d. | Detox only | 4 |
| e. | Not referred to in-patient unit | 5 |

---
**Substance Abuse Outcomes Module,** *See Chapter 14*
---

Substance Abuse Outcomes Module:
# Patient Follow-up Assessment

Name _____     Clinician_____

ID#_____     Site _____

Date Completed _____/_____/_____
           Month    Day    Year

**Mode of Collection**

| | |
|---|---|
| Self-administered .................................................................................. | 1 |
| Personal Interview ............................................................................... | 2 |
| Telephone Interview ............................................................................ | 3 |
| Mail ....................................................................................................... | 4 |
| Other..................................................................................................... | 5 |

**INSTRUCTIONS:** This survey asks for your views about your health. This information will help keep track of how you feel and how well you are able to do your usual activities.

Answer every question by marking the answer as indicated. If you are unsure about how to answer a question, please give the best answer you can.

1. In general, would you say your health is:

                                                                           **(circle one)**

| | |
|---|---|
| Excellent ............................................................................................ | 1 |
| Very Good ........................................................................................... | 2 |
| Good .................................................................................................... | 3 |
| Fair...................................................................................................... | 4 |
| Poor ..................................................................................................... | 5 |

2. **Compared to one year ago,** how would you rate your health in general **now**?

                                                                           **(circle one)**

| | |
|---|---|
| Much better now than one year ago ........................................................ | 1 |
| Somewhat better now than one year ago................................................. | 2 |
| About the same........................................................................................ | 3 |
| Somewhat worse now than one year ago .................................................. | 4 |
| Much worse now than one year ago ......................................................... | 5 |

3. The following items are about activities you might do during a typical day. Does **your health now limit you** in these activities? If so, how much?

(**circle one number on each line**)

| ACTIVITIES | Yes, Limited A Lot | Yes, Limited A Little | No, Not Limited At All |
|---|---|---|---|
| a. Vigorous activities, such as running, lifting heavy objects, participating in strenuous sports | 1 | 2 | 3 |
| b. **Moderate activities,** such as moving a table, pushing a vacuum cleaner, bowling, or playing golf | 1 | 2 | 3 |
| c. Lifting or carrying groceries | 1 | 2 | 3 |
| d. Climbing **several** flights of stairs | 1 | 2 | 3 |
| e. Climbing **one** flight of stairs | 1 | 2 | 3 |
| f. Bending, kneeling, or stooping | 1 | 2 | 3 |
| g. Walking **more than a mile** | 1 | 2 | 3 |
| h. Walking **several blocks** | 1 | 2 | 3 |
| i. Walking **one block** | 1 | 2 | 3 |
| j. Bathing or dressing yourself | 1 | 2 | 3 |

The following questions ask about problems and experiences during the **past 4 weeks**. Remember, **past 4 weeks** means in the **4 weeks before** entering treatment this time.

4. **During the past 4 weeks,** have you had any of the following problems with your work or other regular daily activities **as a result of your physical health**?

(**circle one number on each line**)

| | YES | NO |
|---|---|---|
| a. Cut down on the **amount of time** you spent on work or other activities | 1 | 2 |
| b. **Accomplished less** than you would like | 1 | 2 |
| c. Were limited in the **kind** of work or other activities | 1 | 2 |
| d. Had **difficulty** performing the work or other activities (for example, it took extra effort) | 1 | 2 |

5. **During the past 4 weeks,** have you had any of the following problems with your work or other regular daily activities **as a result of any emotional problems** (such as feeling depressed or anxious)?

(**circle one number on each line**)

| | YES | NO |
|---|---|---|
| a. Cut down on the **amount of time** you spent on work or other activities | 1 | 2 |
| b. **Accomplished less** than you would like | 1 | 2 |
| c. Didn't do work or other activities as **carefully** as usual | 1 | 2 |

6. **During the past 4 weeks,** to what extent has your physical health or emotional problems interfered with your normal social activities with family, friends, neighbors, or groups?

**(circle one)**

| | |
|---|---|
| Not at all | 1 |
| Slightly | 2 |
| Moderately | 3 |
| Quite a bit | 4 |
| Extremely | 5 |

7. How much **bodily** pain have you had **during the past 4 weeks**?

**(circle one)**

| | |
|---|---|
| None | 1 |
| Very mild | 2 |
| Mild | 3 |
| Moderate | 4 |
| Severe | 5 |
| Very Severe | 6 |

8. **During the past 4 weeks,** how much did **pain** interfere with your normal work (including both work outside the home and housework)?

**(circle one)**

| | |
|---|---|
| Not at all | 1 |
| A little bit | 2 |
| Moderately | 3 |
| Quite a bit | 4 |
| Extremely | 5 |

9. These questions are about how you feel and how things have been with you **during the past 4 weeks.** For each question, please give the one answer that comes closest to the way you have been feeling. How much of the time during the **past 4 weeks . . .**

**(circle one number on each line)**

| | All of the Time | Most of the Time | A Good Bit of the Time | Some of the Time | A Little of the Time | None of the Time |
|---|---|---|---|---|---|---|
| a. Did you feel full of pep? | 1 | 2 | 3 | 4 | 5 | 6 |
| b. Have you been a very nervous person? | 1 | 2 | 3 | 4 | 5 | 6 |
| c. Have you felt so down in the dumps that nothing could cheer you up? | 1 | 2 | 3 | 4 | 5 | 6 |
| d. Have you felt calm and peaceful? | 1 | 2 | 3 | 4 | 5 | 6 |
| e. Did you have a lot of energy? | 1 | 2 | 3 | 4 | 5 | 6 |
| f. Have you felt downhearted and blue? | 1 | 2 | 3 | 4 | 5 | 6 |
| g. Did you feel worn out? | 1 | 2 | 3 | 4 | 5 | 6 |
| h. Have you been a happy person? | 1 | 2 | 3 | 4 | 5 | 6 |
| i. Did you feel tired? | 1 | 2 | 3 | 4 | 5 | 6 |

10. During the **past 4 weeks,** how much of the time has your **physical health or emotional problems** interfered with your social activities (like visiting with friends, relatives, etc.)?

(circle one)

| | |
|---|---|
| All of the time | 1 |
| Most of the time | 2 |
| Some of the time | 3 |
| A little of the time | 4 |
| None of the time | 5 |

11. How **TRUE** OR **FALSE** is *each* of the following statements for you?

**(circle one number on each line)**

| | Definitely True | Mostly True | Don't Know | Mostly False | Definitely False |
|---|---|---|---|---|---|
| a. I seem to get sick a little easier than other people | 1 | 2 | 3 | 4 | 5 |
| b. I am as healthy as anybody I know | 1 | 2 | 3 | 4 | 5 |
| c. I expect my health to get worse | 1 | 2 | 3 | 4 | 5 |
| d. My health is excellent | 1 | 2 | 3 | 4 | 5 |

12. **During the past 4 weeks,** how many days did your physical health or emotional problems keep you in bed **all or most of the day? (Your answer may range from 0-28 days.)** ............................................................ _____days
(If none, enter 0)

13. **During the past 4 weeks,** how many days did you cut down on things you usually do for **one-half day or more** because of physical health or emotional problems, NOT counting days spent in bed? **(Your answer may range from 0-28 days. Do not include days already counted in Question 12.)** ............................................................ _____days
(If none, enter 0)

(circle one)
YES     NO

14. **During the past four weeks,** did you work at any time at a job or business not counting work around the house? ................................................. 1     2
(If no, skip
to Quesion 20.)

15. **During the past 4 weeks,** how many days did you miss more than half of the day from your job or business because of illness or injury? **(Your answer may range from 0 to 28 days.)** ......................................................... _____days
(If none, enter 0)

16. **During the past 4 weeks,** how many days did you fail to do what was expected of you at work, school, or home **because of drinking or drug use? (Your answer may range from 0 to 28 days.)** ..................................... _____days
(If none, enter 0)

The following question asks about your legal status.

(circle one)
YES     NO

17. Are you **now** on **probation** or **parole**? .............................................................. 1     2

18. Since the last time you completed these forms, have you been involved in or received:

**(circle one on each line)**

|  | | YES | NO |
|---|---|---|---|
| a. | Alcoholics Anonymous/12 Step Program | 1 | 2 |
|  | If yes, how many sessions? | \_\_\_\_\_sessions | |
| b. | Job Training | 1 | 2 |
|  | If yes, how many hours? | \_\_\_\_\_hours | |
| c. | Nutritional Counseling | 1 | 2 |
|  | If yes, how many sessions? | \_\_\_\_\_sessions | |
| d. | Housing Assistance | 1 | 2 |
|  | If yes, how much assistance? $\_\_\_\_\_or \_\_\_\_nights | | |
| e. | Income Assistance | 1 | 2 |
|  | If yes, how much assistance? $_____ | | |

The next question asks you about services that you received that were NOT provided by (insert name of health care system) or that were NOT paid for by (insert name of insurer).

19. Since you finished or left the program where you last completed these forms, have you

**(circle one on each line)**

|  | | YES | NO |
|---|---|---|---|
| a. | been admitted to detox | 1 | 2 |
|  | If yes, how many times? | \_\_\_\_\_admissions | |
| b. | been admitted to a chemical dependency program where you stayed overnight in a hospital or health facility | 1 | 2 |
|  | If yes, how many times? | \_\_\_\_\_admissions | |
| c. | been admitted to a chemical dependency program where you did *not* stay overnight | 1 | 2 |
|  | If yes, how many times? | \_\_\_\_\_admissions | |
| d. | gotten counseling from a mental health professional | 1 | 2 |
|  | If yes, how many sessions? | \_\_\_\_\_sessions | |
| e. | visited a medical doctor | 1 | 2 |
|  | If yes, how many visits? | \_\_\_\_\_visits | |
| f. | used an emergency room | 1 | 2 |
|  | If yes, how many times? | \_\_\_\_\_times | |
| g. | been admitted to a hospital for medical or surgical problems | 1 | 2 |
|  | If yes, how many admissions? | \_\_\_\_\_admissions | |

**REMEMBER**—None of the information you give us regarding drugs taken or alcohol consumed will be reported to anyone connected with your treatment, family or friends, or law enforcement agencies.

A DRINK means a can or bottle of beer, a glass of wine, a wine cooler, or a shot of hard liquor (like scotch, gin, vodka), including a mixed drink.

BEER (12 oz.) = WINE (4 oz.) = WINE COOLERS (4 oz.) = MIXED DRINK (with 1 shot)

**(circle one)**

| | YES | NO |
|---|---|---|
| 20. **During the past 6 months,** have you had any alcohol to drink?.................... | 1 | 2 |

21. **During the past 4 weeks,** how many days have you had any alcohol to drink? **(Your answer may range from 0 to 28 days.)**................................. _____days

22. **During the past 4 weeks,** on the days that you drank, how much did you usually drink?................................................................................................ _____drinks

23. **During the past 4 weeks,** how many heavy drinking days have you had? Heavy drinking means 6 drinks or more in one day. **(Your answer may range from 0 to 28 days.)** .............................................................. _____days

24. **During the past 4 weeks,** on the days you drank heavily, how much did you usually drink?................................................................................................ _____drinks

25. How does your **DRINKING AND DRUG USE in the 4 weeks before you came here this time** compare to your **DRINKING AND DRUG USE during the past 6 months**?

**(circle one)**

| | |
|---|---|
| Much less ................................................................................................ | 1 |
| Less ........................................................................................................ | 2 |
| About the same....................................................................................... | 3 |
| More ........................................................................................................ | 4 |
| Much more ............................................................................................. | 5 |

26. Please indicate how many days you have used each of the following drugs **on your own in the past 4 weeks**. **(Each answer may range from 0 - 28).**

| | **(Number of days used in the past 4 weeks)** **(Each answer may range from 0-28)** |
|---|---|
| a.  marijuana or hash (grass, pot, ganja) | _____ Number of days used in past 4 weeks |
| b.  cocaine or crack (rock, coca leaves, blow, snow) | _____ Number of days used in past 4 weeks |
| c.  heroin (skag, speedballs) | _____ Number of days used in past 4 weeks |
| d.  hallucinogens (like LSD, PCP, sherms, acid, TKO, DMT) | _____ Number of days used in past 4 weeks |
| e.  inhalants (whippets, glue, amyl nitrite, popper) | _____ Number of days used in past 4 weeks |
| f.  methadone **prescribed to you** | _____ Number of days used in past 4 weeks |
| g.  methadone **prescribed to others** | _____ Number of days used in past 4 weeks |
| h.  other opiates and analgesics **prescribed to you** (morphine, demerol) | _____ Number of days used in past 4 weeks |
| i.  other opiates and analgesics **prescribed to others or street drugs** | _____ Number of days used in past 4 weeks |
| j.  barbiturates **prescribed to you** (reds, yellows, downers) | _____ Number of days used in past 4 weeks |
| k.  barbiturates **prescribed to others or street drugs** | _____ Number of days used in past 4 weeks |
| l.  other sedatives, hypnotics, or tranquilizers, **prescribed to you** (Zanax, Librium, Valium, Quaaludes, Halcion) | _____ Number of days used in past 4 weeks |
| m.  other sedatives, hypnotics, or tranquilizers, **prescribed to others or street drugs** | _____ Number of days used in past 4 weeks |
| n.  amphetamines **prescribed to you** (black beauties, crank, bennies, speed, crystal) | _____ Number of days used in past 4 weeks |
| o.  amphetamines **prescribed to others or street drugs** | _____ Number of days used in past 4 weeks |

27. **In the past 4 weeks,** how many days did you use more than one drug a day? COUNT ALCOHOL AS A DRUG, BUT DO **NOT** INCLUDE DRUGS PRESCRIBED TO YOU TAKEN AS YOUR DOCTOR RECOMMENDED. **Your answer may range from 0-28)** ............................................................ _____days

(If none, enter 0)

28. Which **one** of the following is your **biggest** problem now?

**(circle one number)**

| | |
|---|---|
| Alcohol................................................................................................... | 01 |
| Marijuana or hash (grass, pot, ganja)..................................................... | 02 |
| Cocaine or crack (rock, coca leaves, blow, snow).................................... | 03 |
| Hallucinogens (LSD, PCP, sherms, acid, TKO, DMT)............................. | 04 |
| Inhalants (whippets, glue, amyl nitrite, poppers)................................... | 05 |
| Heroin (skag, speedballs)........................................................................ | 06 |
| Methadone............................................................................................... | 07 |
| Other opiates/analgesics (morphine, demerol)....................................... | 08 |
| Barbiturates (reds, yellows, downers).................................................... | 09 |
| Other sedatives, hypnotics, or tranquilizers (Zanax, Librium, | |
| Valium, Quaaludes, Halcion)............................................................... | 10 |
| Amphetamines (black beauties, crank, bennies)..................................... | 11 |

Please indicate if each of the following statements have been true for you in the **PAST 6 MONTHS**. For those statements that are true for you in the **PAST 6 MONTHS** please indicate if it was due primarily to alcohol, drugs other than alcohol or both.

| | Was this true in the **PAST 6 MONTHS?** | | | Was this due primarily to alcohol, drugs or both? | | |
|---|---|---|---|---|---|---|
| | No | Yes | | Alcohol | Drugs | Both |
| 29. I was arrested, questioned or warned by the police as a result of using alcohol or drugs. | No | Yes | If Yes → | 1 | 2 | 3 |
| 30. I neglected family or friends for two or more days in a row as a result of alcohol or drugs. | No | Yes | If Yes → | 1 | 2 | 3 |
| 31. My alcohol or drug use caused arguments or fights with others. | No | Yes | If Yes → | 1 | 2 | 3 |
| 32. I used alcohol or drugs the first thing when I got up in the morning. | No | Yes | If Yes → | 1 | 2 | 3 |
| 33. I used alcohol or drugs before going to a party to make sure I had enough. | No | Yes | If Yes → | 1 | 2 | 3 |
| 34. After several hours without alcohol or drugs, I had to get more to "fortify" myself. | No | Yes | If Yes → | 1 | 2 | 3 |
| 35. I needed more and more alcohol or drugs to get the same effect as before. | No | Yes | If Yes → | 1 | 2 | 3 |
| 36. I found I was getting less effect from using the same amount of drugs or alcohol. | No | Yes | If Yes → | 1 | 2 | 3 |
| 37. Stopping or cutting down on my alcohol or drugs made me sick (vomiting, cramps, head spinning, the shakes) or gave me withdrawal symptoms. | No | Yes | If Yes → | 1 | 2 | 3 |
| 38. I used alcohol or drugs to keep from having withdrawal symptoms. | No | Yes | If Yes → | 1 | 2 | 3 |
| 39. I used alcohol or drugs to get rid of a hangover or the shakes. | No | Yes | If Yes → | 1 | 2 | 3 |
| 40. Without realizing it, I ended up using more alcohol or drugs than I planned. | No | Yes | If Yes → | 1 | 2 | 3 |

| | Was this true in the **PAST 6 MONTHS?** | | | Was this due primarily to alcohol, drugs or both? | | |
|---|---|---|---|---|---|---|
| | No | Yes | | Alcohol | Drugs | Both |
| 41. Once I started using alcohol or drugs it was difficult for me to stop before becoming "drunk or wasted." | No | Yes | If Yes → | 1 | 2 | 3 |
| 42. I kept on using alcohol or drugs even after I promised myself not to. | No | Yes | If Yes → | 1 | 2 | 3 |
| 43. I found it difficult to stop using alcohol or drugs, even for a single day. | No | Yes | If Yes → | 1 | 2 | 3 |
| 44. I tried to cut down on alcohol or drugs but couldn't. | No | Yes | If Yes → | 1 | 2 | 3 |
| 45. I spent a great deal of time getting, using, or getting over the effects of alcohol or drugs. | No | Yes | If Yes → | 1 | 2 | 3 |
| 46. I gave up or cut way back on important activities in order to use alcohol or drugs (activities like sports, work, or associating with friends or relatives). | No | Yes | If Yes → | 1 | 2 | 3 |
| 47. I had difficulty doing my work, inside and outside the house, because of physical problems resulting from alcohol or drug use. | No | Yes | If Yes → | 1 | 2 | 3 |
| 48. I continued using alcohol or drugs even though they caused repeated problems (like problems with my health, emotional or mental state, family or friends, school, or the law). | No | Yes | If Yes → | 1 | 2 | 3 |
| 49. I continued to use alcohol or drugs in dangerous situations, like driving a car, operating a machine. | No | Yes | If Yes → | 1 | 2 | 3 |
| 50. My family has objected strongly to my alcohol or drug use. | No | Yes | If Yes → | 1 | 2 | 3 |
| 51. My friends, doctor, or clergyman have objected strongly to my alcohol or drug use. | No | Yes | If Yes → | 1 | 2 | 3 |
| 52. My boss or people at work or school have objected strongly to my alcohol or drug use. | No | Yes | If Yes → | 1 | 2 | 3 |
| 53. I got into physical fights while using alcohol or drugs. | No | Yes | If Yes → | 1 | 2 | 3 |

54. Here are a number of events that people who use alcohol or drugs sometimes experience. Read each one carefully, and indicate **how often** each one has happened to you **DURING THE PAST 4 WEEKS** by circling the appropriate number (**0 = Never, 1 = Once or a few times, 2 = Once or twice a week, 3 = Daily or almost daily, etc.). If an item does not apply to you, circle zero (0).**

During the past **4 weeks** , about how often has this happened to you?

**(Circle one number on each line)**

| | Never | Once or a few times | Once or twice a week | Daily or almost daily |
|---|---|---|---|---|
| a. I have been unhappy because of my drinking or use of drugs. | 0 | 1 | 2 | 3 |
| b. Because of my drinking or use of drugs, I have not eaten properly. | 0 | 1 | 2 | 3 |
| c. I have failed to do what is expected of me because of my drinking or use of drugs. | 0 | 1 | 2 | 3 |
| d. I have felt guilty or ashamed because of drinking or drug use. | 0 | 1 | 2 | 3 |
| e. I have taken foolish risks when I have been drinking or using drugs. | 0 | 1 | 2 | 3 |
| f. When drinking or using drugs, I have done impulsive things that I regretted later. | 0 | 1 | 2 | 3 |
| g. My physical health has been harmed by my drinking or use of drugs. | 0 | 1 | 2 | 3 |
| h. I have had money problems because of my drinking or use of drugs. | 0 | 1 | 2 | 3 |
| i. My physical appearance has been harmed by my drinking or use of drugs. | 0 | 1 | 2 | 3 |
| j. My family has been hurt by my drinking or use of drugs. | 0 | 1 | 2 | 3 |
| k. A friendship or close relationship has been damaged by my drinking or use of drugs. | 0 | 1 | 2 | 3 |
| l. My drinking or use of drugs has gotten in the way of my growth as a person. | 0 | 1 | 2 | 3 |
| m. My drinking or use of drugs has damaged my social life, popularity, or reputation. | 0 | 1 | 2 | 3 |
| n. I have spent too much time or lost a lot of money because of my drinking or use of drugs. | 0 | 1 | 2 | 3 |
| o. I have had an accident while drinking or using drugs. | 0 | 1 | 2 | 3 |

55. Which of the following best describes your current marital status?

|  | (circle one) |
|---|---|
| Married ........................................................................................................... | 1 |
| Widowed............................................................................................................ | 2 |
| Separated........................................................................................................... | 3 |
| Divorced ........................................................................................................... | 4 |
| Never married ................................................................................................. | 5 |

56. What is the highest grade you completed in school?

|  | (circle one) |
|---|---|
| 8th grade or less ............................................................................................. | 1 |
| Some high school ............................................................................................. | 2 |
| High school graduate ....................................................................................... | 3 |
| Some college...................................................................................................... | 4 |
| College graduate............................................................................................... | 5 |
| Any post-graduate work.................................................................................... | 6 |

57. How many people *other than yourself* live in your household?
(fill in the blanks)

Number of adults:.................................................................................... _____

Number of children: ............................................................................... _____

58. Which of the following categories best describes your household's total income before taxes last year? Please include income from all sources such as salaries and wages, Social Security, retirement income, investments, and other sources.

|  | (circle one) |
|---|---|
| Less than $20,000............................................................................................... | 1 |
| $20,000 - $39,999............................................................................................... | 2 |
| $40,000 - $59,999............................................................................................... | 3 |
| $60,000 - $79,999............................................................................................... | 4 |
| $80,000 or more ................................................................................................ | 5 |

59. What is your zip code? _____

60. Since you last completed this questionnaire,

|  | (circle one) | |
|---|---|---|
|  | **YES** | **NO** |
| a. enrolled in any vocational or technical schools?......................................... | 1 | 2 |
| b. enrolled in any college or other school? ...................................................... | 1 | 2 |
| c. received any job training?............................................................................. | 1 | 2 |

61. Since you last completed this questionnarie, how many **weeks** have you been unemployed? ........................................................................................ _____weeks
(If none, enter 0 and skip to Question 62)

    a. If employed in the past 6 months, how many **hours per week** did you usually work? ..................................................................................... _____hours/week
(If none, enter 0)

    b. If employed in the past 6 months, what was your **average hourly wage**? ............................................................................................... _____wage $___.00

    c. If employed in the past 6 months, how many sick days did you take due to problems using alcohol or drugs? ............................................................ _____sick days due to alcohol or drugs (If none, enter 0)

    d. If employed in the past 6 months, how many sick days have you taken for other reasons? ...................................................................................... _____sick days due to other reasons (If none, enter 0)

(circle one)

| | YES | NO |
|---|---|---|

    e. If employed in the past 6 months, were you employed in the **month** before entering this program? ................................................................... 1      2

    f. If employed in the past 6 months, were you employed **when you entered this program**? .......................................................................... 1      2
(If no, skip to Question 62)

    g. If employed before you entered this program do you plan to return to this job? ............................................................................................... 1      2

62. If unemployed, what is the **main** reason you are not currently employed? (If employed, skip to Question 64.)

(circle one)

| | |
|---|---|
| Student ................................................................................................ | 1 |
| Poor health or disabled .................................................................... | 2 |
| Retired ................................................................................................ | 3 |
| Homemaker ......................................................................................... | 4 |
| Laid off................................................................................................ | 5 |
| Jail........................................................................................................ | 6 |
| Other (please specify)........................................................................ | 7 |

63. If unemployed, how long have you been without steady or regular work?

(circle one)

| | |
|---|---|
| Less than one month........................................................................... | 1 |
| Less than 3 months ............................................................................ | 2 |
| 4 to 6 months ...................................................................................... | 3 |
| 7 to 9 months ...................................................................................... | 4 |
| 10 to 12 months .................................................................................. | 5 |
| More than a year ................................................................................ | 6 |

64. Do you have a valid driver's license?

(circle one)

| | |
|---|---|
| Yes...................................................................................................... | 1 |
| No ....................................................................................................... | 2 |

65. Do you have an automobile available for your use?

(circle one)

| | |
|---|---|
| Yes...................................................................................................... | 1 |
| No ....................................................................................................... | 2 |

66. Which category **best** describes your living situation?

(circle one)

A house or apartment ............................................................................... 1
A rooming house or hotel ....................................................................... 2
A halfway house or group home ........................................................... 3
A hospital or other inpatient treatment facility ..................................... 4
In jail or prison ....................................................................................... 5
A shelter or domiciliary ......................................................................... 6
On the streets, in a park, a car or a vacant building .............................. 7

67. What type of residence was typical for **you since you last completed this questionnaire?**

(circle one)

A house or apartment ............................................................................... 1
A rooming house or hotel ....................................................................... 2
A halfway house or group home ........................................................... 3
A hospital or other inpatient treatment facility ..................................... 4
In jail or prison ....................................................................................... 5
A shelter or domiciliary ......................................................................... 6
On the street, in a park, a car, or a vacant building .............................. 7

68. **Since you last completed this questionnaire,** how many times have you moved?

(circle one)

None .......................................................................................................... 1
Once .......................................................................................................... 2
Two to five times ..................................................................................... 3
More than five times ............................................................................... 4

69. **In the past 4 weeks,** please indicate if you received money from any of the following sources. (For those marked **YES,** please indicate if this made up most of your support).

| | Received money from this source | | IF YES, Did this make up most of your support? | |
|---|---|---|---|---|
| | NO | YES | NO | YES |
| Employment | ——— | ——⌐→ If yes → | ——— | ——— |
| Investments | ——— | ——⌐→ If yes → | ——— | ——— |
| Unemployment Compensation | ——— | ——⌐→ If yes → | ——— | ——— |
| Public Assistance including welfare, food stamps | ——— | ——⌐→ If yes → | ——— | ——— |
| Pension benefits or social security (Including SSI, VA benefits, worker's compensation, pensions for disability and retirement) | ——— | ——⌐→ If yes → | ——— | ——— |
| Mate, family or friends | ——— | ——⌐→ If yes → | ——— | ——— |
| Other (for example: tax returns, donating blood, selling drugs, prostitution, and pan handling, recycling) | ——— | ——⌐→ If yes → | ——— | ——— |

70. Who completed this form?

|  | (circle one) |
|---|---|
| I filled it out with no help ........................................................................... | 1 |
| I filled it out with help from family or friends......................................... | 2 |
| I filled it out with help from a health care provider................................ | 3 |
| Family or friends................................................................................ | 4 |
| Health care provider ............................................................................ | 5 |

---

**Substance Abuse Outcomes Module,** *See Chapter 14*

---

Substance Abuse Outcomes Module:
# Medical Record Review

---

Name _____     Clinician_____

ID#_____     Site _____

Date Completed _____/_____/_____     Date of Initial Assessment/or
                                               Last Follow-up _____/_____/_____
                                                              Month     Day     Year

INDEX CHEMICAL DEPENDENCY TREATMENT

1. Please complete the following information about the chemical dependency program the patient
   participated in *at the time of baseline assessment.*

| | | *Index Treatment* | *Length of treatment* | *Completed program* | |
|---|---|---|---|---|---|
| YES | NO | | | YES | NO |
| a. [ ] | [ ] | Outpatient program ............................ | _____days ...... | [ ] | [ ] |
| b. [ ] | [ ] | Day treatment program ...................... | _____days ...... | [ ] | [ ] |
| c. [ ] | [ ] | Chemical dependency unit in hospital.............................................. | _____days ...... | [ ] | [ ] |
| d. [ ] | [ ] | Chemical dependency unit NOT hospital-based............................. | _____days ...... | [ ] | [ ] |
| e. [ ] | [ ] | General psychiatry, inpatient............. | _____days ...... | [ ] | [ ] |
| f. [ ] | [ ] | Detox unit, inpatient........................... | _____days ...... | [ ] | [ ] |
| g. [ ] | [ ] | Other (specify)_____ . | _____days ...... | [ ] | [ ] |

2. Please check whether the patient received any of the following services as part of the index
   treatment program.

   YES     NO
   a. [ ]   [ ]   Alcoholics Anonymous/12 Step
   b. [ ]   [ ]   Job training
   c. [ ]   [ ]   Nutritional counseling
   d. [ ]   [ ]   Housing assistance after discharge
   e. [ ]   [ ]   Income assistance after discharge

CHEMICAL DEPENDENCY TREATMENT AFTER DISCHARGE FROM INDEX TREATMENT

3. Please complete the following information about chemical dependency services the patient participated in *after discharge from index treatment.*

| | Subsequent Treatments | Total Number | Total Length of Treatment |
|---|---|---|---|
| | YES NO | | |
| a. | [ ] [ ] Outpatient programs .................... | _____admissions . . . . . | _____ days |
| b. | [ ] [ ] Day treatment program................ | _____admissions . . . . . | _____ days |
| c. | [ ] [ ] Chemical dependency unit in hospital......................................... | _____admissions . . . . . | _____ days |
| d. | [ ] [ ] Chemical dependency unit NOT hospital-based ...................... | _____admissions . . . . . | _____ days |
| e. | [ ] [ ] General psychiatry, inpatient ...... | _____admissions . . . . . | _____ days |
| f. | [ ] [ ] Detox unit, inpatient.................... | _____admissions . . . . . | _____ days |
| g. | [ ] [ ] Other ............................................ (specify)_____ | _____admissions . . . . . | _____ days |

4. Please check whether the patient received any of the following services as part of chemical dependency programs s/he participated in after discharge from index treatment or on her/his own.

YES NO
a. [ ] [ ] Alcoholics Anonymous/12 Step
b. [ ] [ ] Job training
c. [ ] [ ] Nutritional counseling
d. [ ] [ ] Housing assistance
e. [ ] [ ] Income assistance

5. Please complete the following information about other health services the patient received after discharge from index treatment. Do **NOT** include visits that were part of programs listed in questions 1-4 above.

YES NO
a. [ ] [ ] Visits to medical doctors............ _____visits
b. [ ] [ ] Counseling with mental health professional..................... _____visits
c. [ ] [ ] Emergency room visits............... _____visits
d. [ ] [ ] Medical or surgical hospitalizations.......................... _____admissions.................. _____nights in hospital

|  | YES | NO |
|---|---|---|
| 6. Is patient deceased? | [ ] | [ ] |

    If yes, please record cause of death_____

> ## The Child Behavior Checklist and Related Instruments, *See Chapter 17*

## CHILD BEHAVIOR CHECKLIST FOR AGES 4–18

For office use only
ID #

CHILD'S NAME

| SEX | AGE | ETHNIC GROUP OR RACE |
|---|---|---|
| ☐ Boy ☐ Girl | | |

TODAY'S DATE

Mo. _____ Date _____ Yr. _____

CHILD'S BIRTHDATE

Mo. _____ Date _____ Yr. _____

GRADE IN SCHOOL _____

NOT ATTENDING SCHOOL ☐

Please fill out this form to reflect *your* view of the child's behavior even if other people might not agree. Feel free to write additional comments beside each item and in the spaces provided on page 2.

PARENTS' USUAL TYPE OF WORK, even if not working now. *(Please be specific — for example, auto mechanic, high school teacher, homemaker, laborer, lathe operator, shoe salesman, army sergeant.)*

FATHER'S TYPE OF WORK: _____

MOTHER'S TYPE OF WORK: _____

THIS FORM FILLED OUT BY:

☐ Mother (name): _____

☐ Father (name): _____

☐ Other — name & relationship to child: _____

---

**I.** Please list the sports your child most likes to take part in. For example: swimming, baseball, skating, skate boarding, bike riding, fishing, etc.

☐ None

Compared to others of the same age, about how much time does he/she spend in each?

Compared to others of the same age, how well does he/she do each one?

| | Don't Know | Less Than Average | Average | More Than Average | Don't Know | Below Average | Average | Above Average |
|---|---|---|---|---|---|---|---|---|
| a. _____ | ☐ | ☐ | ☐ | ☐ | ☐ | ☐ | ☐ | ☐ |
| b. _____ | ☐ | ☐ | ☐ | ☐ | ☐ | ☐ | ☐ | ☐ |
| c. _____ | ☐ | ☐ | ☐ | ☐ | ☐ | ☐ | ☐ | ☐ |

---

**II.** Please list your child's favorite hobbies, activities, and games, other than sports. For example: stamps, dolls, books, piano, crafts, cars, singing, etc. (Do **not** include listening to radio or TV.)

☐ None

Compared to others of the same age, about how much time does he/she spend in each?

Compared to others of the same age, how well does he/she do each one?

| | Don't Know | Less Than Average | Average | More Than Average | Don't Know | Below Average | Average | Above Average |
|---|---|---|---|---|---|---|---|---|
| a. _____ | ☐ | ☐ | ☐ | ☐ | ☐ | ☐ | ☐ | ☐ |
| b. _____ | ☐ | ☐ | ☐ | ☐ | ☐ | ☐ | ☐ | ☐ |
| c. _____ | ☐ | ☐ | ☐ | ☐ | ☐ | ☐ | ☐ | ☐ |

---

**III.** Please list any organizations, clubs, teams, or groups your child belongs to.

☐ None

Compared to others of the same age, how active is he/she in each?

| | Don't Know | Less Active | Average | More Active |
|---|---|---|---|---|
| a. _____ | ☐ | ☐ | ☐ | ☐ |
| b. _____ | ☐ | ☐ | ☐ | ☐ |
| c. _____ | ☐ | ☐ | ☐ | ☐ |

---

**IV.** Please list any jobs or chores your child has. For example: paper route, babysitting, making bed, working in store, etc. (Include **both** paid and unpaid jobs and chores.)

☐ None

Compared to others of the same age, how well does he/she carry them out?

| | Don't Know | Below Average | Average | Above Average |
|---|---|---|---|---|
| a. _____ | ☐ | ☐ | ☐ | ☐ |
| b. _____ | ☐ | ☐ | ☐ | ☐ |
| c. _____ | ☐ | ☐ | ☐ | ☐ |

---

**V.** 1. About how many close friends does your child have? ☐ None ☐ 1 ☐ 2 or 3 ☐ 4 or more
(Do not include brothers & sisters)

2. About how many times a week does your child do things with any friends outside of regular school hours?
(Do not include brothers & sisters) ☐ Less than 1 ☐ 1 or 2 ☐ 3 or more

**VI.** Compared to others of his/her age, how well does your child:

| | | Worse | About Average | Better | |
|---|---|:---:|:---:|:---:|---|
| a. | Get along with his/her brothers & sisters? | ☐ | ☐ | ☐ | ☐ Has no brothers or sisters |
| b. | Get along with other kids? | ☐ | ☐ | ☐ | |
| c. | Behave with his/her parents? | ☐ | ☐ | ☐ | |
| d. | Play and work by himself/herself? | ☐ | ☐ | ☐ | |

**VII.** 1. For ages 6 and older — performance in academic subjects. If child is not being taught, please give reason _____

| | Failing | Below average | Average | Above average |
|---|:---:|:---:|:---:|:---:|
| a. Reading, English, or Language Arts | ☐ | ☐ | ☐ | ☐ |
| b. History or Social Studies | ☐ | ☐ | ☐ | ☐ |
| c. Arithmetic or Math | ☐ | ☐ | ☐ | ☐ |
| d. Science | ☐ | ☐ | ☐ | ☐ |
| e. _____ | ☐ | ☐ | ☐ | ☐ |
| f. _____ | ☐ | ☐ | ☐ | ☐ |
| g. _____ | ☐ | ☐ | ☐ | ☐ |

Other academic subjects — for example: computer courses, foreign language, business. Do *not* include gym, shop, driver's ed., etc.

2. Is your child in a special class or special school? ☐ No ☐ Yes — what kind of class or school?

3. Has your child repeated a grade? ☐ No ☐ Yes — grade and reason

4. Has your child had any academic or other problems in school? ☐ No ☐ Yes — please describe

When did these problems start?

Have these problems ended? ☐ No ☐ Yes — when?

Does your child have any illness, physical disability, or mental handicap? ☐ No ☐ Yes — please describe

What concerns you most about your child?

Please describe the best things about your child:

Below is a list of items that describe children and youth. For each item that describes your child **now or within the past 6 months**, please circle the **2** if the item is **very true** or **often true** of your child. Circle the **1** if the item is **somewhat** or **sometimes true** of your child. If the item is **not true** of your child, circle the **0**. Please answer all items as well as you can, even if some do not seem to apply to your child.

**0 = Not True (as far as you know)       1 = Somewhat or Sometimes True       2 = Very True or Often True**

| | | | |
|---|---|---|---|
| 0 1 2 | 1. | Acts too young for his/her age |
| 0 1 2 | 2. | Allergy (describe): _____ |
| | | _____ |
| 0 1 2 | 3. | Argues a lot |
| 0 1 2 | 4. | Asthma |
| 0 1 2 | 5. | Behaves like opposite sex |
| 0 1 2 | 6. | Bowel movements outside toilet |
| 0 1 2 | 7. | Bragging, boasting |
| 0 1 2 | 8. | Can't concentrate, can't pay attention for long |
| 0 1 2 | 9. | Can't get his/her mind off certain thoughts; obsessions (describe): _____ |
| | | _____ |
| 0 1 2 | 10. | Can't sit still, restless, or hyperactive |
| 0 1 2 | 11. | Clings to adults or too dependent |
| 0 1 2 | 12. | Complains of loneliness |
| 0 1 2 | 13. | Confused or seems to be in a fog |
| 0 1 2 | 14. | Cries a lot |
| 0 1 2 | 15. | Cruel to animals |
| 0 1 2 | 16. | Cruelty, bullying, or meanness to others |
| 0 1 2 | 17. | Day-dreams or gets lost in his/her thoughts |
| 0 1 2 | 18. | Deliberately harms self or attempts suicide |
| 0 1 2 | 19. | Demands a lot of attention |
| 0 1 2 | 20. | Destroys his/her own things |
| 0 1 2 | 21. | Destroys things belonging to his/her family or others |
| 0 1 2 | 22. | Disobedient at home |
| 0 1 2 | 23. | Disobedient at school |
| 0 1 2 | 24. | Doesn't eat well |
| 0 1 2 | 25. | Doesn't get along with other kids |
| 0 1 2 | 26. | Doesn't seem to feel guilty after misbehaving |
| 0 1 2 | 27. | Easily jealous |
| 0 1 2 | 28. | Eats or drinks things that are not food— *don't* include sweets (describe): _____ |
| | | _____ |
| 0 1 2 | 29. | Fears certain animals, situations, or places, other than school (describe): _____ |
| | | _____ |
| 0 1 2 | 30. | Fears going to school |

| | | | |
|---|---|---|---|
| 0 1 2 | 31. | Fears he/she might think or do something bad |
| 0 1 2 | 32. | Feels he/she has to be perfect |
| 0 1 2 | 33. | Feels or complains that no one loves him/her |
| 0 1 2 | 34. | Feels others are out to get him/her |
| 0 1 2 | 35. | Feels worthless or inferior |
| 0 1 2 | 36. | Gets hurt a lot, accident-prone |
| 0 1 2 | 37. | Gets in many fights |
| 0 1 2 | 38. | Gets teased a lot |
| 0 1 2 | 39. | Hangs around with others who get in trouble |
| 0 1 2 | 40. | Hears sounds or voices that aren't there (describe): _____ |
| | | _____ |
| 0 1 2 | 41. | Impulsive or acts without thinking |
| 0 1 2 | 42. | Would rather be alone than with others |
| 0 1 2 | 43. | Lying or cheating |
| 0 1 2 | 44. | Bites fingernails |
| 0 1 2 | 45. | Nervous, highstrung, or tense |
| 0 1 2 | 46. | Nervous movements or twitching (describe): |
| | | _____ |
| 0 1 2 | 47. | Nightmares |
| 0 1 2 | 48. | Not liked by other kids |
| 0 1 2 | 49. | Constipated, doesn't move bowels |
| 0 1 2 | 50. | Too fearful or anxious |
| 0 1 2 | 51. | Feels dizzy |
| 0 1 2 | 52. | Feels too guilty |
| 0 1 2 | 53. | Overeating |
| 0 1 2 | 54. | Overtired |
| 0 1 2 | 55. | Overweight |
| | 56. | Physical problems without known medical cause: |
| 0 1 2 | a. | Aches or pains (*not* headaches) |
| 0 1 2 | b. | Headaches |
| 0 1 2 | c. | Nausea, feels sick |
| 0 1 2 | d. | Problems with eyes (describe): _____ |
| | | _____ |
| 0 1 2 | e. | Rashes or other skin problems |
| 0 1 2 | f. | Stomachaches or cramps |
| 0 1 2 | g. | Vomiting, throwing up |
| 0 1 2 | h. | Other (describe): _____ |
| | | _____ |

0 = Not True (as far as you know)     1 = Somewhat or Sometimes True     2 = Very True or Often True

| | | | | |
|---|---|---|---|---|
| 0 | 1 | 2 | 57. | Physically attacks people |
| 0 | 1 | 2 | 58. | Picks nose, skin, or other parts of body (describe): _____ |
| 0 | 1 | 2 | 59. | Plays with own sex parts in public |
| 0 | 1 | 2 | 60. | Plays with own sex parts too much |
| 0 | 1 | 2 | 61. | Poor school work |
| 0 | 1 | 2 | 62. | Poorly coordinated or clumsy |
| 0 | 1 | 2 | 63. | Prefers being with older kids |
| 0 | 1 | 2 | 64. | Prefers being with younger kids |
| 0 | 1 | 2 | 65. | Refuses to talk |
| 0 | 1 | 2 | 66. | Repeats certain acts over and over; compulsions (describe): _____ |
| 0 | 1 | 2 | 67. | Runs away from home |
| 0 | 1 | 2 | 68. | Screams a lot |
| 0 | 1 | 2 | 69. | Secretive, keeps things to self |
| 0 | 1 | 2 | 70. | Sees things that aren't there (describe): _____ |
| 0 | 1 | 2 | 71. | Self-conscious or easily embarrassed |
| 0 | 1 | 2 | 72. | Sets fires |
| 0 | 1 | 2 | 73. | Sexual problems (describe): _____ |
| 0 | 1 | 2 | 74. | Showing off or clowning |
| 0 | 1 | 2 | 75. | Shy or timid |
| 0 | 1 | 2 | 76. | Sleeps less than most kids |
| 0 | 1 | 2 | 77. | Sleeps more than most kids during day and/or night (describe): _____ |
| 0 | 1 | 2 | 78. | Smears or plays with bowel movements |
| 0 | 1 | 2 | 79. | Speech problem (describe): _____ |
| 0 | 1 | 2 | 80. | Stares blankly |
| 0 | 1 | 2 | 81. | Steals at home |
| 0 | 1 | 2 | 82. | Steals outside the home |
| 0 | 1 | 2 | 83. | Stores up things he/she doesn't need (describe): _____ |

| | | | | |
|---|---|---|---|---|
| 0 | 1 | 2 | 84. | Strange behavior (describe): _____ |
| 0 | 1 | 2 | 85. | Strange ideas (describe): _____ |
| 0 | 1 | 2 | 86. | Stubborn, sullen, or irritable |
| 0 | 1 | 2 | 87. | Sudden changes in mood or feelings |
| 0 | 1 | 2 | 88. | Sulks a lot |
| 0 | 1 | 2 | 89. | Suspicious |
| 0 | 1 | 2 | 90. | Swearing or obscene language |
| 0 | 1 | 2 | 91. | Talks about killing self |
| 0 | 1 | 2 | 92. | Talks or walks in sleep (describe): _____ |
| 0 | 1 | 2 | 93. | Talks too much |
| 0 | 1 | 2 | 94. | Teases a lot |
| 0 | 1 | 2 | 95. | Temper tantrums or hot temper |
| 0 | 1 | 2 | 96. | Thinks about sex too much |
| 0 | 1 | 2 | 97. | Threatens people |
| 0 | 1 | 2 | 98. | Thumb-sucking |
| 0 | 1 | 2 | 99. | Too concerned with neatness or cleanliness |
| 0 | 1 | 2 | 100. | Trouble sleeping (describe): _____ |
| 0 | 1 | 2 | 101. | Truancy, skips school |
| 0 | 1 | 2 | 102. | Underactive, slow moving, or lacks energy |
| 0 | 1 | 2 | 103. | Unhappy, sad, or depressed |
| 0 | 1 | 2 | 104. | Unusually loud |
| 0 | 1 | 2 | 105. | Uses alcohol or drugs for nonmedical purposes (describe): _____ |
| 0 | 1 | 2 | 106. | Vandalism |
| 0 | 1 | 2 | 107. | Wets self during the day |
| 0 | 1 | 2 | 108. | Wets the bed |
| 0 | 1 | 2 | 109. | Whining |
| 0 | 1 | 2 | 110. | Wishes to be of opposite sex |
| 0 | 1 | 2 | 111. | Withdrawn, doesn't get involved with others |
| 0 | 1 | 2 | 112. | Worries |
| | | | 113. | Please write in any problems your child has that were not listed above: _____ |

PLEASE BE SURE YOU HAVE ANSWERED ALL ITEMS.     UNDERLINE ANY YOU ARE CONCERNED ABOUT.

# YOUNG ADULT SELF-REPORT

| YOUR FULL NAME | First | Middle | Last |
|---|---|---|---|

**YOUR USUAL TYPE OF WORK**, even if not working now. (Please be specific—for example, auto mechanic, high school teacher, homemaker, laborer, lathe operator, shoe salesman, army sergeant, student.) _____

| YOUR SEX | YOUR AGE | ETHNIC GROUP OR RACE |
|---|---|---|
| ☐ Male ☐ Female | | |

**PLEASE CIRCLE HIGHEST EDUCATION OBTAINED**

1. Grade 1-9
2. Grade 10-12
3. General Equivalence Diploma
4. High School Graduate
5. 1-2 years College
6. Associate's Degree
7. 3-4 years College
8. Bachelor's or RN Degree
9. Some Graduate School
10. Master's Degree
11. Doctoral or Law Degree

Other education (specify): _____

**TODAY'S DATE**

Mo._____ Date_____ Yr._____

**YOUR BIRTHDATE**

Mo._____ Date_____ Yr._____

Please fill out this form to reflect *your* views, even if other people might not agree. Feel free to write additional comments beside each item.

If you attend school, please state type of school and major subject: _____

## I. FRIENDS:

A. About how many close friends do you have?

☐ none    ☐ 1    ☐ 2 or 3    ☐ 4 or more

B. About how many times a month do you have contact with any of your close friends? (including in-person contacts, phone, letters)

☐ less than 1    ☐ 1 or 2    ☐ 3 or more

C. How well do you get along with your close friends?

☐ not well    ☐ average    ☐ very well

D. About how many times a month do you invite any people to your home?

☐ less than 1    ☐ 1 or 2    ☐ 3 or more

## II. EDUCATION:

In the last 6 months, have you attended school, college or any educational institution?

☐ No ☐ Yes--what kind of school? _____

Do you expect to earn a degree? ☐ No ☐ Yes--what kind of degree? _____ When? _____

If you attended any educational institution in the last 6 months, please circle *0, 1,* or *2* beside items A-G to describe your experience:

**0 = Not True       1 = Somewhat or Sometimes True       2 = Very True or Often True**

| | | |
|---|---|---|
| 0 1 2 | A. I get along well with other students | |
| 0 1 2 | B. I have trouble getting along with teachers | |
| 0 1 2 | C. I achieve what I am capable of | |
| 0 1 2 | D. I have trouble studying | |

| | |
|---|---|
| 0 1 2 | E. I am satisfied with my school situation |
| 0 1 2 | F. I do things that may cause me to fail |
| 0 1 2 | G. I skip classes even if I'm not sick |

## III. JOB:

In the last 6 months, have you held any paid jobs (including military service)?

☐ No       ☐ Yes--please describe_____.

If you held any paid job(s) in the last 6 months, please circle *0, 1,* or *2* beside items A-G to describe your work:

**0 = Not True       1 = Somewhat or Sometimes True       2 = Very True or Often True**

| | | |
|---|---|---|
| 0 1 2 | A. I work well with others | |
| 0 1 2 | B. I have trouble getting along with bosses | |
| 0 1 2 | C. I do my work well | |
| 0 1 2 | D. I have trouble getting my work done | |

| | |
|---|---|
| 0 1 2 | E. I am satisfied with my work situation |
| 0 1 2 | F. I do things that may cause me to lose my job |
| 0 1 2 | G. I stay away from my job even if I'm not sick or not on vacation |

## IV. FAMILY:

Compared with others, how well do you:

|  | Worse | About average | Better | No Contact | |
|---|---|---|---|---|---|
| A. Get along with your brothers and sisters? | ☐ | ☐ | ☐ | ☐ | ☐ No living siblings |
| B. Get along with your mother? | ☐ | ☐ | ☐ | ☐ | ☐ Mother is deceased |
| C. Get along with your father? | ☐ | ☐ | ☐ | ☐ | ☐ Father is deceased |

## V. MARRIAGE OR PARTNER:

At any time during the last 6 months, were you married or did you have a similar relationship with a partner (such as living together)? ☐ No ☐ Yes--please describe_____.

If you were married or had a similar relationship in the last 6 months, please circle *0*, *1*, or *2* beside items A-K to describe your relationship:

| 0 = Not True | 1 = Somewhat or Sometimes True | 2 = Very True or Often True |
|---|---|---|

0 1 2   A. I get along well with my partner

0 1 2   B. My partner and I have trouble sharing responsibilities

0 1 2   C. I feel satisfied with my partner

0 1 2   D. My partner and I *dis*agree about money

0 1 2   E. My partner and I *dis*agree about the amount of time we should spend together

0 1 2   F. My partner and I *dis*agree about what to do when we are together

0 1 2   G. My partner and I enjoy similar activities

0 1 2   H. My partner and I *dis*agree about sexual matters

0 1 2   I. My partner and I *dis*agree about living arrangements, such as where we live

0 1 2   J. I have trouble with my partner's family

0 1 2   K. I like my partner's friends

## VI. Below is a list of items that describe people. For each item, please circle *0, 1,* or *2* to describe yourself over the past 6 months. Please answer all items as well as you can, even if some do not seem to apply to you.

| 0 = Not True | 1 = Somewhat or Sometimes True | 2 = Very True or Often True |
|---|---|---|

0 1 2   1. I act too young for my age

0 1 2   2. I make good use of my opportunities

0 1 2   3. I argue a lot

0 1 2   4. I work up to my ability

0 1 2   5. I act like the opposite sex

0 1 2   6. I use drugs (other than alcohol) for nonmedical purposes (describe):_____

0 1 2   7. I brag

0 1 2   8. I have trouble concentrating or paying attention

0 1 2   9. I can't get my mind off certain thoughts (describe): _____

0 1 2   10. I have trouble sitting still

0 1 2   11. I am too dependent on others

0 1 2   12. I feel lonely

0 1 2   13. I feel confused or in a fog

0 1 2   14. I cry a lot

0 1 2   15. I am pretty honest

0 1 2   16. I am mean to others

0 1 2   17. I daydream a lot

0 1 2   18. I deliberately try to hurt or kill myself

0 1 2   19. I try to get a lot of attention

0 1 2   20. I destroy my things

0 1 2   21. I destroy things belonging to others

0 1 2   22. I worry about my future

0 1 2   23. I break rules at school or work

0 1 2   24. I don't eat as well as I should

0 1 2   25. I don't get along with other people

0 1 2   26. I don't feel guilty after doing something I shouldn't

0 1 2   27. I am jealous of others

0 1 2   28. I get along badly with my family

0 1 2   29. I am afraid of certain animals, situations, or places (describe): _____

0 1 2   30. I worry about my relations with the opposite sex

0 1 2   31. I am afraid I might think or do something bad

0 1 2   32. I feel that I have to be perfect

0 1 2   33. I feel that no one loves me

0 1 2   34. I feel that others are out to get me

0 1 2   35. I feel worthless or inferior

0 1 2   36. I accidentally get hurt a lot

0 1 2   37. I get in many fights

0 1 2   38. I get teased a lot

| 0 = Not True | 1 = Somewhat or Sometimes True | 2 = Very True or Often True |
| --- | --- | --- |

0 1 2    39. I hang around with others who get in trouble

0 1 2    40. I hear sounds or voices that other people think aren't there (describe): _____

0 1 2    41. I act without stopping to think

0 1 2    42. I would rather be alone than with others

0 1 2    43. I lie or cheat

0 1 2    44. I bite my fingernails

0 1 2    45. I am nervous or tense

0 1 2    46. Parts of my body twitch or make nervous movements (describe): _____

0 1 2    47. I lack self-confidence

0 1 2    48. I am not liked by others

0 1 2    49. I can do certain things better than other people

0 1 2    50. I am too fearful or anxious

0 1 2    51. I feel dizzy

0 1 2    52. I feel too guilty

0 1 2    53. I eat too much

0 1 2    54. I feel overtired

0 1 2    55. I am overweight

       56. Physical problems without known medical cause:

0 1 2       a. Aches or pains (*not* stomach or headaches)

0 1 2       b. Headaches

0 1 2       c. Nausea, feel sick

0 1 2       d. Problems with eyes (describe): _____

0 1 2       e. Rashes or other skin problems

0 1 2       f. Stomachaches or cramps

0 1 2       g. Vomiting, throwing up

0 1 2       h. Heart pounding

0 1 2       i. Numbness or tingling in body parts

0 1 2       j. Other (describe): _____

0 1 2    57. I physically attack people

0 1 2    58. I pick my skin or other parts of my body (describe): _____

0 1 2    59. I have trouble finishing things I should do

0 1 2    60. There is very little that I enjoy

0 1 2    61. My school work or job performance is poor

0 1 2    62. I am poorly coordinated or clumsy

0 1 2    63. I would rather be with older people than with people of my own age

0 1 2    64. I would rather be with younger people than with people of my own age

0 1 2    65. I refuse to talk

0 1 2    66. I repeat certain actions over and over (describe): _____

0 1 2    67. I have trouble making or keeping friends

0 1 2    68. I scream a lot

0 1 2    69. I am secretive or keep things to myself

0 1 2    70. I see things that other people think aren't there (describe): _____

0 1 2    71. I am self-conscious or easily embarrassed

0 1 2    72. I set fires

0 1 2    73. I meet my responsibilities to my family

0 1 2    74. I show off or clown

0 1 2    75. I am shy or timid

0 1 2    76. My behavior is irresponsible

0 1 2    77. I sleep more than most others during day and/or night (describe): _____

0 1 2    78. I have trouble making decisions

0 1 2    79. I have a speech problem (describe): _____

0 1 2    80. I stand up for my rights

0 1 2    81. I worry about my job or school work (describe): _____

0 1 2    82. I steal

0 1 2    83. I store up things I don't need (describe): _____

0 1 2    84. I do things other people think are strange (describe): _____

0 1 2    85. I have thoughts that other people would think are strange (describe): _____

0 1 2    86. I am stubborn or irritable

0 1 2    87. My moods or feelings change suddenly

0 1 2    88. I enjoy being with other people

0 1 2    89. I am suspicious

0 1 2    90. I drink too much alcohol or get drunk

0 1 2    91. I think about killing myself

0 1 2    92. I do things that may cause me trouble with the law (describe): _____

0 1 2    93. I talk too much

0 1 2    94. I tease others a lot

0 1 2    95. I have a hot temper

0 1 2    96. I think about sex too much

0 1 2    97. I threaten to hurt people

0 1 2    98. I like to help others

0 1 2    99. I am too concerned about being neat or clean

0 1 2    100. I have trouble sleeping (describe): _____

0 1 2    101. I am able to make friends easily

| | | | |
|---|---|---|---|
| **0 = Not True** | **1 = Somewhat or Sometimes True** | **2 = Very True or Often True** | |

0 1 2 102. I don't have much energy

0 1 2 103. I am unhappy, sad, or depressed

0 1 2 104. I am louder than others

0 1 2 105. I like to make others laugh

0 1 2 106. I try to be fair to others

0 1 2 107. I feel that I can't succeed

0 1 2 108. I like to take life easy

0 1 2 109. I get along well with my family

0 1 2 110. I wish I were of the opposite sex

0 1 2 111. I keep from getting involved with others

0 1 2 112. I worry a lot

0 1 2 113. I am too concerned about how I look

0 1 2 114. I wake up too early

0 1 2 115. I fail to pay my debts or meet other financial responsibilities

0 1 2 116. I am too concerned about my health

117. How often did you drink alcohol in the last 6 months?
   □ Never in the last 6 months
   In the items below, "drink" means a glass of wine, shot of liquor, or a can or bottle of beer.
   □ less than 1 drink per week, on average
   □ 1-7 drinks per week, on average
   □ 8-14 drinks per week, on average
   □ 15-21 drinks per week, on average
   □ More than 21 per week--about how many? ____

118. On how many days were you drunk in the last 6 months?
   □ Never in the last 6 months
   □ 1 or 2 days
   □ 3 or 4 days
   □ 5 or 6 days
   □ More than 6--about how many days? _____

119. Are you worried about the amount of alcohol you drink?
   □ No    □ Yes

120. Are your family or friends worried about the amount of alcohol you drink? □ No    □ Yes

121. In the last 6 months, on how many days did you use drugs for nonmedical purposes? Circle drugs used: marijuana, amphetamines, hashish, cocaine, crack, PCP, heroin, LSD, other_____.
   □ Never in the last 6 months
   □ 1 or 2 days
   □ 3 or 4 days
   □ 5 or 6 days
   □ More than 6--about how many days? _____

122. In the last 5 years, have you received traffic tickets (excluding parking) or been convicted of offenses other than traffic violations? □ No □ Yes--please list each type and the number of each:

| A. Traffic | Number | B. Nontraffic | Number |
|---|---|---|---|
| _____ | ____ | _____ | ____ |
| _____ | ____ | _____ | ____ |
| _____ | ____ | _____ | ____ |
| _____ | ____ | _____ | ____ |
| _____ | ____ | _____ | ____ |

**VII.   Do you have any illness, physical disability, or handicap?**   □ No      □ Yes--please describe

**VIII.  Please describe any concerns or worries you have about work, school, or other things:**   □ No concerns

**IX.    Please describe the best things about yourself:**

**X.     Please write down anything else that describes your feelings, behavior, or interests:**

**PLEASE BE SURE YOU HAVE ANSWERED ALL ITEMS**

---

**Brief Psychiatric Rating Scale,** *See Chapter 19*

---

# Brief Psychiatric Rating Scale
# Overall and Gorham

---

**DIRECTIONS:** Circle the appropriate number to represent level of severity of each symptom.

Patient Name: _____  Date: _____

Rate: _____  Score (Sum of all item): _____

Scoring Criteria:
1=Not Present  2=Very Mild  3=Mild  4=Moderate
5=Moderately Severe  6=Severe  7=Extremely Severe

| | | | | | | | |
|---|---|---|---|---|---|---|---|
| SOMATIC CONCERN—preoccupation with physical health, fear of physical illness, hypochondriasis. | 1 | 2 | 3 | 4 | 5 | 6 | 7 |
| ANXIETY—worry, fear, over-concern for present or future, uneasiness. | 1 | 2 | 3 | 4 | 5 | 6 | 7 |
| EMOTIONAL WITHDRAWAL—lack of spontaneous interaction, isolation, deficiency in relating to others. | 1 | 2 | 3 | 4 | 5 | 6 | 7 |
| CONCEPTUAL DISORGANIZATION—thought processes confused, disconnected, disorganized, disrupted. | 1 | 2 | 3 | 4 | 5 | 6 | 7 |
| GUILT FEELINGS—self-blame, shame, remorse for past behavior. | 1 | 2 | 3 | 4 | 5 | 6 | 7 |
| TENSION—physical and motor manifestations of nervousness, over-activation. | 1 | 2 | 3 | 4 | 5 | 6 | 7 |
| MANNERISMS AND POSTURING—peculiar, bizarre, unnatural motor behavior (not including tic). | 1 | 2 | 3 | 4 | 5 | 6 | 7 |
| GRANDIOSITY—exaggerated self-opinion, arrogance, conviction of unusual power or abilities. | 1 | 2 | 3 | 4 | 5 | 6 | 7 |
| DEPRESSIVE MOOD—sorrow, sadness, despondency, pessimism. | 1 | 2 | 3 | 4 | 5 | 6 | 7 |
| HOSTILITY—animosity, contempt, belligerence, disdain for others. | 1 | 2 | 3 | 4 | 5 | 6 | 7 |
| SUSPICIOUSNESS—mistrust, belief other harbor malicious or discriminatory intent. | 1 | 2 | 3 | 4 | 5 | 6 | 7 |
| HALLUCINATORY BEHAVIOR—perceptions without normal external stimulus correspondence. | 1 | 2 | 3 | 4 | 5 | 6 | 7 |
| MOTOR RETARDATION—slowed, weakened movements or speech, reduced body tone. | 1 | 2 | 3 | 4 | 5 | 6 | 7 |
| UNCOOPERATIVENESS—resistance, guardedness, rejection of authority. | 1 | 2 | 3 | 4 | 5 | 6 | 7 |
| UNUSUAL THOUGHT CONTENT—unusual, odd, strange, bizarre thought content. | 1 | 2 | 3 | 4 | 5 | 6 | 7 |
| BLUNTED AFFECT—reduced emotional tone, reduction in formal intensity of feelings, flatness. | 1 | 2 | 3 | 4 | 5 | 6 | 7 |
| EXCITEMENT—heightened emotional tone, agitation, increased reactivity. | 1 | 2 | 3 | 4 | 5 | 6 | 7 |
| DISORIENTATION—confusion or lack of proper association for person, place, or time. | 1 | 2 | 3 | 4 | 5 | 6 | 7 |

**NOTE:** Reprinted with permission from Overall and Gorham (Overall JE Gorham DR). The Brief Psychiatric Rating Scale (BPRS): Recent developments in ascertainment and scaling. Psychopharmacol Bull 1988; 24:97-99.

## BPRS Item Descriptions[1]

**1. Somatic Concern.** The severity of physical complaints should be rated solely on the number and nature of complaints or fears of bodily illness or malfunction, or suspiciousness of them, alleged during the interview period. The evaluation is of the degree to which the patient perceives or suspects physical ailments to play an important part in his total lack of well-being. Worry and concern over physical health is the basis for rating somatic concerns. No consideration of the probability of true organic basis for the complaints is required. Only the frequency and severity of complaints are rated.

**2. Anxiety.** Anxiety is the term restricted to the subjective experience of worry, overconcern, apprehension, or fear. Rating of degree of anxiety should be based upon verbal responses reporting such subjective experiences on the part of the patient. Care should be taken to exclude from consideration in rating anxiety the physical signs which are included in the concept of tension, as defined in the BPRS. The sincerity of the report and the strength of the experiences as indicated by the involvement of the patient may be important in evaluating the degree of anxiety.

**3. Emotional Withdrawal.** This construct is defined solely in terms of the ability of the patient to relate in the interpersonal interview situation. Thus, an attempt is made to distinguish between motor aspects of general retardation, which are rated as "motor retardation," and the more mental-emotional aspects of withdrawal, even though ratings in the two areas may be expected to vary to some extent. In the factor analyses of change in psychiatric ratings, a "general retardation" factor has emerged in several different analyses, and it has included emotional, affective, and motor retardation items. It is difficult to identify the basis for rating of "ability to relate"; however, initial work has indicted that raters achieve reasonably high agreement in rating this quality. Emotional withdrawal is represented by the feeling on the part of the rater that an invisible barrier exists between the patient and other persons in the interview situation. It is suspected that eyes, facial expression, voice quality, and lack of variability and expressive movements all enter into the evaluation of this important but nebulous quality of psychiatric patients.

**4. Conceptual Disorganization.** Conceptual disorganization involves the disruption of normal thought processes and is evidenced in confusion, irrelevance, inconsistency, disconnectedness, disjointedness, blocking, confabulation, autism, and unusual chain of associating. Ratings should be based upon the patient's spontaneous verbal products, especially those longer, spontaneous response sequences, which are likely to be elicited during the initial, nondirective portion of the interview. Attention to the facial expression of the patient during the verbal response may be helpful in evaluation the degree of confusion or blocking.

**5. Guilt Feelings.** The strength of guilt feelings should be judged from the frequency and intensity of reported experiences of remorse for past behavior. The strength of the guilt feelings must be judged in part from the degree of involvement evidenced by the patient in reporting such experiences. Care should be exercised not to infer guilt feelings from signs of depression or generalized anxiety. Guilt feelings relate to specific past behavior which the patient now believes to have been wrong and the memory of which is a source of conscious concern.

**6. Tension.** This construct is restricted in the BPRS to physical and motor signs commonly associated with anxiety. Tension does not involve the subjective experience or mental state of the patient. Although research psychologists, in an effort to attain a high degree of objectivity, frequently define anxiety in terms of physical signs, in the BPRS observable physical signs of tension and subjective experiences of anxiety are rated separately. Although anxiety and tension tend to vary together, developmental research with the BPRS has indicated that the degree of pathology in the two areas may be quite different in specific patients. A patient, especially when under the influence of a drug, may report extreme apprehension but give no external evidence of tension whatsoever, or vice versa. In rating the degree of tension, the rater should attend to the number and nature of signs of abnormally heightened activation level such as nervousness, fidgeting, tremors, twitches, sweating, frequent changing

---

[1] These BPRS items descriptions are reproduced with permission from Overall and Klett (JE Overall, CJ Klett, Applied Multivariate Analysis. New York: McGraw Hill, 1972, pp 6-12).

of posture, hypertonicity of movements, and heightened muscle tone.

**7. Mannerisms and Posturing.** This symptom area includes the unusual and bizarre motor behavior by which a mentally ill person can often be identified in a crowd of normal people. The severity of manneristic behavior depends not upon the nature and number of unusual motor responses. However, it is the unusualness, and not simply the amount of movement, which is to be rated. Odd, indirect, repetitive movements or movements lacking normal coordination and integration are rated on this scale. Strained, distorted, abnormal posture and integration which are maintained for extended periods are rated. Grimaces and unusual movements of lips, tongue, or eyes are considered here also. Tics and twitches which are rated as signs of tension are not rated as manneristic behavior.

**8. Grandiosity.** Grandiosity involves the reported feeling of unusual ability, power, wealth, importance, or superiority. The degree of pathology should be rated relative to the discrepancy between self-appraisal and reality. The verbal report of the patient and not his demeanor in the interview situation should provide the primary basis for evaluation of grandiosity. Care should be taken not to infer grandiosity from suspicious of persecution or from other unfounded beliefs where no explicit reference to personal superiority as the basis for persecution has been elicited. Ratings should be based upon opinion currently held by the patient, even though the unfounded superiority may be claimed to have existed in the past.

**9. Depressive Mood.** Depressive mood includes only the affective component of depression. It should be rated on the basis of expression of discouragement, pessimism, sadness, hopelessness, helplessness, and gloomy thema. Facial expression, weeping, moaning, and other modes of communicating modes should be considered, but motor retardation, guilt, and somatic complaint which are commonly associated with the psychiatric syndrome of depression should not be considered in rating depressive mood.

**10. Hostility.** Hostility is a term reserved for reported feelings of animosity, belligerence, contempt, or hatred toward other people outside the interview situation. The rater may attend to the sincerity and affect present reporting on such experiences when she/he attempts to evaluate the severity of pathology in the symptom area. It should be noted that evidences of hostility toward the interviewer in the interview situation should be rated on the uncooperativeness scale and should not be considered in rating hostility as defined here.

**11. Suspiciousness.** Suspiciousness in a term used to designate a wide range of mental experience in which the patient believes to have been wronged by another person or believes that another person has, or has had, intent to wrong. Since no information is usually available as a basis for evaluating the objectivity of the more plausible suspicions, the term "accusation" might be the degree to which the patient tends to project blame and to accuse other people or forces or maliciousness or discriminatory intent. The pathology in this symptom area may range from mild to suspiciousness through delusions of persecution and ideas of reference.

**12. Hallucinatory Behavior.** The evaluation of hallucinatory experiences frequently requires judgment on the part of the rater whether the reported experience represents hallucination or merely vivid mental imagery. In general, unless the rater is quite convinced that the experiences represent true deviation from normal perceptual and imagery processes, hallucinatory behavior should be rated as *not present.*

**13. Motor Retardation.** Motor retardation involves the general slowing down and weakening of voluntary motor responses. Symptomatology in this area is represented by behavior which might be attributed to the loss of energy and vigor necessary to perform voluntary acts in a normal manner. Voluntary acts which are especially affected by reduced energy level include those related to speech as well as gross muscular behavior. With increased motor retardation, speech is slowed, weakened in volume, and reduced in amount. Voluntary movements are slowed, weakened, and less frequent.

**14. Uncooperativness.** This is the

term adopted to represent signs of hostility and resistance to the interviewer and interview situation. It should be noted that "uncooperativeness" is judged on the basis of response of the patient to the interview situation while "hostility" is rated on the basis of verbal reports and hostile feelings or behavior towards others *outside* the interview situation. It was found necessary to separate the two areas because of an occasional patient who refrains from any reference to hostile feelings and who even denies them while evidencing strong animosity toward the interviewer.

**15. Unusual Thought Content.** This symptom area is concerned solely with the *content* of the patient's verbalization; the extent to which it is unusual, odd, strange, or bizarre. Notice that a delusional or paranoid patient may present bizarre or unbelievable ideas in a perfectly straightforward, clear, and organized fashion. Only the unusualness of content should be rated for this item, not the degree of organization or disorganization.

**16. Blunted Affect.** This symptom area is recognized by reduced emotional tone and apparent lack of normal intensity of feeling or involvement. Emotional expressions are apt to be absent or of marked indifference and apathy. Attempted expressions of feeling may appear to be mimetic and without sincerity.

**17. Excitement.** Excitement refers to the emotional, mental, and psychological aspects of increased activation and heightened reactivity. The excited patient tends to be active, agitated, quick, loud, and emotionally responsive. Whereas tension is a construct concerned with physical or motor manifestations of activation, excitement has reference primarily to the mental and emotional areas. Tension usually implies a binding of the physical activation potential, while excitement is the underlying activation potential. The degree of excitement depends on the strength of arousal and heightened affect.

**18. Disorientation.** This rating construct has been included to provide a place for recording the particular kind of confusion that is evidenced by lack of memory or proper association for persons, places, or times. The disoriented individual may not know where he is, how to relate where he is to other points in the environment, or how to get from one place to another. The identities of persons that should be familiar may be confused. Location in time and place and even personal identity may be confused or unavailable for recall. Distortions in identity such as those that occur in delusional systems should not be rated under disorientation. Disorientation represents the type of confusion that frequently occurs in organic conditions.

**The Family Burden Interview Schedule—Short Form,** *See Chapter 20*

*THE FAMILY BURDEN INTERVIEW SCHEDULE—SHORT FORM (FBIS / SF)*

adapted from the

**Toolkit for Evaluating Family Experiences with Severe Mental Illness**

Prepared for the Evaluation Center @ HSRI

by

Richard Tessler, Ph.D.
and
Gail Gamache, Ph.D.

1994

Department of Sociology
Social and Demographic Research Institute
Machmer Hall
University of Massachusetts
Amherst, Ma 01003-4830

Acknowledgement: The authors wish to thank Professor Gene Fisher of the University of Massachusetts in Amherst who collaborated in the development of the FBIS and did much of the early psychometric work on which the FBIS/SF is based.

## SECTION A: ASSISTANCE IN DAILY LIVING MODULE

It frequently happens that persons who have a mental illness need help or need to be reminded to do everyday things. The next questions are about that. All of them may not apply to (*NAME*), but please try to answer them to the best of your knowledge.

**A1a.** During the past 30 days, how often did you help (*NAME*) with, or remind (*NAME*) to do things like grooming, bathing or dressing? Was it:

| 1 | 2 | 3 | 4 | 5 |
|---|---|---|---|---|
| not at all (GO TO **A2a**.) | less than once a week | 1 or 2 times a week | 3 to 6 times a week | every day? |

A1b. How much did you mind helping (*NAME*) with or reminding about these things? Was it:

| 1 | 2 | 3 | 4 |
|---|---|---|---|
| not at all | very little | some | a lot? |

**A2a.** During the past 30 days, how often did you help, remind, or encourage (*NAME*) to take (his/her) medicine? Was it:

| 1 | 2 | 3 | 4 | 5 |
|---|---|---|---|---|
| not at all doesn't take medication (GO TO **A3a**.) | less than once a week | 1 or 2 times a week | 3 to 6 times a week | every day? |

A2b. How much did you mind helping, reminding, or encourage (*NAME*) to take (his/her) medicine? Was it:

| 1 | 2 | 3 | 4 |
|---|---|---|---|
| not at all | very little | some | a lot? |

**A3a.** During the past 30 days, how often did you help (*NAME*) with, or remind (*NAME*) to do (his/her) housework or laundry? Was it:

| 1 | 2 | 3 | 4 | 5 |
|---|---|---|---|---|
| not at all (GO TO **A4a**.) | less than once a week | 1 or 2 times a week | 3 to 6 times a week | every day? |

A3b. How much did you mind helping (*NAME*) with or reminding him/her about these things? Was it:

| 1 | 2 | 3 | 4 |
|---|---|---|---|
| not at all | very little | some | a lot? |

**A4a.** *During the past 30 days,* how often did you help (*NAME*) with, or remind (*NAME*) to do, shopping for groceries, clothes, and other things? Was it:

| 1 | 2 | 3 | 4 | 5 |
|---|---|---|---|---|
| not at all (GO TO **A5a**.) | less than once a week | 1 or 2 times a week | 3 to 6 times a week | every day? |

A4b. How much did you mind helping (*NAME*) with or reminding (him/her) about these things? Was it:

| 1 | 2 | 3 | 4 |
|---|---|---|---|
| not at all | very little | some | a lot? |

**A5a.** *During the past 30 days,* how often did you cook for (*NAME*) or help (him/her) prepare meals? Was it:

| 1 | 2 | 3 | 4 | 5 |
|---|---|---|---|---|
| not at all (GO TO **A6a**.) | less than once a week | 1 or 2 times a week | 3 to 6 times a week | every day? |

**A5b.** How much did you mind cooking for (*NAME*) or helping (him/her) prepare meals? Was it:

| 1 | 2 | 3 | 4 |
|---|---|---|---|
| not at all | very little | some | a lot? |

**A6a.** *During the past 30 days,* how often did you give (*NAME*) a ride, or help (him/her) to use public transportation? Was it:

| 1 | 2 | 3 | 4 | 5 |
|---|---|---|---|---|
| not at all (GO TO **A7a**.) | less than once a week | 1 or 2 times a week | 3 to 6 times a week | every day? |

**A6b.** How much did you mind helping (*NAME*) with (his/her) transportation needs? Was it:

| 1 | 2 | 3 | 4 |
|---|---|---|---|
| not at all | very little | some | a lot? |

**A7a.** *During the past 30 days,* how often did you help (*NAME*) to manage (his/her) money, or manage it for (him/her)? Was it:

| 1 | 2 | 3 | 4 | 5 |
|---|---|---|---|---|
| not at all (GO TO **A8a**.) | less than once a week | 1 or 2 times a week | 3 to 6 times a week | every day? |

**A7b.** How much did you mind helping (*NAME*) manage (his/her) money? Was it:

| 1 | 2 | 3 | 4 |
|---|---|---|---|
| not at all | very little | some | a lot? |

**A8a.** During the past 30 days, how often did you help, remind, or urge (*NAME*) to make use of (his/her) time such as going to work, or school, or aftercare, or visiting with friends? Was it:

| 1 | 2 | 3 | 4 | 5 |
|---|---|---|---|---|
| not at all (GO TO **B1a**.) | less than once a week | 1 or 2 times a week | 3 to 6 times a week | every day? |

**A8b.** How much did you mind helping (*NAME*) make use of (his/her) time? Was it:

| 1 | 2 | 3 | 4 |
|---|---|---|---|
| not at all | very little | some | a lot? |

## SECTION B. SUPERVISION MODULE

Less frequently, persons with mental illness can require some assistance when certain troublesome behaviors occur. The next questions may not apply to (*NAME*), but please try to answer them to the best of your knowledge.

**B1a.** *During the past 30 days,* how often did you try to prevent or stop (*NAME*) from doing something embarrassing? Was it:

| 1 | 2 | 3 | 4 | 5 |
|---|---|---|---|---|
| not at all (GO TO **B2a**.) | less than once a week | 1 or 2 times a week | 3 to 6 times a week | every day? |

**B2b.** How much did you mind dealing with (*NAME*)'s embarrassing behavior? Was it:

| 1 | 2 | 3 | 4 |
|---|---|---|---|
| not at all | very little | some | a lot? |

**B2a.** *During the past 30 days,* how often did you try to prevent or stop (*NAME*) from making excessive demands for attention? Was it:

| 1 | 2 | 3 | 4 | 5 |
|---|---|---|---|---|
| not at all (GO TO **B3a**.) | less than once a week | 1 or 2 times a week | 3 to 6 times a week | every day? |

B2b. How much did you mind dealing with (*NAME*)'s attention-seeking behavior? Was it:

| 1 | 2 | 3 | 4 |
|---|---|---|---|
| not at all | very little | some | a lot? |

**B3a.** During the past 30 days, how often did you try to prevent or stop (*NAME*) from keeping anyone up at night? Was it:

| 1 | 2 | 3 | 4 | 5 |
|---|---|---|---|---|
| not at all (GO TO **B4a.**) | less than once a week | 1 or 2 times a week | 3 to 6 times a week | every day? |

B3b. How much did you mind having to deal with (*NAME*)'s disturbing behavior? Was it:

| 1 | 2 | 3 | 4 |
|---|---|---|---|
| not at all | very little | some | a lot? |

**B4a.** In the past 30 days, how often did you try to prevent or stop (*NAME*) from injuring or threatening to injure anyone? Was it:

| 1 | 2 | 3 | 4 | 5 |
|---|---|---|---|---|
| not at all (GO TO **B5a.**) | less than once a week | 1 or 2 times a week | 3 to 6 times a week | every day? |

B4b. How much did you mind doing that? Was it:

| 1 | 2 | 3 | 4 |
|---|---|---|---|
| not at all | very little | some | a lot? |

**B5a.** In the past 30 days, how often did you try to prevent or stop (*NAME*) from talking about, threatening, or attempting suicide? Was it:

| 1 | 2 | 3 | 4 | 5 |
|---|---|---|---|---|
| not at all (GO TO **B6a.**) | less than once a week | 1 or 2 times a week | 3 to 6 times a week | every day? |

B5b. How much did you mind dealing with (*NAME*)'s suicidal (talk/threats/attempts)? Was it:

| 1 | 2 | 3 | 4 |
|---|---|---|---|
| not at all | very little | some | a lot? |

**B6a.** During the past 30 days, how often did you try to prevent or stop (*NAME*) from drinking too much? Was it:

| 1 | 2 | 3 | 4 | 5 |
|---|---|---|---|---|
| not at all (GO TO **B7a.**) | less than once a week | 1 or 2 times a week | 3 to 6 times a week | every day? |

B6b. How much did you mind having to deal with (*NAME*)'s drinking? Was it:

| 1 | 2 | 3 | 4 |
|---|---|---|---|
| not at all | very little | some | a lot? |

**B7a.** During the past 30 days, how often did you try to prevent or stop (*NAME*) from using drugs? Was it:

| 1 | 2 | 3 | 4 | 5 |
|---|---|---|---|---|
| not at all (GO TO **C1a.**) | less than once a week | 1 or 2 times a week | 3 to 6 times a week | every day? |

B7b. How much did you mind having to deal with (*NAME*) using drugs? Was it:

| 1 | 2 | 3 | 4 |
|---|---|---|---|
| not at all | very little | some | a lot? |

## SECTION C.  FINANCIAL EXPENDITURES MODULE

C1. *During the past 30 days,* have you *personally* paid for, or given (*NAME*) money for any of the following for which (*NAME*) has not paid you back?

    (IF YES, IMMEDIATELY ASK Q. C2.)

C2. How much money was that?

| | Q. C1 | | Q. C2 AMOUNT IN PAST 30 DAYS |
|---|---|---|---|
| | YES | NO | |
| a. transportation expenses, carfare, gas, taxi, etcetera? | 1 | 2 | $_____ |
| b. clothing? | 1 | 2 | $_____ |
| c. pocket money? | 1 | 2 | $_____ |
| d. food? (IF [*NAME*] LIVES WITH R ASK R TO ESTIMATE [*NAME*]'S SHARE OF GROCERY BILL) | 1 | 2 | $_____ |
| e. shelter (rent, mortgage)? (IF [*NAME*] LIVES WITH R ASK R TO ESTIMATE [*NAME*]'S SHARE OF RENT/MORTGAGE | 1 | 2 | $_____ |
| f. medication? | 1 | 2 | $_____ |
| g. mental health treatment? | 1 | 2 | $_____ |
| h. other medical expenses? | 1 | 2 | $_____ |
| i. cigarettes? | 1 | 2 | $_____ |
| j. personal items? | 1 | 2 | $_____ |
| k. other expenses (SPECIFY):_____ | 1 | 2 | $_____ |

C3. Was (*NAME*) a financial burden to you during the past 12 months? Was it:

| | |
|---|---|
| constantly or almost constantly, | 1 |
| often, | 2 |
| sometimes, | 3 |
| seldom, or | 4 |
| never? | 5 |

## SECTION D.  IMPACT ON DAILY ROUTINES MODULE

D1a. *During the past 30 days* how often did you miss, or were you late for (school/[and] work) because of your involvement with (*NAME*)? Was it:

| 1 | 2 | 3 | 4 | 5 |
|---|---|---|---|---|
| not at all | less than once a week | 1 or 2 times a week | 3 to 6 times a week | every day? |

D1b. *During the past 30 days,* how often were your social and leisure activities changed or disrupted because of (*NAME*)? Was it:

| 1 | 2 | 3 | 4 | 5 |
|---|---|---|---|---|
| not at all | less than once a week | 1 or 2 times a week | 3 to 6 times a week | every day? |

D1c. *During the past 30 days,* how often was your usual housework or domestic routine disrupted or changed because of (*NAME*)? Was it:

| 1 | 2 | 3 | 4 | 5 |
|---|---|---|---|---|
| not at all | less than once a week | 1 or 2 times a week | 3 to 6 times a week | every day? |

D1d. *During the past 30 days,* how often did taking care of (*NAME*) prevent you from giving other family members as much time and attention as they needed? Was it:

| 1 | 2 | 3 | 4 | 5 |
|---|---|---|---|---|
| not at all | less than once a week | 1 or 2 times a week | 3 to 6 times a week | every day? |

D2  Has (*NAME*)'s illness caused you to make more or less permanent changes in your daily routine, work, or social life such as:

> (YOU MAY CIRCLE MORE THAN ONE RESPONSE)
> working less or quitting job,          1
> retiring earlier than you planned,     2
> having no social life,                 3
> losing friendships, or                 4
> not taking vacations?                  5

## SECTION E: WORRY

E1. (Even when people have not seen each other for a period of time, sometimes they worry anyway about the other person.) I would like to ask you about concerns or worries you may have about (*NAME*).

a. Do you worry about (*NAME*)'s safety:

| 1 | 2 | 3 | 4 | 5 |
|---|---|---|---|---|
| constantly or almost constantly | often | sometimes | seldom | never? |

b. Do you worry about the kind of help and treatment (*NAME*) is receiving:

| 1 | 2 | 3 | 4 | 5 |
|---|---|---|---|---|
| constantly or almost constantly | often | sometimes | seldom | never? |

c. Do you worry about (*NAME*)'s social life:

| 1 | 2 | 3 | 4 | 5 |
|---|---|---|---|---|
| constantly or almost constantly | often | sometimes | seldom | never? |

d. Do you worry about (*NAME*)'s physical health:

| 1 | 2 | 3 | 4 | 5 |
|---|---|---|---|---|
| constantly or almost constantly | often | sometimes | seldom | never? |

e. Do you worry about (*NAME*)'s current living arrangements:

| 1 | 2 | 3 | 4 | 5 |
|---|---|---|---|---|
| constantly or almost constantly | often | sometimes | seldom | never? |

f. Do you worry about how (*NAME*) would manage financially if you were not there to help (him/her):

| 1 | 2 | 3 | 4 | 5 |
|---|---|---|---|---|
| constantly or almost constantly | often | sometimes | seldom | never? |

g. Do you worry about (*NAME*)'s future prospects:

| 1 | 2 | 3 | 4 | 5 |
|---|---|---|---|---|
| constantly or almost constantly | often | sometimes | seldom | never? |

---

**Alcohol Use Scale,** *See Chapter 21*

---

Client Name: _____

Date of Rating: _____

### CLINICIAN ALCOHOL USE SCALE

Please rate your client's use of alcohol over the past six months according to the following scale. If the person is in an institution, the reporting interval is the time period prior to institutionalization. You should weight evidence from self-report, interviews, behavioral observations, and collateral reports (family, day center, community, etc.) in making this rating.

_____ 1 = **ABSTINENT** Client has not used alcohol during this time interval.

_____ 2 = **USE WITHOUT IMPAIRMENT** Client has used alcohol during this time interval, but there is no evidence of persistent or recurrent social, occupational, psychological, or physical problems related to use and no evidence of recurrent dangerous use.

_____ 3 = **ABUSE** Client has used alcohol during this time interval and there is evidence of persistent or recurrent social, occupational, psychological, or physical problems related to use or evidence of recurrent dangerous use. For example, recurrent alcohol use leads to disruptive behavior and housing problems. Problems have persisted for at least one month.

_____ 4 = **DEPENDENCE** Meets criteria for moderate plus at least three of the following: greater amounts or intervals of use than intended, much of time used obtaining or using substance, frequent intoxication or withdrawal interferes with other activities, important activities given up because of alcohol use, continued use despite knowledge of substance-related problems, marked tolerance, characteristic withdrawal symptoms, alcohol taken to relieve or avoid withdrawal symptoms. For example, drinking binges and preoccupation with drinking have caused client to drop out of job training and non-drinking social activities.

_____ 5 = **DEPENDENCE WITH INSTITU-TIONALIZATION** Meets criteria for severe plus related problems are so severe that they make noninstitutional living difficult. For example, constant drinking leads to disruptive behavior and inability to pay rent so that client is frequently reported to police and seeking hospitalization.

---

**Drug Use Scale,** *See Chapter 21*

---

Client Name: _____

Date of Rating: _____

### *CLINICIAN DRUG USE SCALE*

Please rate your client's use of drugs over the past six months according to the following scale. If the person is in an institution, the reporting interval is the time period prior to institutionalization. You should weight evidence from self-report, interviews, behavioral observations, and collateral reports (family, day center, community, etc.) in making this rating.

_____ 1 = ***ABSTINENT*** Client has not used drugs during this time interval.

_____ 2 = ***USE WITHOUT IMPAIRMENT*** Client has used drugs during this time interval, but there is no evidence of persistent or recurrent social, occupational, psychological, or physical problems related to use and no evidence of recurrent dangerous use.

_____ 3 = ***ABUSE*** Client has used drugs during this time interval and there is evidence of persistent or recurrent social, occupational, psychological, or physical problems related to use or evidence of recurrent dangerous use. For example, recurrent drug use leads to disruptive behavior and housing problems. Problems have persisted for at least one month.

_____ 4 = ***DEPENDENCE*** Meets criteria for moderate plus at least three of the following: greater amounts or intervals of use than intended, much of time used obtaining or using substance, frequent intoxication or withdrawal interferes with other activities, important activities given up because of drug use, continued use despite knowledge of substance-related problems, marked tolerance, characteristic withdrawal symptoms, drugs taken to relieve or avoid withdrawal symptoms. For example, binges and preoccupation with drugs have caused client to drop out of job training and non-drug social activities.

_____ 5 = ***DEPENDENCE WITH INSTITUTIONALIZATION*** Meets criteria for severe plus related problems are so severe that they make noninstitutional living difficult. For example, constant drug use leads to disruptive behavior and inability to pay rent so that client is frequently reported to police and seeking hospitalization.

*Circle drugs used:* cannabis  cocaine  hallucinogens  opiates  PCP  sedatives/hypnotics/anxiolytics  stimulants  over-the-counter

Other_____

**Substance Abuse Treatment Scale,** *See Chapter 21*

---

## Substance Abuse Treatment Scale

*Instructions:* This scale is for assessing a person's stage of substance abuse treatment, not for determining diagnosis. The reporting interval is the last *six months*. If the person is in an institution, the reporting interval is the time period prior to institutionalization.

**1. Pre-engagement.** The person (not client) does not have contact with a case manager, mental health counselor or substance abuse conselor.

**2. Engagement.** The client has had contact with an assigned case manager or counselor but does not have regular contacts. The lack of regular contact implies lack of a working alliance.

**3. Early Persuasion.** The client has regular contacts with a case manager or counselor but has not reduced substance use more than a month. Regular contacts imply a working alliance and a relationship in which substance abuse can be discussed.

**4. Late Persuasion.** The client is engaged in a relationship with case manager or counselor, is discussing substance use or attending a group, and shows evidence of reduc-

tion in use for at least one month (fewer drugs, smaller quantities, or both). External controls (e.g., Antabuse) may be involved in reduction.

**5. Early Active Treatment.** The client is engaged in treatment, is discussing substance use or attending a group, has reduced use for at least one month, and is working toward abstinence (or controlled use without associated problems) as a goal, even though he or she may still be abusing.

**6. Late Active Treatment.** The person is engaged in treatment, has acknowledged that substance abuse is a problem, and has achieved abstinence (or controlled use without associated problems), but for less than six months.

**7. Relapse Prevention.** The client is engaged in treatment, has acknowledged that substance abuse is a problem, and has achieved abstinence (or controlled use without associated problems) for at least six months. Occasional lapses, not days of problematic use, are allowed.

**8. In Remission or Recovery.** The client has had *no* problems related to substance use for over one year and is no longer in any type of substance abuse treatment.

---

**Quality of Life Interview,** *See Chapter 22*

---

# Quality of Life Interview
# Full Version

---

### SECTION A: DEMOGRAPHICS

**Time Began (military time):** ___ ___ : ___ ___

First, I'm going to ask you a few background questions.

1. SEX OF RESPONDENT (CODE BY OBSERVATION)

   Male ....................................1
   Female ...............................2

2. What is your date of birth?

   ___ ___ / ___ ___ / ___ ___
   m  m     d   d     y   y

3. How old are you?

   Age ...........................___ ___
   Missing ............................99

4. What is your marital status?

   Married..............................1
   Separated ..........................2
   Divorced............................3
   Widowed ...........................4
   Never married...................5
   Co-habitating ....................6
   Missing .............................9

5. A. How many children do you have?

   No. of children ..........___ ___
   None.................................00
   Missing .............................99

   B. How many of your children are under 18 years of age?

   No...............................___ ___

6. What is the highest grade in school or year of college you have completed?

   Grade .......................___ ___
   None.................................00
   Missing .............................99

   IF Q6 CODED 12 OR MORE GO TO Q8

7. Did you pass a high school equivalency test?

   No.......................................0
   Yes .....................................1
   Missing .............................9

8. Do you have a college degree?

   No (go to Q10) ....................0
   Yes .....................................1
   Missing .............................9

9. What degree is that?

   Associate............................1
   Bachelors............................2
   Masters...............................3
   Doctorate ...........................4
   Other (specify)...................5

SPECIFY_____

10. Do you have any other training?

No (go to Q12) ....................0
Yes .....................................1
Missing ..............................9

11. What kind of training?

_____

_____ __ __

12. Which of the following best describes your race?

Caucasian (not Hispanic).......................1
African-American (not Hispanic)............2
Hispanic ...................................................3
American Indian.....................................4
Asian ......................................................5
Other (specify) ......................................6
Missing...................................................9

SPECIFY_____

13. Did you ever serve in the Armed Forces of the United States?

No (go to next section).............0
Yes............................................1
Missing......................................9

14. What branch of the Armed Forces?

Army .........................................1
Navy..........................................2
Marines.....................................3

15. What type of discharge did you receive when you left the armed forces?

Honorable ...............................1
General ....................................2
Undesirable .............................3
Bad conduct ............................4
Dishonorable or dismissal ......5
Other........................................6

## SECTION B:  GENERAL LIFE SATISFACTION

Please look at this card. (HAND SUBJECT THE DELIGHTED-TERRIBLE SCALE.) This is called the Delighted-Terrible Scale (D/T Scale).

The scale goes from terrible, which is the lowest ranking of 1, to delighted, which is the highest ranking of 7. There are also points 2 through 6 with descriptions below them. (READ POINTS ON THE SCALE.)

During the interview we'll be using this scale from time to time to help you tell me how you feel about different things in your life. All you have to do is tell me what on the scale best describes how you feel. For example, if I ask, "how do you feel about chocolate ice cream" and you are someone who loves chocolate ice cream, you might point to "delighted." On the other hand, if you hate chocolate ice cream, you might point to "terrible." If you feel about equally satisfied and dissatisfied with chocolate ice cream, then you would point to the middle of the scale.

Do you have any questions about the scale? Please show me how you feel about chocolate ice cream. Let's begin.

The first question is a very general one.

1.   How do you feel about your life in general?
     **D-T SCALE:**

Missing        _____  9

Now, set the scale aside. I'll let you know when we need it again.

## SECTION C:  LIVING SITUATION

Now I am going to ask you some questions about your living situation.

1.  What is your *current* living situation? ...................................................................\_\_\_\_\_  \_\_\_\_\_

(IF RESPONDENT IS CURRENTLY IN THE HOSPITAL, AND THIS HOSPITALIZATION HAS LASTED LESS THAN 3 MONTHS, LIVING SITUATION = LIVING SITUATION JUST PRIOR TO THE HOSPITALIZATION. IF THE HOSPITALIZATION HAS BEEN FOR 3 MONTHS OR MORE, CODE "HOSPITAL".)

01  Hospital
02  Skilled nursing facility — 24 hour nursing service
03  Intermediate care facility — less than 24 hour nursing facility
04  Supervised group living (generally long term)
05  Transitional group home (halfway or quarterway house)
06  Family foster care
07  Cooperative apartment, supervised (staff on premises)
08  Cooperative apartment, unsupervised (staff not on premises)
09  Board and care home (private proprietary home for adults, with program and supervision)
10  Boarding house (includes meals, no program or supervision)
11  Rooming or boarding house or hotel (includes single room occupancy, no meals are provided, cooking facilities may be available)
12  Private house or apartment
13  Shelter
14  Jail
15  No current residence (including the streets, bus stations, missions, etc.)
16  Other_____
99  No information

2.  Have you lived any place else during the past <year>? (including hospital)

No (go to Q5) ......................0
Yes (go to Q3) .....................1
Missing (go to Q5) ..............9

3.  List in order the places you have lived during the past <year>, including hospitalizations, beginning with your *current* living situation. (USE CODES IN Q.1 ABOVE)

| *CODE* | *DESCRIPTION* |
|---|---|
| a. \_\_\_\_ \_\_\_\_ | _____ |
| b. \_\_\_\_ \_\_\_\_ | _____ |
| c. \_\_\_\_ \_\_\_\_ | _____ |
| d. \_\_\_\_ \_\_\_\_ | _____ |
| e. \_\_\_\_ \_\_\_\_ | _____ |
| f. \_\_\_\_ \_\_\_\_ | _____ |
| g. \_\_\_\_ \_\_\_\_ | _____ |
| h. \_\_\_\_ \_\_\_\_ | _____ |

Total number of different, non-hospital residences, during past <year>?    \_\_\_\_ \_\_\_\_

4.  Which of these was your usual residence during the past <year>?
(use codes in Q1 above)    \_\_\_\_ \_\_\_\_

5.  During the past <year> did you sleep in any of the following locations?

| *LOCATION* | *NO* | *YES* | *MISSING* |
|---|---|---|---|
| a.  outside without shelter | 0 | 1 | 9 |
| b.  inside an empty building | 0 | 1 | 9 |
| c.  in a public shelter | 0 | 1 | 9 |
| d.  in a church/mission | 0 | 1 | 9 |

6. Do you *currently* have a regular place to live where you spend at least 5 out of 7 nights on the average?

No..........................................0
Yes .......................................1
Missing ..............................9

7. **NOW LOOK AT THE D-T SCALE AGAIN AND ANSWER THE FOLLOWING: (HAND RESPONDENT THE D-T SCALE. IF RESPONDENT IS CURRENTLY IN THE HOSPITAL FOR LESS THAN 3 MONTHS, USE MOST RECENT RESIDENCE PRIOR TO HOSPITALIZATION. IF RESPONDENT IS IN THE HOSPITAL 3 MONTHS OR MORE, USE HOSPITAL AS THE RESIDENCE. SKIP IF HOMELESS).**

How do you feel about:

A. The living arrangements where you live? ...................................................... _____
B. The food there? ........................................................................................... _____
C. The rules there? ......................................................................................... _____
D. The privacy you have there? ....................................................................... _____
E. The amount of freedom you have? ............................................................... _____
F. The prospect of staying on where you currently live for a long period of time?........ _____

8. **STILL USING THE D-T SCALE, ANSWER THE FOLLOWING: (IF RESPONDENT IS IN THE HOSPITAL FOR LESS THAN 3 MONTHS, USE MOST RECENT RESIDENCE PRIOR TO HOSPITALIZATION. IF RESPONDENT IS IN THE HOSPITAL 3 MONTHS OR MORE, USE HOSPITAL AS THE RESIDENCE. SKIP IF HOMELESS).**

How do you feel about:

A. The people who live in the houses and apartments near yours? ............................... _____
B. People who live in this community? ............................................................. _____
C. The outdoor space there is for you to use outside your home?................................ _____
D. The particular neighborhood as a place to live? ............................................. _____
E. This community as a place to live? ............................................................... _____
F. How safe you feel in this neighborhood? ....................................................... _____

## SECTION D: DAILY ACTIVITIES AND FUNCTIONING

1. Now let's talk about some of the things you did with your time in the *past week*. I'm going to read you a list of things people may do with their free time. For each of these, please tell me if you did it during the past week. Did you . . . (READ OPTIONS A-P)?

|  | NO | YES | MISS |
|---|---|---|---|
| A. Go for a walk? | 0 | 1 | 9 |
| B. Go to a movie or play? | 0 | 1 | 9 |
| C. Watch television? | 0 | 1 | 9 |
| D. Go shopping? | 0 | 1 | 9 |
| E. Go to a restaurant or coffee shop? | 0 | 1 | 9 |
| F. Go to a bar? | 0 | 1 | 9 |
| G. Read a book, magazine or newspaper? | 0 | 1 | 9 |
| H. Listen to a radio? | 0 | 1 | 9 |
| I. Play cards? | 0 | 1 | 9 |
| J. Go for a ride in a bus or car? | 0 | 1 | 9 |
| K. Prepare a meal? | 0 | 1 | 9 |
| L. Work on a hobby? | 0 | 1 | 9 |
| M. Play a sport? | 0 | 1 | 9 |
| N. Go to a meeting of some organization or social group? (INCLUDE PROGRAM-RELATED MEETINGS) | 0 | 1 | 9 |
| O. Go to a park? | 0 | 1 | 9 |
| P. Go to a library? | 0 | 1 | 9 |

2. Overall, how would you rate your functioning in home, social, school, and work settings at the present time? Would you say your functioning in these areas is excellent, good, fair or poor?

EXCELLENT............................................1
GOOD......................................................2
FAIR........................................................3
POOR .....................................................4
Missing...................................................9

3. **NOW PLEASE LOOK AT THE D-T SCALE AGAIN.**

How do you feel about: (READ OPTIONS A-F)?

A. The way you spend your spare time? ................................................................. _____
B. The amount of time you have to do the things you want to do?............................... _____
C. The chance you have to enjoy pleasant or beautiful things?.................................... _____
D. The amount of fun you have?................................................................................ _____
E. The amount of relaxation in your life? ................................................................. _____
F. The pleasure you get from the television or radio?................................................. _____

**SECTION E:  FAMILY**

The next few questions are about your relationship with your family including any relatives with whom you live.

1. In the past <year>, how often did you talk to a member of your family on the telephone? Would you say at least once a day, at least once a week, at least once a month, less than once a month but at least once during the year, or not at all?

AT LEAST ONCE A DAY..........................5
AT LEAST ONCE A WEEK ......................4
AT LEAST ONCE A MONTH ...................3
LESS THAN ONCE A MONTH ................2
NOT AT ALL.............................................1
NO FAMILY (GO TO SECTION F) ..........0
Missing .....................................................9

2. In the past <year>, how often did you get together with a member of your family—at least once a day, at least once a week, at least once a month, less than once a month but at least once during the year, or not at all?

AT LEAST ONCE A DAY..........................5
AT LEAST ONCE A WEEK ......................4
AT LEAST ONCE A MONTH ...................3
LESS THAN ONCE A MONTH ................2
NOT AT ALL.............................................1
NO FAMILY (GO TO SECTION F) ..........0
Missing .....................................................9

3. **PLEASE LOOK AT THE D-T SCALE AGAIN.**

How do you feel about: (READ OPTIONS A-D)?

A. Your family in general? .......................................................................................... _____
B. How often you have contact with your family?......................................................... _____
C. The way you and your family act toward each other?............................................... _____
D. The way things are in general between you and your family?................................... _____

## SECTION F: SOCIAL RELATIONS

Now I'd like to know about other people in your life, that is, people who are not in your family.

1.  About how often do you do the following? Would you say, at least once a day, once a week, once a month, less than once a month or not at all?

    AT LEAST ONCE A DAY ......................5
    AT LEAST ONCE A WEEK...................4
    AT LEAST ONCE A MONTH................3
    LESS THAN ONCE A MONTH .............2
    NOT AT ALL .........................................1
    Missing................................................9

    A.  Do things with a close friend?...............................................................  _____
    B.  Visit with someone who does not live with you?.........................................  _____
    C.  Telephone someone who does not live with you?.........................................  _____
    D.  Write a letter to someone? ......................................................................  _____
    E.  Do something with another person that you planned ahead of time?.......................  _____
    F.  Spend time with someone you consider more than a friend, like a spouse, boyfriend or girlfriend?...................................................................................  _____

2.  **PLEASE LOOK AT THE D-T SCALE AGAIN.**

    How do you feel about:

    A.  The things you do with other people?.........................................................  _____
    B.  The amount of time you spend with other people?.......................................  _____
    C.  The people you see socially?....................................................................  _____
    D.  How you get along with other people in general?.......................................  _____
    E.  The chance you have to know people with whom you really feel comfortable?.........  _____
    F.  The amount of friendship in your life? ....................................................  _____

## SECTION G: FINANCES

A few questions about money.

1.  In the past <year> have you had any financial support from the following sources?

    |  | YES | NO | MISS |
    |---|---|---|---|
    | A.  Earned income | 1 | 0 | 9 |
    | B.  Social Security Benefits (SSA) | 1 | 0 | 9 |
    | C.  Social Security Disability Income (SSDI) | 1 | 0 | 9 |
    | D.  Supplemental Security Income (SSI) | 1 | 0 | 9 |
    | E.  Armed Service connected disability payments | 1 | 0 | 9 |
    | F.  Other Social Welfare benefits—state or county (general welfare, Aid to Families with Dependent Children (AFDC)) | 1 | 0 | 9 |
    | G.  Vocational program (Comprehensive Employment and Training Act (CETA), Vocational Rehabilitation, sheltered workshop | 1 | 0 | 9 |
    | H.  Unemployment compensation | 1 | 0 | 9 |
    | I.  Retirement, investment or savings income | 1 | 0 | 9 |
    | J.  Rent supplements (including HUD, Section 8 certificates, living programs receiving public assistance support) | 1 | 0 | 9 |
    | K.  Alimony and child support | 1 | 0 | 9 |
    | L.  Food stamps | 1 | 0 | 9 |
    | M.  Family and/or spouse contribution | 1 | 0 | 9 |
    | N.  Other source(s) **(SPECIFY):** | 1 | 0 | 9 |

    _____

2.  How much money did you receive during the *past month* from all of these sources?

    $_____ _____ _____ _____
    Missing                    9999

2A. Was this a usual *month* in terms of the amount of money you received?

    Yes (go to Q3)....................1
    No (go to Q2B)...................0
    Missing (go to Q2B) ...........9

2B. Would you say that the amount of money you received during the *past month* was more than or less than usual?

    More than usual.................1
    Less than usual..................2
    Missing ..............................9

2C. How much would you say that you have usually received *per month* during the past *year*?

    $_____ _____ _____ _____
    Missing                    9999

3.  On the average, how much money did you have to spend on yourself in the *past month,* not counting money for room and meals?

    $_____ _____ _____ _____
    Missing                    9999

INTERVIEWER RATING:

HOW RELIABLE DO YOU THINK R'S RESPONSES WERE TO Q1,

    VERY RELIABLE.........................4
    GENERALLY RELIABLE ...........3
    GENERALLY UNRELIABLE......2
    VERY UNRELIABLE...................1

4.  Is there anyone who handles your money for you?

    No  (Go to Q5)....................0
    Yes ......................................1

    A. Are your checks mailed directly to this person?

    No.........................................0
    Yes ......................................1

5.  During the past <year>, did you generally have enough money each month to cover (READ OPTIONS A-F)?

    |  | YES | NO | MISS |
    |---|---|---|---|
    | A. Food? | 0 | 1 | 9 |
    | B. Clothing? | 0 | 1 | 9 |
    | C. Housing? | 0 | 1 | 9 |
    | D. Medical care? | 0 | 1 | 9 |
    | E. Traveling around the city for things like shopping, medical appointments, or visiting friends and relatives? | 0 | 1 | 9 |
    | F. Social activities like movies or eating in restaurants? | 0 | 1 | 9 |

6.  **NOW, I'D LIKE YOU TO USE THE D-T SCALE AGAIN.** In general, how do you feel about: (READ OPTIONS A-D)?
    A. The amount of money you get? ................................................................................  _____
    B. The amount of money you have to cover basic necessities such as food, housing, and clothes?................................................................................................................  _____
    C. How comfortable and well-off you are financially?......................................................  _____
    D. The amount of money you have available to spend for fun? ......................................  _____

## SECTION H:  WORK AND SCHOOL

1. During a usual week, what do you do *most of the time?*

   Work at a job for pay (go to Q3)...........................1
   Go to a structured day program ........................2
   Go to school.........................................................3
   Do volunteer work...............................................4
   Keep house...........................................................5
   Nothing much (e.g., drink coffee, smoke
     cigarettes, watch TV)......................................6
   Something else (specify)....................................7
   Missing..................................................................9

   SPECIFY_____

2. Are you currently working in a job for pay?

   No (Go Q11)........................0
   Yes ......................................1
   Missing ...............................9

3. I'd like to know about the job you have now. What kind of business or industry do you work in?

   (IF MORE THAN ONE JOB, USE THE JOB AT WHICH THE PERSON EARNS THE HIGHER
   WEEKLY SALARY)

   DESCRIBE_____  ____ ____

   A.  What kind of work do you do?

   SPECIFY:_____  ____ ____

   B.  What are your most important activities or duties?

   SPECIFY:_____  ____ ____

4. How long have you been working at this job?

   # of months.........___ ___ ___
   Less than one month .....995
   Less than one week........996
   Missing ...........................999

5. Is this job in a sheltered workshop?

   No.........................................0
   Yes ......................................1
   Missing ...............................9

6. Do you have a special supervisor or a job coach?

   No.........................................0
   Yes ......................................1
   Missing ...............................9

7. Is this a job you can keep as long as you wish?

   No.........................................0
   Yes (go to Q9) .....................1
   Missing ...............................9

8. Is this a job that ends after a certain period of time when you are
   expected to find another job at another place of work?

   No.........................................0
   Yes ......................................1
   Missing ...............................9

9. How many hours a week do you usually work?

   # of hours............___ ___ ___
   Missing ...........................999

10. How much do you earn per hour/week at this job?
    (CHOOSE ONE)

$ per hour ...........___ ___ ___
$ per week ..........___ ___ ___

**SKIP TO Q17**

11. Have you *ever* worked in the past <year>?

No........................................0
Yes ......................................1
Missing ...............................9

12. How long has it been since you had a job for pay?

# of years ..................___ ___
Less than a year...............01
Missing ..............................99

13. What do you think is the main reason that you don't have
    a steady job right now?

Psychiatric reasons............1
Physical problems ..............2
Laid off ...............................3
Looking/can't find a job .....4
Other reason ......................5
Missing ...............................9

14. Are you looking for work right now?

No (go to Q18) ....................0
Yes, full-time.....................1
Yes, part-time ...................2
Yes, casual.........................3
Missing (go to Q18)...........9

15. How long have you been looking?

< 1 month ...........................0
1-3 months.........................1
4-6 months.........................2
7-12 months.......................3
1-5 years ............................4
5-10 years ..........................5
> 10 years ..........................6
Missing (go to Q18)...........9

16. During the past <year> have you either:
    A. Filled out an application for a job?

No........................................0
Yes ......................................1
Missing ...............................9

    B. Interviewed for a job?

No........................................0
Yes ......................................1
Missing ...............................9

**SKIP TO Q18**

17. **JOB SATISFACTION (USE D-T SCALE) (SKIP IF UNEMPLOYED)**

How do you feel about:

A. Your job? ....................................................................................................... _____
B. The people you work with?........................................................................... _____
C. What it is like where you work (the physical surroundings) .................... _____
D. The number of hours you work? ................................................................. _____
E. The amount you get paid?............................................................................ _____

18. Have you been a student during the past <year>?

No (go to next section).............0
Yes..........................................1
Missing (go to next section) ....9

19. At what level was the schooling?

High School (grades 9 - 12, including GED) .....1
Adult Education ................................................2
College (undergraduate) ...................................3
Graduate school................................................4
Vocational/technical school...............................5
Job Training .....................................................6
Other (specify)_____7

20. Did you carry a full-time load of studies?

No.........................................0
Yes .......................................1
Missing ................................9

21. Are you attending now?

No.........................................0
Yes .......................................1
Missing ................................9

22. **USING THE D-T SCALE AGAIN,** how do you feel about:
A. Being a student? ........................................................................................... _____
B. Your school? ................................................................................................. _____
C. The other students at your school?............................................................. _____

## SECTION I:  LEGAL AND SAFETY ISSUES

1. In the past <year>, were you a victim of:

A. Any violent crimes such as assault, rape, mugging, or robbery?

No........................................0
Yes .......................................1
Missing ................................9

B. Any nonviolent crimes such as burglary, theft of your property or money, or being cheated?

No........................................0
Yes .......................................1
Missing ................................9

2. Have you been arrested or picked-up for any crimes in the past <year>?

# ARRESTS ____ ____

3. Have you spent any nights in jail in the past <year>?

# NIGHTS ____ ____ ____

4. **PLEASE LOOK AT THE D-T SCALE AGAIN.**

How do you feel about: (READ OPTIONS A-E)?

A. Your personal safety? .................................................................................... _____
B. How safe you are on the streets in your neighborhood? ........................... _____
C. How safe you are where you live? ................................................................ _____
D. The protection you have against being robbed or attacked? ..................... _____
E. Your chance of finding a policeman if you need one? ................................ _____

## SECTION J:  HEALTH

**NOW I'D LIKE TO ASK YOU ABOUT YOUR HEALTH.**

1. In general, would you say your health is:

Excellent ............................. 1
Very Good ........................... 2
Good .................................... 3
Fair ...................................... 4
Poor ..................................... 5
Missing ................................ 9

2. *Compared to six months ago,* how would you rate your health in general *now*?

Much better now than six months ago ............. 1
Somewhat better now than six months ago ..... 2
About the same ................................................ 3
Somewhat worse now than six months ago ..... 4
Much worse now than six months ago ............. 5
Missing .............................................................. 9

3. How do you feel about: **(USE THE D/T SCALE)**
A. Your health in general? .............................................................................. _____
B. The medical care available to you if you need it? ...................................... _____
C. How often you see a doctor? ........................................................................ _____
D. The chance you have to talk with a therapist? ........................................... _____
E. Your physical condition? .............................................................................. _____
F. Your emotional well-being? .......................................................................... _____

## SECTION K:  GLOBAL RATING

1. And a very general question again. **USING THE D-T SCALE AGAIN,** how do
you feel about your life in general? ................................................................... _____

Time Ended (military time): \_\_\_ \_\_\_ : \_\_\_ \_\_\_

## CARD I:  DELIGHTED— TERRIBLE SCALE

| 1 | 2 | 3 | 4 | 5 | 6 | 7 |
|---|---|---|---|---|---|---|
| Terrible | Unhappy | Mostly Dissatisfied | Mixed (about equally satisfied and dissatisfied) | Mostly Satisfied | Pleased | Delighted |

---

**The Client Satisfaction Questionnaire,** *See Chapter 23*

---

**CSQ-8**
**CLIENT SATISFACTION QUESTIONNAIRE**

Please help us improve our program by answering some questions about the services you have received. We are interested in your honest opinions, whether they are positive or negative. *Please answer all of the questions.* We also welcome your comments and suggestions. Thank you very much, we really appreciate your help.

**CIRCLE YOUR ANSWERS**

1. How would you rate the quality of service you have received?

| 4 | 3 | 2 | 1 |
|---|---|---|---|
| *Excellent* | *Good* | *Fair* | *Poor* |

2. Did you get the kind of service you wanted?

| 4 | 3 | 2 | 1 |
|---|---|---|---|
| *No, definitely not* | *No, not really* | *Yes, generally* | *Yes, definitely* |

3. To what extent has our program met your needs?

| 4 | 3 | 2 | 1 |
|---|---|---|---|
| *Almost all of my needs have been met* | *Most of my needs have been met* | *Only a few of my needs have been met* | *None of my needs have been met* |

4. If a friend were in need of similar help, would you recommend our program to him or her?

| 4 | 3 | 2 | 1 |
|---|---|---|---|
| *No, definitely not* | *No, I don't think so* | *Yes, I think so* | *Yes, definitely* |

5. How satisfied are you with the amount of help you have received?

| 4 | 3 | 2 | 1 |
|---|---|---|---|
| *Quite dissatisfied* | *Indifferent or mildly dissatisfied* | *Mostly satisfied* | *Very satisfied* |

6. Have the services you received helped you to deal more effectively with your problems?

| 4 | 3 | 2 | 1 |
|---|---|---|---|
| *Yes, they helped a great deal* | *Yes, they helped somewhat* | *No, they really didn't help* | *No, they seemed to make things worse* |

7. In an overall, general sense, how satisfied are you with the service you have received?

| 4 | 3 | 2 | 1 |
|---|---|---|---|
| *Very satisfied* | *Mostly satisfied* | *Indifferent or mildly dissatisfied* | *Quite dissatisfied* |

8. If you were to seek help again, would you come back to our program?

| 1 | 2 | 3 | 4 |
|---|---|---|---|
| *No, definitely not* | *No, I don't think so* | *Yes, I think so* | *Yes, definitely* |

---

## The Service Satisfaction Scale-30, *See Chapter 23*

---

SERVICES EVALUATION

## *CONFIDENTIAL*

Please read the following statements carefully. Indicate the answer that best describes your feeling about each aspect of the services you have received. We are interested in your *overall experience* based on all visits or contacts you have had *during the last year.* By "practitioner" we mean the one or more doctors, psychologists, counselors, clinicians, etc. who have worked with you.

**What is your overall feeling about the . . .**

1. Kinds of services offered

| ☐ | ☐ | ☐ | ☐ | ☐ |
|---|---|---|---|---|
| *DELIGHTED* | *MOSTLY SATISFIED* | *MIXED* | *MOSTLY DISSATISFIED* | *TERRIBLE* |

2. Opportunity to choose which practitioner you see

| ☐ | ☐ | ☐ | ☐ | ☐ |
|---|---|---|---|---|
| *TERRIBLE* | *MOSTLY DISSATISFIED* | *MIXED* | *MOSTLY SATISFIED* | *DELIGHTED* |

3. Effect of services in helping you deal with your problems

| ☐ | ☐ | ☐ | ☐ | ☐ |
|---|---|---|---|---|
| *DELIGHTED* | *MOSTLY SATISFIED* | *MIXED* | *MOSTLY DISSATISFIED* | *TERRIBLE* |

4. Office personnel (receptionists, clerks) on the telephone or in person

| ☐ | ☐ | ☐ | ☐ | ☐ |
|---|---|---|---|---|
| *TERRIBLE* | *MOSTLY DISSATISFIED* | *MIXED* | *MOSTLY SATISFIED* | *DELIGHTED* |

5. Office procedures (scheduling, forms, tests, etc.)

| ☐ | ☐ | ☐ | ☐ | ☐ |
|---|---|---|---|---|
| *DELIGHTED* | *MOSTLY SATISFIED* | *MIXED* | *MOSTLY DISSATISFIED* | *TERRIBLE* |

**What is your overall feeling about the . . .**

6. Professional knowledge and competence of the main practitioner(s)

| ☐ | ☐ | ☐ | ☐ | ☐ |
|---|---|---|---|---|
| *TERRIBLE* | *MOSTLY DISSATISFIED* | *MIXED* | *MOSTLY SATISFIED* | *DELIGHTED* |

7. Location and accessibility of the services (distance, parking, public transportation, etc.)

| ☐ | ☐ | ☐ | ☐ | ☐ |
|---|---|---|---|---|
| *DELIGHTED* | *MOSTLY SATISFIED* | *MIXED* | *MOSTLY DISSATISFIED* | *TERRIBLE* |

8. Appearance and physical layout of the facility (e.g., waiting area)

| □ | □ | □ | □ | □ |
|---|---|---|---|---|
| TERRIBLE | MOSTLY DISSATISFIED | MIXED | MOSTLY SATISFIED | DELIGHTED |

9. Ability of your practitioner(s) to listen to and understand your problems

| □ | □ | □ | □ | □ |
|---|---|---|---|---|
| DELIGHTED | MOSTLY SATISFIED | MIXED | MOSTLY DISSATISFIED | TERRIBLE |

10. Personal manner of the main practitioner(s) seen

| □ | □ | □ | □ | □ |
|---|---|---|---|---|
| TERRIBLE | MOSTLY DISSATISFIED | MIXED | MOSTLY SATISFIED | DELIGHTED |

11. Waiting time between asking to be seen and the appointment (date and time) given

| □ | □ | □ | □ | □ |
|---|---|---|---|---|
| DELIGHTED | MOSTLY SATISFIED | MIXED | MOSTLY DISSATISFIED | TERRIBLE |

12. Waiting time when you come to be seen or keep an appointment made

| □ | □ | □ | □ | □ |
|---|---|---|---|---|
| TERRIBLE | MOSTLY DISSATISFIED | MIXED | MOSTLY SATISFIED | DELIGHTED |

**What is your overall feeling about the . . .**

13. Availability of appointment times that fit your schedule

| □ | □ | □ | □ | □ |
|---|---|---|---|---|
| DELIGHTED | MOSTLY SATISFIED | MIXED | MOSTLY DISSATISFIED | TERRIBLE |

14. Cost of services to me

| □ | □ | □ | □ | □ |
|---|---|---|---|---|
| TERRIBLE | MOSTLY DISSATISFIED | MIXED | MOSTLY SATISFIED | DELIGHTED |

15. Effect of services in maintaining well-being and preventing relapse

| □ | □ | □ | □ | □ |
|---|---|---|---|---|
| DELIGHTED | MOSTLY SATISFIED | MIXED | MOSTLY DISSATISFIED | TERRIBLE |

16. Confidentiality and respect for your rights as an individual

| □ | □ | □ | □ | □ |
|---|---|---|---|---|
| TERRIBLE | MOSTLY DISSATISFIED | MIXED | MOSTLY SATISFIED | DELIGHTED |

17. Amount of help you have received

| □ | □ | □ | □ | □ |
|---|---|---|---|---|
| DELIGHTED | MOSTLY SATISFIED | MIXED | MOSTLY DISSATISFIED | TERRIBLE |

18. Availability of information on how to get the most out of the services

| □ | □ | □ | □ | □ |
|---|---|---|---|---|
| TERRIBLE | MOSTLY DISSATISFIED | MIXED | MOSTLY SATISFIED | DELIGHTED |

19. Prescription (or nonprescription) of medications

☐ | ☐ | ☐ | ☐ | ☐
*DELIGHTED* | *MOSTLY SATISFIED* | *MIXED* | *MOSTLY DISSATISFIED* | *TERRIBLE*

**What is your overall feeling about the . . .**

20. Explanations of specific procedures and approaches used

☐ | ☐ | ☐ | ☐ | ☐
*TERRIBLE* | *MOSTLY DISSATISFIED* | *MIXED* | *MOSTLY SATISFIED* | *DELIGHTED*

21. Effect of services in helping relieve symptoms or reduce problems

☐ | ☐ | ☐ | ☐ | ☐
*DELIGHTED* | *MOSTLY SATISFIED* | *MIXED* | *MOSTLY DISSATISFIED* | *TERRIBLE*

22. Response to crises or urgent needs during office hours

☐ | ☐ | ☐ | ☐ | ☐
*TERRIBLE* | *MOSTLY DISSATISFIED* | *MIXED* | *MOSTLY SATISFIED* | *DELIGHTED*

23. Arrangements made for after hours emergencies or urgent help

☐ | ☐ | ☐ | ☐ | ☐
*DELIGHTED* | *MOSTLY SATISFIED* | *MIXED* | *MOSTLY DISSATISFIED* | *TERRIBLE*

24. Thoroughness of the main practitioner(s) you have seen

☐ | ☐ | ☐ | ☐ | ☐
*TERRIBLE* | *MOSTLY DISSATISFIED* | *MIXED* | *MOSTLY SATISFIED* | *DELIGHTED*

25 Appropriate use of referrals to other practitioners or services when needed

☐ | ☐ | ☐ | ☐ | ☐
*DELIGHTED* | *MOSTLY SATISFIED* | *MIXED* | *MOSTLY DISSATISFIED* | *TERRIBLE*

26. Collaboration between service providers (if more than one)

☐ | ☐ | ☐ | ☐ | ☐
*TERRIBLE* | *MOSTLY DISSATISFIED* | *MIXED* | *MOSTLY SATISFIED* | *DELIGHTED*

**What is your overall feeling about the . . .**

27. Publicity or information about programs and services offered

☐ | ☐ | ☐ | ☐ | ☐
*DELIGHTED* | *MOSTLY SATISFIED* | *MIXED* | *MOSTLY DISSATISFIED* | *TERRIBLE*

28. Handling and accuracy of your records (as best you can tell)

☐ | ☐ | ☐ | ☐ | ☐
*TERRIBLE* | *MOSTLY DISSATISFIED* | *MIXED* | *MOSTLY SATISFIED* | *DELIGHTED*

29. Contribution of services to achievement of your life goals

☐ | ☐ | ☐ | ☐ | ☐
*DELIGHTED* | *MOSTLY SATISFIED* | *MIXED* | *MOSTLY DISSATISFIED* | *TERRIBLE*

30. In an overall general sense, how satisfied are you with the service you have received?

☐      ☐      ☐      ☐      ☐
*TERRIBLE*    *MOSTLY*    *MIXED*    *MOSTLY*    *DELIGHTED*
     *DISSATISFIED*      *SATISFIED*

31 (If applicable) Support of the group as a whole, helpfulness and caring of its members

☐      ☐      ☐      ☐      ☐
*DELIGHTED*    *MOSTLY*    *MIXED*    *MOSTLY*    *TERRIBLE*
     *SATISFIED*      *DISSATISFIED*

It is important to know something about our clients as a whole, so we request some demographic information. Only grouped data will be used, and you will never be identified. However, if you prefer not to answer any or all questions, you may freely do so.

32. About how many miles (one way) from the facility do you live?

☐    ☐    ☐    ☐    ☐    ☐
5 or less    6-10    11-15    16-20    20-25    26 or more

33. Approximately how many *weeks* have you been involved with this program?

☐    ☐    ☐    ☐    ☐    ☐
Less than 1    1-2    3-4    5-6    7-12    more than 12

34. Including today's, approximately how many sessions have you had in this program?

☐   ☐   ☐   ☐   ☐   ☐   ☐   ☐   ☐   ☐   ☐
0   1   2   3   4   5   6-10   11-20   21-30   31-50   51+

35 Your Sex:     MALE ☐     FEMALE ☐

36. Your Age:   ☐   ☐   ☐   ☐   ☐   ☐   ☐   ☐   ☐
    UNDER 20   21-25   26-35   36-45   46-55   56-65   66-75   76-85   86+

37. Yearly Family Income:
| | | | |
|---|---|---|---|
| Under $10,000 | ☐ | $10,000 - $20,000 | ☐ |
| $20,001 - $40,000 | ☐ | $40,001 - $60,000 | ☐ |
| $60,001 - $80,000 | ☐ | Over $80,000 | ☐ |

38. Your Education:
| | | | |
|---|---|---|---|
| Grade 8 or less | ☐ | Some high school | ☐ |
| High school grad. | ☐ | Some college | ☐ |
| College grad. | ☐ | Some post grad. | ☐ |
| Masters | ☐ | Ph.D., M.D., etc. | ☐ |

39. Ethnic Background:
| | | | |
|---|---|---|---|
| Caucasian/White | ☐ | Asian/Pacific American | ☐ |
| Native American/Indian | ☐ | Hispanic/Latino | ☐ |
| African American/Black | ☐ | Other (Specify) | ☐ |
| Prefer not to answer | ☐ | _____ | |

40. In general these days, how do you feel about your life as a whole?

☐   ☐   ☐   ☐   ☐   ☐   ☐
TERRIBLE   UNHAPPY   MOSTLY   MIXED   MOSTLY   PLEASED   DELIGHTED
    DISSATISFIED     SATISFIED

41. In general these days, how do you feel about your health?

☐   ☐   ☐   ☐   ☐   ☐   ☐
TERRBLE   UNHAPPY   MOSTLY   MIXED   MOSTLY   PLEASED   DELIGHTED
    DISSATISFIED     SATISFIED

# CONFIDENTIAL

*THANK YOU VERY MUCH FOR YOUR HELP WITH THIS SURVEY. WE WOULD APPRECIATE ANY ADDITIONAL COMMENTS ABOUT THIS SERVICE YOU WOULD CARE TO ADD. YOU MAY WRITE THEM BELOW.*

41. The thing I have liked best about my experience here is:

42. What I liked least was:

43. If I could change one thing about this service it would be:

# INDEX